Nuclear Cardiology—From Perfusion to Tissue Biology

Guest Editor

FRANK M. BENGEL, MD

CARDIOLOGY CLINICS

www.cardiology.theclinics.com

Consulting Editor

MICHAEL H. CRAWFORD, MD

May 2009 • Volume 27 • Number 2

SAUNDERS an imprint of ELSEVIER, Inc.

W.B. SAUNDERS COMPANY
A Division of Elsevier Inc.

Elsevier, Inc. • 1600 John F. Kennedy Blvd. • Suite 1800 • Philadelphia, Pennsylvania 19103-2899

http://www.theclinics.com

CARDIOLOGY CLINICS Volume 27, Number 2
May 2009 ISSN 0733-8651, ISBN-13: 978-1-4377-0457-0, ISBN-10: 1-4377-0457-3

Editor: Barbara Cohen-Kligerman

Cardiology Clinics (ISSN 0733-8651) is published quarterly by Elsevier Inc., 360 Park Avenue South, New York, NY 10010-1710. Months of issue are February, May, August, and November. Business and editorial Offices: 1600 John F. Kennedy Blvd., Suite 1800, Philadelphia, PA 19103-2899. Customer Service Office: 11830 Westline Industrial Drive, St. Louis, MO 63146. Periodicals postage paid at New York, NY, and additional mailing offices. Subscription prices are $244.00 per year for US individuals, $378.00 per year for US institutions, $122.00 per year for US students and residents, $298.00 per year for Canadian individuals, $470.00 per year for Canadian institutions, $346.00 per year for international individuals, $470.00 per year for international institutions and $173.00 per year for Canadian and foreign students/residents. To receive student/resident rate, orders must be accompanied by name of affiliated institution, data of term, and the signature of program/residency coordinator on institution letterhead. Orders will be billed at individual rate until proof of status is received. Foreign air speed delivery is included in all Clinics subscription prices. All prices are subject to change without notice. **POSTMASTER:** Send address changes to Cardiology Clinics, Elsevier Periodicals Customer Service, 11830 Westline Industrial Drive, St. Louis, MO 63146. **Customer Service: 1-800-654-2452 (US). From outside of the US, call 314-453-7041. Fax: 314-453-5170. E-mail: JournalsCustomer Service-usa@elsevier.com (for print support); JournalsOnlineSupport-usa@elsevier.com (for online support).**

Reprints. For copies of 100 or more, of articles in this publication, please contact the Commercial Reprints Department, Elsevier Inc., 360 Park Avenue South, New York, NY 10010-1710. Tel.: 212-633-3812; Fax: 212-462-1935; Email: reprints@elsevier.com.

Cardiology Clinics is also published in Spanish by McGraw-Hill Interamericana Editores S. A., P.O. Box 5-237, 06500, Mexico D. F., Mexico; in Portuguese by Reichmann and Alfonso Editores Rio de Janeiro, Brazil; and in Greek by Dimitrios P. Lagos, 8 Pondon Street, GR115-28 Ilissia, Greece.

Cardiology Clinics is covered in *MEDLINE/PubMed (Index Medicus), Excerpta Medica, The Cumulative Index to Nursing and Allied Health Literature* (CINAHL).

Printed and bound by CPI Group (UK) Ltd, Croydon, CR0 4YY
Transferred to Digital Print 2011

Contributors

CONSULTING EDITOR

MICHAEL H. CRAWFORD, MD
Professor of Medicine, University of California
San Francisco; Lucie Stern Chair in Cardiology,
and Interim Chief of Cardiology, University of
California, San Francisco Medical Center,
San Francisco, California

GUEST EDITOR

FRANK M. BENGEL, MD
Director of Cardiovascular Nuclear Medicine,
Division of Nuclear Medicine, Russell H.
Morgan Department of Radiology and
Radiological Science, Johns Hopkins
University, Baltimore, Maryland

AUTHORS

ADIL BASHIR, PhD
Research Instructor, Division of Radiological
Sciences, Cardiovascular Imaging Laboratory,
Edward Mallinckrodt Institute of Radiology,
St. Louis, Missouri

JEROEN J. BAX, MD, PhD
Department of Cardiology, Leiden University
Medical Center, Leiden, The Netherlands

ROB BEANLANDS, MD
Chief of Cardiac Imaging, Division of Cardiology,
Department of Medicine, Molecular Function
and Imaging Program, National Cardiac PET
Centre, University of Ottawa Heart Institute,
Ottawa, Ontario, Canada

FRANK M. BENGEL, MD
Director of Cardiovascular Nuclear Medicine,
Division of Nuclear Medicine, Russell H.
Morgan, Department of Radiology and
Radiological Science, Johns Hopkins
University, Baltimore, Maryland

MARK M. BOOGERS, MD
Department of Cardiology, Leiden University
Medical Center, Leiden, The Netherlands

MARCELO F. DI CARLI, MD
Noninvasive Cardiovascular Imaging Program,
Departments of Medicine (Cardiology) and
Radiology; and Division of Nuclear Medicine
and Molecular Imaging, Department of
Radiology, Brigham and Women's Hospital,
Harvard Medical School, Boston,
Massachusetts

**MAYSOON ELKHAWAD, MA, MB,
BChir, MRCS**
Clinical Research Fellow, Division of
Cardiovascular Medicine, Addenbrooke's
Hospital, Cambridge, United Kingdom

TRACY L. FABER, PhD
Associate Professor, Department of Radiology,
Emory University Hospital, Emory University
School of Medicine, Atlanta, Georgia

ERNEST V. GARCIA, PhD
Professor, Department of Radiology, Emory
University Hospital, Emory University School
of Medicine, Atlanta, Georgia

ROBERT J. GROPLER, MD
Professor of Radiology, Medicine, and Biomedical Engineering, Division of Radiological Sciences, Cardiovascular Imaging Laboratory, Edward Mallinckrodt Institute of Radiology, St. Louis; Cardiovascular Division, Department of Medicine, Washington University School of Medicine, St. Louis, Missouri

LUCILLE LALONDE, MD
Associate Professor of Medicine, Medical Director of Nuclear Cardiac Imaging, Division of Cardiology, Department of Medicine, Mazinkowski Alberta Heart Institute, University of Alberta, Walter Mackenzie Health Sciences Centre, Edmonton, Alberta, Canada

RIIKKA LAUTAMÄKI, MD, PhD
Turku PET Centre, Turku University Hospital, Turku, Finland; Division of Nuclear Medicine, Department of Radiology, Johns Hopkins Medical Institutions, Baltimore, Maryland

ALAN R. MORRISON, MD, PhD
Clinical Fellow, Section of Cardiovascular Medicine, Yale University School of Medicine, New Haven, Connecticut

JAMES H.F. RUDD, PhD, MRCP
BHF Clinical Lecturer and Honorary Specialist Registrar, Division of Cardiovascular Medicine, Addenbrooke's Hospital, Cambridge, United Kingdom

HEINRICH R. SCHELBERT, MD, PhD
Department of Molecular and Medical Pharmacology, David Geffen School of Medicine at University of California at Los Angeles, Los Angeles, California

JOANNE D. SCHUIJF, PhD
Department of Cardiology, Leiden University Medical Center, Leiden, The Netherlands

ALBERT J. SINUSAS, MD
Professor of Medicine and Diagnostic Radiology, Director of Cardiovascular Imaging, Yale University School of Medicine, New Haven, Connecticut

MARK I. TRAVIN, MD
Professor of Clinical Nuclear Medicine and Clinical Medicine, Department of Nuclear Medicine, Montefiore Medical Center, Albert Einstein College of Medicine, Bronx, New York

MARIA CECILIA ZIADI, MD
Clinical Research Fellow, Division of Cardiology, Department of Medicine, Molecular Function and Imaging Program, National Cardiac PET Centre, University of Ottawa Heart Institute, Ottawa, Ontario, Canada

Contents

Foreword   ix

Michael H. Crawford

Preface   xi

Frank M. Bengel

New Trends in Camera and Software Technology in Nuclear Cardiology   227

Ernest V. Garcia and Tracy L. Faber

> This article describes advancements in hardware and software for myocardial
> perfusion imaging that are becoming commercialized today and their implication
> in clinical practice.

Cardiac Positron Emission Tomography: Current Clinical Practice   237

Lucille Lalonde, Maria Cecilia Ziadi, and Rob Beanlands

> In the last two decades, the field of nuclear cardiology has experienced significant
> progress. The introduction of positron emission tomography (PET) imaging repre-
> sented a major breakthrough that has significantly contributed to a better under-
> standing of physiology and pathophysiology of several heart diseases. Currently,
> PET imaging is recognized as a well-established method to assess cardiac perfu-
> sion, function, metabolism, and viability. This article summarizes the main clinical
> applications of state-of-the art cardiac PET technology.

Hybrid Imaging: Integration of Nuclear Imaging and Cardiac CT   257

Marcelo F. Di Carli

> The integration of nuclear medicine cameras with multidetector CT scanners pro-
> vides a unique opportunity to delineate cardiac and vascular anatomic abnormalities
> and their physiologic consequences in a single setting. By revealing the burden of
> anatomic coronary artery disease and its physiologic significance, hybrid imaging
> can provide unique information that may improve noninvasive diagnosis, risk
> assessment, and management of coronary artery disease. By integrating the
> detailed anatomic information from CT with the high sensitivity of radionuclide imag-
> ing to evaluate targeted molecular and cellular abnormalities, hybrid imaging may
> play a key role in shaping the future of molecular diagnostics and therapeutics.
> This article reviews potential clinical applications of hybrid imaging in cardiovascular
> disease.

Nuclear Imaging in Heart Failure   265

Jeroen J. Bax, Mark M. Boogers, and Joanne D. Schuijf

> Heart failure is becoming the main clinical challenge in cardiology in the twenty-first
> century and is associated with high morbidity and mortality. Currently, several

therapeutic options are available for heart failure patients, including medical therapy, revascularization, advanced cardiac surgery, device therapy, and cardiac transplantation. Future therapies are directed at cell and gene therapy. In this article the role of nuclear imaging in the management of heart failure patients is discussed.

Quantification of Myocardial Blood Flow: What is the Clinical Role?   277

Heinrich R. Schelbert

Quantification of regional myocardial blood flow and of its responses to targeted physiologic and pharmacologic interventions, which is now available with positron emitting tracers of blood flow and positron emission tomography (PET), extends the diagnostic potential of standard myocardial perfusion imaging. These noninvasive flow measurements serve as tools for quantifying functional consequences of epicardial coronary artery disease, as well as of impairments in microcirculatory reactivity that escape detection by standard perfusion imaging. Flow measurements are clinically useful for more comprehensively assessing the extent and severity of coronary vascular disease or impairments in microcirculatory function in noncoronary cardiac disease. Flow estimates in these disorders contain independent or unique prognostic information about future major cardiac events. Flow measurements are also useful for assessing the coronary risk, for predicting long-term cardiovascular events, and for monitoring the effectiveness of risk reduction strategies.

Translation of Myocardial Metabolic Imaging Concepts into the Clinics   291

Adil Bashir and Robert J. Gropler

Flexibility in myocardial substrate metabolism for energy production is fundamental to cardiac health. This loss in plasticity or flexibility leads to overdependence on the metabolism of an individual category of substrates, with the predominance in fatty acid metabolism characteristic of diabetic heart disease and the accelerated glucose use associated with pressure-overload left ventricular hypertrophy being prime examples. There is a strong demand for accurate noninvasive imaging approaches of myocardial substrate metabolism that can facilitate the crosstalk between the bench and the bedside, leading to improved patient management paradigms. In this article potential future applications of metabolic imaging, particularly radionuclide approaches, for assessment of cardiovascular disease are discussed.

Cardiac Neuronal Imaging at the Edge of Clinical Application   311

Mark I. Travin

Cardiac neuronal innervation plays an important role in normal cardiac function and is adversely affected in the presence of disease. In particular, radiotracer imaging of cardiac sympathetic function has been extensively investigated and not only provides a method of assessing the severity of disease but also has repeatedly been shown to be prognostically useful with a potential for helping to guide patient management. SPECT imaging of myocardial uptake of ^{123}I-mIBG, an analog of the sympathetic neurotransmitter norepinephrine, has been the most studied, but PET neurotracers, such as ^{11}C-HED, are also under investigation. The ability of cardiac neuronal imaging to visualize and measure underlying molecular processes should allow it to provide a perspective on cardiac disease that other testing modalities cannot.

New Molecular Imaging Targets to Characterize Myocardial Biology 329

Alan R. Morrison and Albert J. Sinusas

Molecular imaging represents a targeted approach to noninvasively assess biologic (both physiologic and pathologic) processes in vivo. Ideally the goal of molecular imaging is not just to provide diagnostic and prognostic information based on identification of the molecular events associated with a pathologic process but rather to guide individually tailored pharmacologic, cell-based, or genetic therapeutic regimens. This article reviews the recent advances in myocardial molecular imaging in the context of the cardiovascular processes of angiogenesis, apoptosis, inflammation, and ventricular remodeling. The focus is on radiotracer-based single photon emission computed tomography and positron emission tomography molecular imaging approaches.

Radiotracer Imaging of Atherosclerotic Plaque Biology 345

Maysoon Elkhawad and James H.F. Rudd

Traditional imaging modalities used in the assessment of atherosclerotic plaque have focused on anatomic characteristics of size, location and luminal encroachment. The ability to identify plaques that are at risk for rupture, and thus may go on to cause clinical events, remains limited, however. By labeling tracer compounds capable of identifying important cellular or molecular processes involved in plaque vulnerability with radioactive isotopes, there is now potential for the noninvasive identification of vulnerable plaques. This article discusses several radiotracers that can report on high-risk plaque pathophysiology.

Role of Nuclear Imaging in Regenerative Cardiology 355

Riikka Lautamäki and Frank M. Bengel

Advances in noninvasive imaging techniques may aid in the understanding of cardiac stem cell therapy. Nuclear imaging enables in vivo evaluation of myocardial perfusion, metabolism, and function, in addition to the stem cell fate. This article summarizes recent clinical and experimental nuclear imaging studies in cardiac stem cell therapy.

Index 369

Cardiology Clinics

FORTHCOMING ISSUES

August 2009

Advances in Coronary Angiography
John D. Carroll, MD, and S. James Chen, PhD,
Guest Editors

November 2009

Advances in Cardiac Computed Tomography
Mario J. Garcia, MD, FACC, *Guest Editor*

February 2010

Advanced Applied Interventional Cardiology
Samin Sharma, MD, and
Annapoorna Kini, MD, *Guest Editors*

RECENT ISSUES

February 2009

Atrial Fibrillation
Ranjan K. Thakur, MD, MPH, and
Andrea Natale, MD, FACC, FHRS,
Guest Editors

November 2008

Cardiology Drug Update
JoAnne M. Foody, *Guest Editor*

August 2008

Ventricular Arrhythmias
John M. Miller, MD, *Guest Editor*

ISSUES OF RELATED INTEREST

Heart Failure Clinics, April 2009 (Vol. 5, No. 2)
Hemodynamic Monitoring in the Diagnosis and Management of Heart Failure
Ragavendra R. Baliga, MD, MBA, and William T. Abraham, MD, *Guest Editors*
Available at: http://www.heartfailure.theclinics.com/

Anesthesiology Clinics, September 2008 (Vol. 26, No. 3)
Cardiac Anesthesia: Today and Tomorrow
Davy C.H. Cheng, MD, MSc, FRCPC, FCAHS, *Guest Editor*
Available at: http://www.anesthesiology.theclinics.com/

VISIT THE CLINICS ONLINE!

Access your subscription at:
www.theclinics.com

Foreword

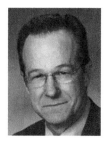

Michael H. Crawford, MD
Consulting Editor

The nuclear technique most frequently used by cardiologists is nuclear perfusion imaging, which is a fairly mature technology. However, mature technologies can be tweaked, as is demonstrated by the first three articles in this issue. The combination of a nuclear camera with CT allows for the attainment of coronary anatomic, cardiac functional, and myocardial perfusion imaging from one piece of equipment. Also, nuclear processing software continues to improve. PET scanning has now entered the mainstream with smaller equipment and the use of rubidium as a tracer. PET/SPECT cameras can now assess perfusion, function, and metabolism. Assessing cardiac viability is now fairly routine with these enhancements to cardiac imaging.

Most of this issue is devoted to new applications of nuclear imaging, which have variably penetrated the clinical arena at this time. Imaging cardiac nerves has tremendous potential given the tight link between the heart and the nervous system. Of course the Holy Grail of imaging is atherosclerotic plaque imaging, which will detect the vulnerable plaque. Perfection of this imaging challenge will revolutionize how we treat coronary artery disease. As stem cell therapies become a reality,

imaging information on cardiac cell biology will become important. Accurate quantitation of myocardial blood flow has many clinical applications. For example, it could be used to determine the functional significance of borderline lesions seen on CT angiography. Finally, nuclear imaging techniques to assess cardiac dyssynchrony and its response to resynchronization therapy show great promise, and an accurate technique to guide this therapy is desperately needed.

Cardiac nuclear imaging shows great promise for solving all these clinical cardiac imaging problems. These topics are fully discussed by the world's leading experts, who have been assembled by Dr. Bengel in this superb issue of *Cardiology Clinics*. Get ready to be wowed.

Michael H. Crawford, MD
Division of Cardiology
Department of Medicine
University of California, San Francisco Medical Center
505 Parnassus Avenue, Box 0124
San Francisco, CA 94143-0124, USA

E-mail address:
crawfordm@medicine.ucsf.edu (M.H. Crawford)

Cardiol Clin 27 (2009) ix
doi:10.1016/j.ccl.2009.02.001

Preface
The Changing Face of Nuclear Cardiology

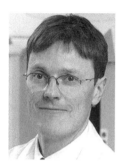

Frank M. Bengel, MD
Guest Editor

The field of cardiovascular imaging is changing. On one hand, myocardial perfusion imaging is a well-established clinical technique for the diagnostic and prognostic workup of coronary artery disease.[1,2] It has been the mainstay of nuclear cardiology for decades. On the other hand, several alternative imaging methodologies for noninvasive functional assessment of ischemic heart disease have emerged, and noninvasive coronary angiography is becoming a clinical reality.[3] As a consequence of the general increase of imaging procedures and associated overall costs, pressure is increasing for individual modalities regarding their cost-effectiveness and appropriateness.[4] Also, there is intense scrutiny by healthcare providers concerning coverage, and there is scrutiny by referring physicians and patients concerning safety, comfort and information content of a test. Therefore, a specific imaging modality requires excellent professional structure, but at the same time requires a constant influx of innovation for continuous improvement of imaging algorithms, minimization of risk, and maximization of clinically relevant information, as well as specificity of the readout for the respective clinical question.

This issue of *Cardiology Clinics* is devoted to the current state of cardiovascular nuclear imaging. It does not focus on the outstanding and well-established professional structure and scientific evidence for its mainstay, myocardial perfusion imaging,[5–7] which is one important component to sustain success in today's competitive imaging environment. Instead, the issue focuses on novel developments in the discipline, which have been made more rapidly in recent years. Nuclear imaging technology has progressed significantly toward higher sensitivity and resolution, and novel, highly specific radiotracers have been introduced. These developments are indicators of a steady evolution of nuclear cardiology beyond the assessment of myocardial perfusion and toward characterization of biologic events on the tissue level.[8] It is hoped that radiotracer techniques, with their unique translational potential and their superior detection sensitivity, will take a leading role in personalized cardiovascular medicine, in which therapeutic and/or preventive strategies are based on individual disease biology.

This issue includes state-of-the-art reviews by leading international experts that focus on novel imaging technology, novel compounds and novel biologic targets, as well as their current and future clinical relevance. Articles on the promises and potential of new technology, including new cameras and data processing for single-photon emission computed tomography (SPECT), high-end positron emission tomography (PET), and hybrid nuclear/CT systems are included. Also, the value of more specific imaging targets that are increasingly entering clinical practice is reviewed. This includes imaging of heart failure, absolute quantification of myocardial blood flow, imaging of myocardial metabolism, and imaging of the cardiac autonomic nervous system. Finally,

Cardiol Clin 27 (2009) xi–xii
doi:10.1016/j.ccl.2009.01.002

cardiology.theclinics.com

novel paradigms for imaging of early disease and monitoring of high-end therapy, which are on the edge of being translated to the clinics, are reviewed. This includes imaging of atherosclerotic plaque biology and imaging of regenerative therapies, as well as a general overview of biology-targeted novel imaging approaches.

The goal of this issue of *Cardiology Clinics* is to provide the reader with a comprehensive overview of the most recent developments in nuclear cardiology. Clearly, this field has produced a significant amount of innovation within recent years, suggesting that it is flexible, and moving forward from perfusion imaging toward imaging of tissue biology. It is hoped that the reader, after going through the included review articles, will share the enthusiasm of the editor and authors for this discipline, which holds the potential to be a key component in the new paradigm of early disease detection, molecular medicine and individualized therapeutic decision making.

Frank M. Bengel, MD
Division of Nuclear Medicine
Russell H. Morgan Department of Radiology
and Radiological Science
Johns Hopkins University
601 N. Caroline Street / JHOC 3225
Baltimore, MD 21287, USA

E-mail address:
fbengel1@jhmi.edu

REFERENCES

1. Berman DS, Shaw LJ, Hachamovitch R, et al. Comparative use of radionuclide stress testing, coronary artery calcium scanning, and noninvasive coronary angiography for diagnostic and prognostic cardiac assessment. Semin Nucl Med 2007;37(1):2–16.

2. Marcassa C, Bax JJ, Bengel F, et al. Clinical value, cost-effectiveness, and safety of myocardial perfusion scintigraphy: a position statement. Eur Heart J 2008;29(4):557–63.

3. Gibbons RJ, Araoz PA, Williamson EE. The year in cardiac imaging. J Am Coll Cardiol 2009;53(1):54–70.

4. Hendel RC. The revolution and evolution of appropriateness in cardiac imaging. J Nucl Cardiol 2008; 15(4):494–6.

5. Brindis RG, Douglas PS, Hendel RC, et al. ACCF/ASNC appropriateness criteria for single-photon emission computed tomography myocardial perfusion imaging (SPECT MPI): a report of the American College of Cardiology Foundation Quality Strategic Directions Committee Appropriateness Criteria Working Group and the American Society of Nuclear Cardiology endorsed by the American Heart Association. J Am Coll Cardiol 2005;46(8):1587–605.

6. Douglas PS, Hendel RC, Cummings JE, et al. ACCF/ACR/AHA/ASE/ASNC/HRS/NASCI/RSNA/SAIP/SCAI/SCCT/SCMR 2008 Health Policy Statement on Structured Reporting in Cardiovascular Imaging. J Am Coll Cardiol 2009;53(1):76–90.

7. Klocke FJ, Baird MG, Lorell BH, et al. ACC/AHA/ASNC guidelines for the clinical use of cardiac radionuclide imaging–executive summary: a report of the American College of Cardiology/American Heart Association Task Force on Practice Guidelines (ACC/AHA/ASNC Committee to Revise the 1995 Guidelines for the Clinical Use of Cardiac Radionuclide Imaging). J Am Coll Cardiol 2003;42(7): 1318–33.

8. Higuchi T, Bengel FM. Cardiovascular nuclear imaging: from perfusion to molecular function: noninvasive imaging. Heart 2008;94(6):809–16.

New Trends in Camera and Software Technology in Nuclear Cardiology

Ernest V. Garcia, PhD[1],*, Tracy L. Faber, PhD

KEYWORDS

- Myocardial perfusion imaging • Ultrafast nuclear cameras
- Solid state cameras • Resolution recovery
- Wide beam reconstruction • Iterative reconstruction

Myocardial perfusion imaging (MPI) with single-photon emission computed tomography (SPECT) has enjoyed widespread clinical use because of its well-documented diagnostic accuracy for detecting coronary artery disease. Despite its success, current clinical, scientific, and financial needs require further improvements in hardware and software to bring MPI SPECT to the next level. It is difficult to realize these improvements with the imaging hardware and software used in most nuclear cardiology laboratories today. The basic SPECT camera design is over 50 years old[1] and is limited by standard parallel-hole collimators to image the heart which use only a small portion of the available sodium iodide (NaI) crystal detector area (**Fig. 1**). The basic filtered backprojection (FBP) reconstruction algorithm used by most SPECT systems today is even older, dating to over 90 years ago.[2]

This article describes advancements in imaging hardware and software that are becoming commercialized today and their implication in clinical practice.

NEW ULTRAFAST CAMERAS

Several manufacturers have begun to break away from the conventional SPECT imaging approach to create innovative designs of dedicated cardiac scanners. In all of these designs, all available detectors are constrained to imaging just the cardiac field of view. **Fig. 2** shows how eight detectors surrounding the patient are all simultaneously imaging the heart. These new designs vary in the number and type of scanning or stationary detectors and in whether NaI or cadmium zinc telluride (CZT) solid state detectors are used. They all have in common the potential for a fivefold to tenfold increase in count sensitivity at no loss or even a gain in resolution, resulting in the potential for acquiring a stress myocardial perfusion scan injected with a standard dose in 2 minutes or less.

D-SPECT System

The first SPECT system to offer a totally different design is the D-SPECT (Spectrum Dynamics, Haifa, Israel).[3–5] This system uses solid state detectors in the form of CZT mounted on nine vertical columns and placed in a 90-degree geometry as shown in **Fig. 3**.[4] Each of the nine detector assemblies is equipped with a tungsten, square, parallel-hole collimator. Each collimator square hole is 2.46 mm on its side, which is large in

Department of Radiology, Emory University Hospital, Emory University School of Medicine, Room E163, 1364 Clifton Road, Atlanta, GA 33022, USA

[1]Dr. Garcia is the principal investigator of a research effort funded by GE Healthcare to evaluate the ultrafast cardiac camera described in this article. Emory University also has received funding to evaluate the CardiArc device described in this article. Both Drs. Garcia and Faber are consultants and shareholders of Syntermed which at this time is pursuing a business venture with Eagle Heart Imaging, developers of the 18 multi-pinhole SPECT imaging approach described herein.

* Corresponding author.
E-mail address: ernest.garcia@emory.edu (E.V. Garcia).

Cardiol Clin 27 (2009) 227–236
doi:10.1016/j.ccl.2008.12.002

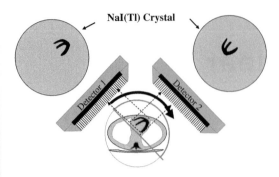

Fig. 1. Limitations of conventional SPECT imaging. The conventional camera design used in dual-detector SPECT systems is over 50 years old and limited when using standard parallel-hole collimators to image the heart and only a small portion of the available NaI(Tl) crystal detector area.

comparison with conventional collimators, which accounts, in part, for the increased count sensitivity. Each detector assembly is made to fan in synchrony with the other eight detector assemblies while all nine are simultaneously imaging the heart. The patient is imaged sitting in a reclining position, similar to a dentist's chair, with the patient's left arm placed on top of the detector housing.

Data acquisition is performed by first obtaining a 1-minute scout scan for the nine detectors to identify the location of the heart to set the limits of each detector's fanning motion. The actual

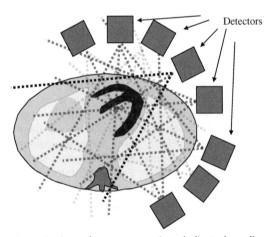

Fig. 2. Design of new generation dedicated cardiac ultrafast acquisition scanners. This diagram shows how eight detectors surrounding the patient are all simultaneously imaging the heart. These new designs vary in the number and type of scanning or stationary detectors and in whether NaI or CZT solid state detectors are used. They have in common the potential for a fivefold to tenfold increase in count sensitivity at no loss or even a gain in resolution.

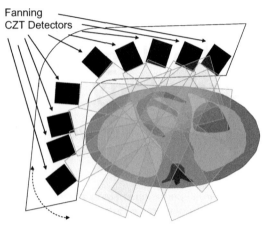

Fig. 3. D-SPECT system configuration. Diagram of the nine-CZT detector column configuration of the D-SPECT system. Each detector column uses a tungsten parallel-hole collimator fanned back and forth and constrained angularly to the heart's field of view.

diagnostic scan is then performed with each detector assembly fanning within the limits set from the scout scan. Reconstruction is performed using a modified iterative algorithm which compensates for the loss of spatial resolution that results from using large square holes in the collimator by mathematically modeling the acquisition and collimator geometry.

In a recent single-center clinical trial publication, it was concluded that using a stress/rest MPI protocol and 4- and 2-minute D-SPECT acquisitions, respectively, yielded studies that highly correlated with 16- and 12-minute stress/rest conventional SPECT with an equivalent level of diagnostic performance.[5] In a preliminary report on a multicenter trial using D-SPECT, the use of normal database quantitative analysis and a comparison protocol similar to the previous report correlated well to the quantitative analysis of conventional SPECT MPI.[6] Another preliminary multicenter trial reported the potential for the D-SPECT device to perform simultaneous Tl-201 (rest)/Tc-99m sestamibi (stress) 15-minute acquisitions.[7]

CardiArc System

The second SPECT system to offer a totally new design is the CardiArc (CardiArc, Lubbock, Texas).[4,8] This system uses three detectors, similar to conventional scintillation cameras, that are curved side-by-side to cover a 180-degree angle. Each detector consists of a curved NaI(Tl) crystal covered by an array of photomultiplier tubes as shown in **Fig. 4**. Horizontal collimation is defined using a series of thin lead sheets which

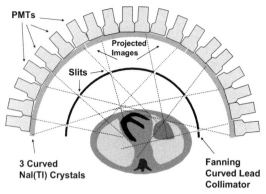

Fig. 4. CardiArc system configuration. Top view of the CardiArc system showing how imaging is performed using a stationary assembly of three curved NaI(Tl) crystals covered by an array of photomultiplier tubes (PMTs). Collimation uses a curved lead sheet with six slits which fans back and forth during acquisition.

are stacked vertically, leaving a gap between sheets that defines the hole aperture. Vertical collimation is achieved using a curved lead sheet with six vertical slits which fan back and forth during acquisition to obtain 180-degree worth of data from multiple projections. The movement of these six slits is synchronized electronically with the six areas of the crystal that are imaging the photons passing through the slits.[4] This synchronization helps eliminate the overlap in acquisition from adjacent slits.

Ultrafast AT Cardiac System

A third SPECT system to offer a revolutionary new design has been developed by GE Healthcare (Haifa, Israel).[9,10] This design uses Alcyone technology (AT), consisting of an array of solid state CZT pixilated detectors which simultaneously image all cardiac views with no moving parts during data acquisition (**Fig. 5**). Iterative reconstruction adapted to this camera's geometry is used to create transaxial slices of the heart. The use of CZT improves the energy and spatial (contrast) resolution, which among other benefits facilitates the development of simultaneous dual-isotope imaging protocols. The use of simultaneously acquired views improves the overall sensitivity and gives complete and consistent angular data needed for dynamic studies and the reduction of motion artifacts.

In a recent preliminary report on a multicenter trial, it was demonstrated that using a rest/stress MPI protocol and 4- and 2-minute AT acquisitions, respectively, yielded studies that diagnostically agreed 90% of the time with 14- and 12-minute rest/stress conventional SPECT acquisitions.[10] **Fig. 6** compares AT versus conventional SPECT images in a normal patient acquired with this protocol. Importantly, this trial also showed excellent left ventricular ejection fraction correlations between the AT and conventional SPECT for the rest (r = .93, P<.001) and stress (r = .91, P<.001) gated MPI studies.[10]

ROTATING CAMERA DEVELOPMENTS

In addition to the radically new camera designs described previously, other manufacturers and investigators have modified the electronics, system geometry, or collimation to significantly

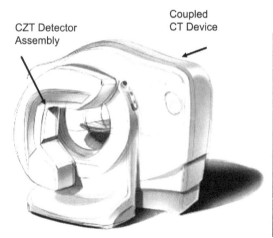

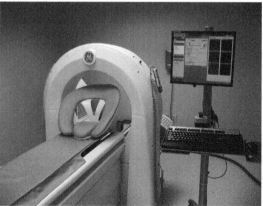

Fig. 5. Ultrafast AT cardiac system. Left panel shows a cartoon of the CZT detector assembly physically coupled to a conventional CT machine for a fast SPECT/CT system configuration. The AT detector assembly may be rotated for patient positioning (supine or prone) but is totally stationary with no moving parts during acquisition. Right panel shows the stand-alone AT cardiac system at Emory University. The detector assembly is on the far end of the photograph.

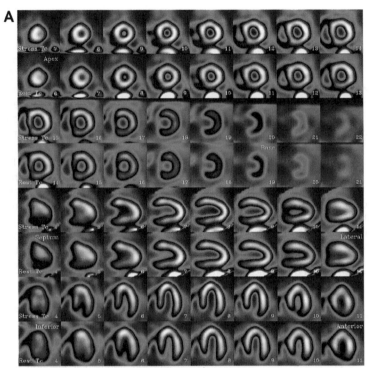

UFC 2/4 min images

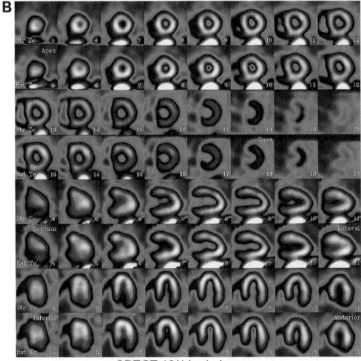

SPECT 12/14 min images

Fig. 6. Normal patient images used to illustrate advantage of the AT cardiac system. Results from a normal patient who underwent rest/stress Tc-99m tetrofosmin MPI using 10 mCi for rest and 30 for stress. (*A*) AT images. Rest and stress acquisitions were 4 and 2 minutes, respectively. The figure shows short, vertical, and horizontal oblique axis slices starting with stress images in the first row and immediately below the corresponding resting images. (*B*) Standard SPECT images. Results from the same normal patient who underwent rest/stress Tc-99m tetrofosmin MPI using 10 mCi for rest and 30 for stress. Rest and stress acquisitions were 14 and 12 minutes, respectively. A conventional CardioMD SPECT system was used to acquire this study.

improve the imaging performance of rotating SPECT cameras.

Cardius 3 XPO System

One of the first systems developed to take advantage of solid state electronics and to use more than two detectors simultaneously imaging the heart is the Cardius 3 XPO (Digirad, Poway, California). This commercial system uses 768 pixilated, thallium-activated cesium iodide [CsI(Tl)] crystals coupled to individual silicon photodiodes and digital Anger electronics to create the planar projection images used for reconstruction.[4] **Fig. 7** shows how the three detectors are fixed using a 67.5-degree angular separation while the patient is rotated through an arc of 202.5 degrees while sitting on a chair with the arms resting above the detectors. The typical acquisition time for a study is 7.5 minutes. Manufacturers of this device claim up to 38% more count sensitivity when compared with conventional dual-head systems while maintaining comparable image quality.[11]

IQ SPECT Collimation

Siemens (Hoffman Estates, Illinois) has reintroduced to the field the use of confocal collimators (now called IQ SPECT). Previously used in single-head SPECT systems, two collimators are mounted on conventional dual-detector SPECT

cameras, separated by 90 degrees and rotated around the patient to obtain a 180-degree reconstruction arc.[12] **Fig. 8** shows how the field of view of these collimators is most convergent at their center for increased sensitivity and resolution while the convergence is relaxed toward the edge of the field of view. The advantage of this approach is that it can be used by existing dual-detector systems. Typical MPI acquisition times range from 4 to 5 minutes.

Multi-Pinhole SPECT System

Another technology that has seen resurgence is the coded aperture technique known as multi-pinhole imaging. The first practical implementation for MPI imaging was the use of the seven-pinhole collimator in 1978.[13] In this approach, a collimator with seven pinholes mounted on a stationary camera was used to simultaneously generate seven projections of the heart. In its most recent implementation, two nine-pinhole collimators are mounted on conventional dual-detector SPECT system to simultaneously generate 18 angular projections (**Fig. 9**). These 18 projections are sufficient to generate diagnostic quality images without the need to rotate the gantry and with five times the efficiency of a rotating SPECT system.[14] This approach also has the advantage that it can be used in existing dual-detector systems. The multi-pinhole approach has also been implemented and validated in SPECT

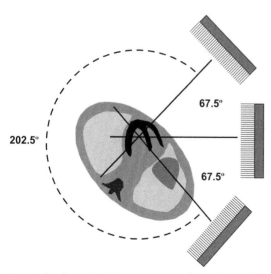

Fig. 7. Cardius 3 XPO system configuration. This diagram shows how patient data are acquired with the Cardius 3 XPO camera by keeping the three detectors stationary and simultaneously imaging the heart while the chair the patients sits on is rotated through a 202.5-degree arc.

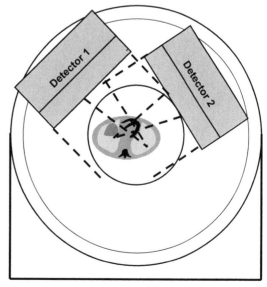

Fig. 8. IQ SPECT system. This diagram shows how patient data are acquired using two confocal collimators mounted on a conventional dual-detector SPECT system by rotating the gantry in the usual fashion through a 90-degree arc.

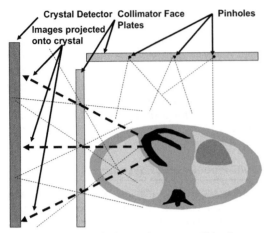

Fig. 9. 18 multi-pinhole SPECT system. This diagram shows how patient data are acquired using two nine-pinhole collimators mounted on a conventional SPECT system. Because 18 simultaneous pinhole projections are obtained during acquisition, there is no need to rotate the detector to obtain sufficient angular sampling.

systems with three heads.[15] The system was modified so that the three detectors have a 67.5-degree angular separation between the center detector and the two lateral detectors.

FASTER ACQUISITION VIA IMAGE RECONSTRUCTION ADVANCEMENTS

The time of acquisition of an MPI study depends on the resolution required to resolve perfusion

defects in the myocardium above the inherent noise due to limited count sensitivity. The resolution and sensitivity of parallel-hole collimators depends on the shape, length, and size of the holes. Each hole in the collimator restricts the photons that may strike the crystal to those that originate within the arc φ. Lengthening the holes of the collimator reduces φ and the area exposed through each hole at a given distance. The longer the length of the collimator hole or smaller the diameter of the hole, the greater the resolution and the lower the count sensitivity obtained by the imaging system. Regardless of the length of the hole, the resolution degrades with the distance from the collimator (**Fig. 10**).

Conventional FBP reconstruction assumes that the photons counted in a voxel over a collimator's parallel hole emanated in a straight line from a radioactive source perpendicular to the detector surface and aligned with the hole (**Fig. 11**). It assumes that all other photons counted from this source are either image noise or counts from other sources positioned in a very narrow line parallel to and directly in front of the hole.

Resolution Recovery

Recent software improvements in image reconstruction take into account the loss of resolution with the distance inherent in parallel-hole collimators, depicted in **Fig. 11** by the cone drawn as a dashed line. Using this knowledge in conjunction with the imaging properties of the system allows for a mathematical correction of this resolution

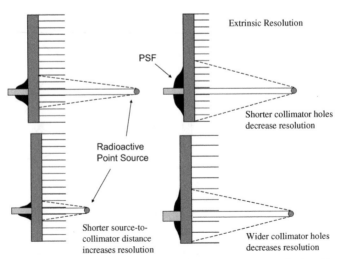

Fig.10. Effect of collimator design and source-to-detector distance on system resolution. The resolution and sensitivity of parallel-hole collimators depends on the shape, length, and size of the holes. Note that regardless of the length of the hole, the resolution degrades with the distance from the collimator. Also note how the response of the system to imaging a radioactive point source (point spread function, PSF) spreads or degrades as resolution is lost.

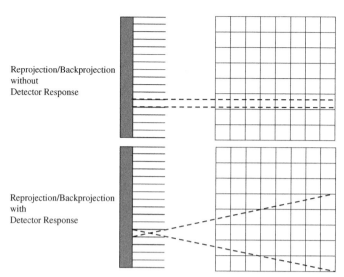

Reprojection/Backprojection
without
Detector Response

Reprojection/Backprojection
with
Detector Response

Fig. 11. Image reconstruction advances allow half-time acquisition. The top panel shows how conventional FBP reconstruction assumes that the photons counted in a voxel over a collimator's parallel hole emanated in a straight (dashed) line from a radioactive source perpendicular to the detector surface and aligned with the hole. It assumes that all other photons counted from this source are either image noise or counts from other sources positioned in a very narrow line parallel to and directly in front of the hole. Bottom panel shows how recent software improvements in image reconstruction take into account the loss of resolution with the distance inherent in parallel home collimators, depicted here by the triangle drawn as a dashed line.

degradation known as resolution recovery. At the same time, noise is suppressed because additional counts are now correctly considered rather than treated as noise. Because resolution recovery actually reduces noise while improving spatial resolution as compared with FBP, resolution recovery can yield reconstructed images from studies acquired in less time with the same signal/noise as FBP images reconstructed from studies acquired for longer times.

Because resolution recovery requires specific information on the imaging properties of the system, the recovery algorithm must accurately account for the physical characteristics of the detector, the collimator, and the patient. These recovery algorithms use a database of known detectors and collimator characteristics. Recovery also requires a specific description of the orbit shape, radius, or distance from the patient to the detector. All of this information is usually found in the study (dicom) header.

Iterative Reconstruction Techniques

Reconstruction that performs resolution recovery is inherently iterative. Iterative reconstruction techniques require more calculations and more computer time to create a transaxial image than does FBP; however, their great advantage is their ability to incorporate corrections for the factors

that degrade SPECT images in the reconstruction process. Iterative techniques use the original projections and models of the acquisition process to predict a reconstruction. The predicted reconstruction is then used again with the models to recreate new predicted projections. If the predicted projections are different from the actual projections, these differences are used to modify the reconstruction. This process is continued until the reconstruction is such that the predicted projections match the actual projections. The primary differences between various iterative methods are how the predicted reconstructions and projections are created and how they are modified at each step. Practically speaking, the more theoretically accurate the iterative technique is, the more time-consuming the process. Maximum likelihood methods allow the noise to be modeled. The most widely used iterative reconstruction method is maximum-likelihood expectation maximization (MLEM).[16] The MLEM algorithm attempts to determine the tracer distribution that would most likely yield the measured projections given the imaging model. To speed up reconstruction, developers have implemented a short-cut to the MLEM algorithm that uses only a subset of the projections for each iteration rather than the entire set of projections. This approach is known as ordered subset expectation maximization (OSEM) and is commonly implemented in most commercial systems. **Fig. 12** shows a patient example of how applying the OSEM algorithm with resolution recovery yields comparable image quality to studies acquired in twice the time but reconstructed without resolution recovery.

A more recent approach at optimizing the MLEM reconstruction has been the use of a priori information in the form of bayesian priors that constraints the reconstruction variables to yield an image with higher signal/noise while using fewer acquired counts, thus having the effect of a noise reduction technique. This approach uses the maximum a posteriori (MAP) principle and is sometimes known as MAP reconstruction.[17]

Commercial Implementations

Various manufacturers have implemented different versions of resolution recovery algorithms which model detector and collimator physics that couple improved resolution with associated noise reduction techniques. These algorithms include Wide Beam Reconstruction (WBR) from UltraSPECT (Haifa, Israel),[18] Astonish from Philips Medical Systems (Milpitas, CA),[19] Evolution from GE Healthcare (Haifa, Israel),[20] Flash3D from Siemens Medical Solutions (Hoffman Estates, IL),[21] and nSPEED from DIGIRAD Corporation (Poway, CA).[22]

Although disclosure of how these resolution recovery algorithms work varies greatly from company to company, the algorithms' general properties are known and can be compared. All five of these algorithms include detector- and collimator-specific modeling using a database of known devices and information from the dicom header. All five algorithms also incorporate into their calculations the patient-to-detector distance using information found in the study's dicom header. The WBR algorithm is the only one known to estimate the patient-to-detector distance if this information is not available in the dicom header. For noise reduction, Evolution adds a filter to the MLEM iterations to approach a MAP reconstruction, whereas the Flash3D and nSPEED algorithms add a post-filter after the MLEM reconstruction. The Astonish algorithm uses the same smoothing Hanning filter applied to the original projections, the reprojections, and the backprojected ratio determination during each MLEM iteration. Although WBR also includes a noise reduction filter, the exact details of this approach remain unpublished. All five resolution recovery algorithms model the imaging system to recover resolution and use some form of noise reduction technique. In addition, the Astonish, Evolution, and Flash3D algorithms can include both compton scatter and attenuation correction as part of modeling the imaging system. Because processing with these algorithms is time consuming, most implementations include simplifying assumptions to obtain speed. Because these simplifications vary from company to company,

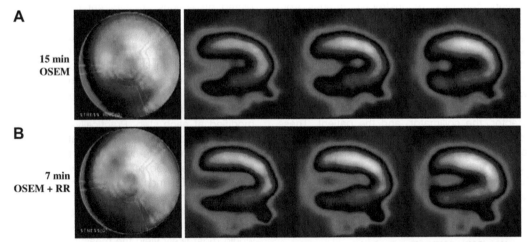

Fig. 12. Normal patient images used to illustrate advantage of resolution recovery (RR) reconstruction. Results are shown from a normal patient who underwent Tc-99m MPI. (*A*) OSEM reconstruction without RR. This panel shows a polar map representation of the left ventricle and typical vertical long axis tomograms for a study acquired at 30 s/projection for a total of 15 minutes and reconstructed without RR. (*B*) OSEM reconstruction with RR. This panel shows for the same patient a polar map representation of the left ventricle and corresponding vertical long axis tomograms for a study acquired at 15 s/projection for a total of 7.5 minutes and reconstructed using RR. Note how the RR half-time acquisition is comparable in both resolution and noise to the full-time acquisition reconstructed without RR.

there is no reason to believe all algorithms perform similarly; therefore, each should be independently validated.

Clinical Trials

SPECT MPI may be performed with the WBR resolution recovery algorithm using half the conventional scan time without compromising perfusion imaging results.[23] In another study, it was shown that the WBR or Evolution algorithm applied to half-time ECG-gated MPI SPECT acquisitions compared favorably with FBP of full-time acquisitions in image quality and correlation of functional parameters, although systematic offsets in end-diastolic and end-systolic volumes and ejection fraction were reported due to the increase in contrast of the resolution recovered gated images over FBP images.[24] In another clinical trial it was shown that the normal myocardial perfusion distribution did not change significantly between half-time and full-time acquisition when reconstructed using Flash3D resolution recovery, whereas two of nine regions were statistically different with FBP.[25]

Results obtained from a multicenter trial also concluded that half-time MPI acquisition and simultaneously acquired radioactive line source transmission images for attenuation correction reconstructed with Astonish improved image quality and interpretative certainty over FBP while preserving diagnostic accuracy.[26] In another large multicenter trial using half-time upright SPECT acquisition reconstructed with nSPEED, this methodology yielded results similar to conventional full acquisition times without compromising perfusion and function information.[27]

It can be concluded from the results of these and other clinical trials that half-time acquisitions reconstructed with resolution recovery improve image quality over FBP and provide perfusion information which is very similar to FBP. Regarding myocardial function, the results from these trials indicate that left ventricular end-diastolic volumes and ejection fraction can be significantly reduced when compared with FBP due to the higher chamber contrast generated by resolution recovery. This finding also appears to enhance detection of wall motion abnormalities.

FAST-SPEED MYOCARDIAL PERFUSION IMAGING: CLINICAL IMPLICATIONS

The camera design and software improvements reviewed in this article result in a reduction of acquisition time for MPI ranging from half of the conventional acquisition time to a minimum 2-minute acquisition. Clinically, these fast acquisitions would allow flexibility of acquisition protocols, reducing camera and patient total time and cost and increasing patient comfort.[28] Reduced acquisition times would also lead to decreased patient motion which results from translation, smearing, and breathing. These more efficient imaging systems would also allow a decrease in the radiation dose absorbed by the patient and staff by generating the same or better diagnostic images than what is obtained today at a much lower radiopharmaceutical dose. High count efficiency would allow true stress acquisitions of myocardial function, as well as dynamic acquisition of SPECT tracers, similar to what is done with PET tracers. Dynamic imaging opens the door to the quantification of blood flow and coronary flow reserve, which could be used to detect disease earlier and to avoid interpretation of three-vessel disease in patients as normal.

SUMMARY

Dedicated cardiac SPECT imagers are undergoing a profound change in design for the first time in 50 years. The Anger camera general purpose design is being replaced with systems with multiple detectors focused on the heart, yielding five to ten times the sensitivity of conventional SPECT. Some of the designs also replace the NaI(Tl) crystal with solid state CZT electronic detectors with superior energy resolution. There are also significant innovations in reconstruction software incorporated into these newly designed systems that take into account the true physics of the SPECT reconstruction geometry to gain at least a factor of 2 in sensitivity. Some of these new systems are ideally suited for dynamic applications facilitating measurements of coronary flow reserve. The fast acquisition also makes the hybrid SPECT/CT systems more practical because it allows the CT scanner to be used for a longer part of the day.

REFERENCES

1. Anger HO. Scintillation camera. Rev Sci Instrum 1958;29(1):27–33.
2. Radon J. [Uber due bestimmung von funktionen durch ihre intergralwerte langsgewisser mannigfaltigkeiten (on the determination of functions from their integrals along certain manifolds)]. Berichte Saechsische Akademie der Wissenschaften 1917;29: 262–77 (In German).
3. Available at: www.spectrum-dynamics.com. Accessed October 29, 2008.
4. Patton JA, Slomka PJ, Germano G, et al. Recent technologic advances in nuclear cardiology. J Nucl Cardiol 2007;14:501–13.

5. Sharir T, Ben-Haim S, Merzon K, et al. High-speed myocardial perfusion imaging: initial clinical comparison with conventional dual detector Anger camera imaging. J Am Coll Cardiol Img 2008;1:156–63.

6. Sharir T, Ben-Haim S, Slomka P, et al. Validation of quantitative analysis of high-speed myocardial perfusion imaging: comparison to conventional SPECT imaging [abstract]. J Nucl Cardiol 2008;15(4):S4–5.

7. Ben-Haim S, Hutton BF, Van Grantberg D, et al. Simultaneous dual isotope myocardial perfusion imaging (DI-MPI) with D-SPECT [abstract]. J Nucl Cardiol 2008;15(4):S2.

8. Available at: http://www.cardiarc.com. Accessed October 29, 2008.

9. Garcia EV, Tsukerman L, Keidar Z. A new solid state ultrafast cardiac multidetector SPECT system [abstract]. J Nucl Cardiol 2008;15(4):S3.

10. Esteves FP, Raggi P, Folks RD, et al. Novel ultrafast cardiac camera in myocardial perfusion SPECT: initial multicenter comparison with standard dual detector cameras. ASNC late breaking clinical trial. Presented at the Program of the 2008 Scientific Session of the American Society of Nuclear Cardiology, Boston, MA. p. 13.

11. Babla H, Bai C, Conwell R, et al. A triple-head solid state camera for cardiac single photon emission tomography (SPECT). Available at: www.digirad.com. Accessed October 29, 2008.

12. IQ-SPECT, Siemens Medical Solutions. Available at: www.usa.siemens.com/mi. Accessed October 29, 2008.

13. Vogel RA, Kirch D, LeFree M, et al. A new method of multiplanar emission tomography using a seven pinhole collimator and an Anger scintillation camera. J Nucl Med 1978;19:648–54.

14. Funk T, Kirch DL, Koss JE, et al. A novel approach to multipinhole SPECT for myocardial perfusion imaging. J Nucl Med 2006;47:595–602.

15. Steele PP, Kirch DL, Koss JE. Comparison of simultaneous dual-isotope multipinhole SPECT with rotational SPECT in a group of patients with coronary artery disease. J Nucl Med 2008;49:1080–9.

16. Shepp LA, Vardi Y. Maximum likelihood reconstruction for emission tomography. IEEE Trans Med Imaging 1982;1:113–22.

17. De Pierro AR, Yamagishi MEB. Fast EM-like methods for maximum a posteriori estimates in emission tomography. IEEE Trans Med Imaging 2001;20(4):280–8.

18. Wide Beam Reconstruction, UltraSPECT Inc. Available at: www.ultraspect.com. Accessed October 29, 2008.

19. Astonish, Philips Medical Systems. Available at: www.medical.philips.com. Accessed October 29, 2008.

20. Evolution, GE Healthcare. Available at: www.gehealthcare.com. Accessed October 29, 2008.

21. Flash 3D, Siemens Medical Solutions. Available at: www.siemens.com/medical. Accessed October 29, 2008.

22. nSPEED, DIGIRAD Corporation. Available at: www.digirad.com. Accessed October 29, 2008.

23. Borges-Neto S, Pagnanelli RA, Shaw LK, et al. Clinical results of a novel wide beam reconstruction method for shortening scan time of Tc-99m cardiac SPECT perfusion studies. J Nucl Cardiol 2007;14:555–65.

24. DePuey EG, Gadraju R, Clark J, et al. Ordered subset expectation maximization and wide beam reconstruction "half-time" gated myocardial perfusion SPECT functional imaging: a comparison to "full-time" filtered backprojection. J Nucl Cardiol 2008;15:547–63.

25. Ficaro EP, Kritzman JN, Corbett JR. Effect of reconstruction parameters and acquisition times on myocardial perfusion distributions in normals [abstract]. J Nucl Cardiol 2008;15(4):S20.

26. Venero CV, Ahlberg AW, Bateman TM, et al. Enhancing nuclear cardiac laboratory efficiency: multicenter evaluation of a new post-processing method with depth-dependent collimator resolution applied to full and half-time acquisitions [abstract]. J Nucl Cardiol 2008;15(4):S4.

27. Maddahi J, Mahmarian J, Mendez R, et al. Prospective multi-center evaluation of rapid gated SPECT myocardial perfusion upright imaging. J Nucl Med 2008;49(Suppl 1):2P.

28. Bonow RO. High-speed myocardial perfusion imaging: dawn of a new era in nuclear cardiology? J Am Coll Cardiol Img 2008;1(2):164–6.

Cardiac Positron Emission Tomography: Current Clinical Practice

Lucille Lalonde, MD[a], Maria Cecilia Ziadi, MD[b],
Rob Beanlands, MD[b],*

KEYWORDS

- PET • Imaging • Myocardial perfusion
- Myocardial viability • Sarcoidosis
- Vasculitis • Medicine • Molecular

With the increase in availability of positron emission tomography (PET), and its clinical growth in other medical fields, the clinical use of PET myocardial imaging has also grown. PET imaging has had two major clinical cardiac applications: (1) cardiac PET imaging is an accurate and well-validated tool for the assessment of myocardial perfusion and blood flow in coronary artery disease (CAD) or suspected CAD and its affect on ventricular function;[1–4] (2) PET is used for the assessment of metabolism and viability of myocardial tissue in the presence of congestive heart failure (CHF) or systolic dysfunction due to CAD, in which fluorodeoxyglucose (FDG) PET is known to be the most sensitive clinical noninvasive method.[1,5] This article focuses on these clinical applications.

MYOCARDIAL PERFUSION TRACERS FOR POSITRON EMISSION TOMOGRAPHY

According to their physical properties, myocardial PET blood flow tracers can be divided into two basic categories: (1) inert freely diffusible tracers, such as ^{15}O-water (H_2^{15}O), and (2) physiologically retained tracers, such as N-13-ammonia ($^{13}NH_3$) and rubidium-82 (^{82}Rb), which are the two most commonly available PET radiotracers used for the clinical assessment of myocardial perfusion.[2–4] The main features of PET flow tracers are summarized in **Table 1**.

^{82}Rb is produced from a strontium-82 (^{82}Sr)/^{82}Rb generator, which can be eluted every 10 minutes. The half-life ($T_{1/2}$) of ^{82}Sr is 25.5 days, which results in a generator life of 4 to 8 weeks. The short $T_{1/2}$ of ^{82}Rb (76 seconds) enables repeated and sequential perfusion studies but requires a delivery system that is linked directly to the patient for tracer administration and then rapid image acquisition shortly after tracer administration. ^{82}Rb has the highest kinetic energy of the commonly used PET tracers but the associated long positron range reduces spatial resolution with PET imaging.

^{82}Rb is a monovalent cationic analog of potassium and has similar biologic activity to thallium-201 (^{201}Tl). Myocardial uptake of ^{82}Rb requires active transport by way of the sodium/potassium adenosine triphosphate transporter. In animal models, the net retention is approximately 50% to 60% at rest and decreases to 30% at peak flow.[6] The retention fraction can be altered by acidosis and acute hypoxia.[7] As a potassium analog, ^{82}Rb is also taken up in the stomach, which can sometimes interfere with interpretation in the inferior wall.

Rob Beanlands is a Career Investigator supported by the Heart and Stroke Foundation of Ontario (HSFO). Maria Cecilia Ziadi is a Research Fellow supported by University of Ottawa International Fellowship Program, the Molecular Function and Imaging Program (HSFO grant #PRG6242) and the Division of Cardiology.

[a] Division of Cardiology, Department of Medicine, Mazinkowski Alberta Heart Institute, University of Alberta, 2C2 Walter Mackenzie Health Sciences Centre, Edmonton, Alberta T6G 2B7, Canada

[b] Division of Cardiology, Department of Medicine, Molecular Function and Imaging Program, National Cardiac PET Centre, University of Ottawa Heart Institute, 40 Ruskin Street, Ottawa, Ontario, K1Y 4W7, Canada

* Corresponding author.

E-mail address: rbeanlands@ottawaheart.ca (R. Beanlands).

Cardiol Clin 27 (2009) 237–255
doi:10.1016/j.ccl.2008.12.003

Table 1
Positron emission tomography myocardial perfusion tracers

Pharmaceutical	Radioisotope	Physical Half-Life	Production Method	Parent Compound Physical Half-Life	Physiology	Primary Application	Average Positron Energy (MeV)[a]	RMS Positron Range (mm)
Water	O-15	122 sec	Cyclotron	—	Diffusible	Perfusion	0.74	1.02
Ammonia	N-13	10 min	Cyclotron	—	Diffusible/ retained	Perfusion	0.49	0.57
Acetate	C-11	20 min	Cyclotron	—	Extracted/ metabolized	Oxidative metabolism	0.39	0.39
FDG	F-18	110 min	Cyclotron	—	Extracted/ retained	Metabolism/ viability	0.25	0.23
Rubidium	Rb-82	76 sec	^{82}Sr/^{82}Rb generator	^{82}Sr = 25.5 d	Extracted/ retained	Perfusion	1.48	2.60

Abbreviation: RMS, Root-mean square.
[a] From www.nndc.bnl.gov/mird (May 2008).
Adapted from Ziadi MC, Beanlands RSB, deKemp RA, et al. Diagnosis and prognosis in cardiac disease using cardiac PET perfusion imaging. In: Clinical nuclear cardiology: state of the art and future directions. Zaret BL, Beller GA (editors). 4th edition. in press; with permission.

Because of its short $T_{1/2}$, clinical stress perfusion studies are usually limited to pharmacologic stress with adenosine, dipyridamole, or dobutamine, although exercise imaging has been performed also.[8] Gated acquisition and analysis of contractility is feasible.[9] List-mode acquisition now enables simultaneous acquisition of dynamic data needed for flow quantification (see later discussion and separate section on flow quantification) and gating for ventricular function.[10]

$^{13}NH_3$ production requires an on-site cyclotron. It has a physical $T_{1/2}$ of 9.96 minutes. As such, transport is only feasible for short distances between production facility and use site.

$^{13}NH_3$ diffuses freely across capillary and cell membranes. Once in the cell, it can either be incorporated into ^{13}N-glutamine, which requires ATP, or it can diffuse back into the vascular space. The initial extraction is high and proportional to flow, even at high flow rates. As such, the uptake rate constant K_1 is a good estimate for quantitative blood flow.[10] The uptake and retention thus depends on both adequate blood flow to the cells and intact metabolism.

$^{13}NH_3$ has a higher first pass extraction than ^{82}Rb. It also has a longer $T_{1/2}$ than ^{82}Rb and a shorter positron range. These advantages improve count statistics and therefore image quality. This improvement is particularly helpful when imaging obese patients.

Myocardial retention of $^{13}NH_3$ may be heterogeneous, and the lateral left ventricular (LV) wall uptake can be 10% lower than other segments in normal subjects.[10,11] This difference must be considered when interpreting images. Also, image quality can sometimes be hampered by uptake in the liver, which could interfere with the evaluation of the inferior wall. Finally, in patients who have severe LV impairment, chronic obstructive pulmonary disease (COPD), or smoking, the sequestration of $^{13}NH_3$ in the lungs can be abnormally increased. Because of this increased lung uptake, static image acquisition may need to be delayed 3 to 4 minutes after the radiopharmaceutical has been injected. The acquisition time is 5 to 20 minutes.[3,4] As with ^{82}Rb, images can be gated to assess myocardial function.[12]

$H_2^{15}O$ ($T_{1/2}$ = 2.04 minutes) production requires a cyclotron. Because $H_2^{15}O$ is a freely diffusible agent, the extraction fraction is not affected by flow rates and is independent of the metabolic state of the myocardium. Because of this property, it has become the gold standard for absolute flow quantification (see later discussion and article by Schelbert elsewhere in this issue). Cardiac imaging with $H_2^{15}O$ can be demanding due to its high concentration in the blood pool that requires subtraction of the blood pool counts from the original image to visualize the myocardium.[10] At the present time its clinical use is limited to a few centers where it is also used in clinical research.[13]

Other tracers that have been used for PET perfusion imaging include ^{11}C-acetate ($T_{1/2}$ = 20.4 minutes), which is used more widely as a research tool to noninvasively measure myocardial oxygen consumption (MVO_2).[14] ^{62}Cu-PTSM (pyruvaldehyde bis [N^4-methylthiosemicarbazone]) ($T_{1/2}$ = 9.7 minutes) is another generator-produced PET perfusion tracer that has been used in the past.[15] The $^{62}Zn/^{62}Cu$ generator $T_{1/2}$ is 9.3 hours, thus requiring daily delivery. Liver uptake seems to be reduced with the newer related tracer ^{62}Cu-ETS.[16] ^{62}Cu also has high positron energy similar to ^{82}Rb, which may affect image resolution. ^{18}F-FBnTP (p-fluorobenzyl triphenyl phosphonium cation) is a member of a new class of positron-emitting lipophilic cations that may act as myocardial perfusion PET tracers.[17] ^{18}F-BMS-747158-02, an inhibitor of mitochondrial complex I (MC-1), is another promising PET myocardial perfusion imaging (MPI) tracer.[18] The longer $T_{1/2}$ of ^{18}F (110 minutes) gives these compounds the potential for wide distribution, but may require reinjection or 2-day stress-rest imaging protocols, as occurs with ^{99m}Tc SPECT agents. On the other hand, this feature may enable routine exercise stress PET MPI, which to date has not been widely applied (recent data notwithstanding).[19]

Gallium-based complexes are also being explored as potential PET perfusion tracers. $^{68}Ge/^{68}Ga$ generators could provide a convenient source of PET tracers because of the long physical $T_{1/2}$ of ^{68}Ge (271 days) and a suitable daughter $T_{1/2}$ (^{68}Ga = 67.7 minutes). Recently, good cardiac uptake has been demonstrated with a ligand labeled with ^{67}Ga for SPECT suggesting potential for these ligands as PET MPI tracers.[20]

MYOCARDIAL METABOLISM TRACERS FOR POSITRON EMISSION TOMOGRAPHY

^{18}F-FDG is a PET metabolism agent used to assess viability of the myocardium. ^{18}F production requires a cyclotron. Its relatively long $T_{1/2}$ of 110 minutes means that ^{18}F-based tracers can be transported significant distances. Most urban centers in the developed world are in proximity to a production source of ^{18}F-FDG. The increased $T_{1/2}$ means lower tracer doses must be administered to keep radiation exposure to a minimum. The radiation burden with a standard dose of ^{18}F is less than ^{201}Tl but greater than that received from a ^{99m}Tc procedure.[21] ^{18}F has the lowest positron range and therefore the highest associated spatial resolution among currently clinically available PET isotopes.[21]

^{18}F-FDG is a glucose analog that enters the myocyte in proportion to glucose uptake and undergoes phosphorylation. Unlike glucose, however, the resulting [18]FDG-6-phosphate becomes metabolically trapped by the myocyte. ^{18}F-FDG uptake thus reflects exogenous glucose use and can be used to identify viable tissue.[22,23]

There is a host of tracers used in research for other aspects of metabolism, including TCA cycle flux and oxidative metabolism (^{11}C-acetate), glucose oxidation (^{11}C-glucose), and fatty acid metabolism (eg, ^{11}C-palmitate, ^{18}F-FTHA). Their clinical application remains to be determined.

POSITRON EMISSION TOMOGRAPHY MYOCARDIAL PERFUSION IMAGING PROTOCOLS

With the short physical $T_{1/2}$ of the PET tracers applied in clinical practice ([13]NH$_3$ and [82]Rb) exercise imaging is not performed in most PET imaging facilities. Maximal coronary flow is therefore usually obtained either by the use of pharmacologic vasodilator agents (adenosine, dipyridamole, and adenosine triphosphate) or inotropic agents (ie, dobutamine).[4,24]

Patient preparation is important. Patients must not eat for at least 6 hours before scanning and must abstain from caffeine-containing products for at least 12 hours before the procedure. In addition, patients must avoid theophylline-containing medications for 48 hours before the test. Patients undergoing dobutamine stress tests should discontinue β-blockers 48 hours before the test (only for diagnostic purposes and if it is clinically safe to do so).

Common protocols used for imaging myocardial perfusion with dedicated PET or PET/CT systems involve the following steps: (1) Scout scanning: to ensure that the patient is correctly positioned. With PET/CT systems, a CT scout scan is routinely used. (2) Transmission scan: for attenuation correction (AC) purposes (before rest and after stress). (3) Emission scans: (both at rest and stress) whereby images are acquired in three different ways: (a) ECG gated imaging, (b) multiframe or dynamic imaging, and (c) list-mode imaging. In patients undergoing a PET/CT study, it is also possible to estimate coronary calcium score, and with 16-slice or greater PET/CT devices it is possible to obtain a coronary CT angiogram (CTA).

Imaging is best obtained with the patient's arms raised above the shoulders (an arm support

is useful). The same position must be maintained during the scout CT/AC and the actual PET scan to avoid artifact. Dynamic acquisition begins immediately with tracer injection. Static acquisition begins after the blood pool has cleared sufficiently (usually 3 minutes). The acquisition time is 6 to 10 minutes for [82]Rb and 5 to 20 minutes for [13]NH$_3$.[3,4,24] The rest image precedes the stress and it is recommended that the patient come out of the gantry between the rest and stress image for patient comfort and to allow the medical staff to interact with the patient. An entire rest/stress [82]Rb study can be completed in 45 minutes in most facilities. For [13]NH$_3$, it is recommended to perform the stress imaging 45 to 50 minutes after the rest injection giving 5 $T_{1/2}$ for decay of [13]NH$_3$. (Further description of PET myocardial perfusion protocols is available in the American Society of Nuclear Cardiology/American College of Cardiology [ASNC/ACC] imaging guidelines).[4]

^{18}F-FLUORODEOXYGLUCOSE POSITRON EMISSION TOMOGRAPHY VIABILITY IMAGING PROTOCOL

Under the fasting state, free fatty acids are the preferred energy source for myocardial cells. After a meal or during ischemia, glucose is the preferred substrate. Accordingly, patients are instructed to fast for at least 6 hours; then, to facilitate ^{18}F-FDG uptake in normal viable myocardial cells, a glucose load is required. ^{18}F-FDG is injected following either an oral glucose load with monitoring of the blood sugar (patients who do not have diabetes) or, for patients who have diabetes, a modified glucose load with supplemental insulin or a glucose-insulin clamp protocol. [8]F-FDG is injected in a dose of 5 MBq/kg intravenous (IV) (<550 MBq maximum). A waiting time of approximately 60 minutes (45–75 minute range) before static PET imaging is essential to ensure appropriate myocardial uptake. The acquisition takes 10 to 30 minutes and is followed by the AC scan.[4] ^{18}F-FDG uptake can be quantified as an estimate of glucose use using Patlak[25] graphical analysis of the time activity data. In this case, acquisition begins at the moment of FDG administration.

A PET perfusion scan is also required for comparison to the viability study to determine regions of reduced perfusion to distinguish perfusion/metabolism match (scar) and mismatch (hibernation). Usually, this is done as outlined earlier and precedes the ^{18}F-FDG protocol. Some centers also routinely perform stress perfusion imaging before FDG to evaluate for reversible stress induced ischemia.

ADVANTAGES AND DISADVANTAGES OF POSITRON EMISSION TOMOGRAPHY PERFUSION IMAGING
Advantages

PET MPI has several advantages over single photon emission computed tomography (SPECT) MPI. Most PET perfusion tracers have better extraction characteristics so that myocardial tracer uptake–flow relationship is more linear at higher flow rates (>2.5 mL/min/g). The technetium-based agents for SPECT can have significant uptake in the liver and bowel, which can increase artifacts and reduce the quality of the images. AC, although available for SPECT, has been problematic and not widely applied. The associated abnormalities reduce the quality of the image and therefore reduce the confidence in the interpretation of the SPECT MPI.

On the other hand, attenuation effects are significantly higher with PET in comparison with SPECT. Nonetheless, AC is relatively straightforward with PET because the length of the path of attenuation for the pair of 511-keV photons (ie, the distance between any two detectors) is constant and known for PET but is variable with SPECT. In addition, the algorithms to correct for attenuation are more accurate with PET.[2,4] AC is routine in PET imaging analysis, which contributes to achieving images of higher quality with fewer attenuation artifacts and fewer false-positive studies. Transmission source AC is used in dedicated PET scanners, but AC is now commonly performed using CT that can be acquired with low radiation to the patient. The increased specificity seen with PET MPI is in part related to better AC.

PET perfusion imaging has high spatial resolution compared with SPECT. Contrast resolution (target-to-background ratio) is also high. Because of this better resolution, there is enhanced detection of milder perfusion abnormalities, which can contribute to superior sensitivity. It has been reported by Bateman and colleagues[9] that PET perfusion images are more often judged to be of excellent quality than SPECT MPI (79% versus 62%) with less gut uptake (5% versus 41%) and fewer artifacts (17% versus 44%). Enhanced image quality leads to more confidence in reporting and less frequent equivocal reports.

Iterative reconstruction is the most commonly used reconstructive algorithm, again an advantage over the commonly used filtered back projection of SPECT imaging. The acquisition is typically done in list mode and can be gated to both cardiac and respiratory cycles. Temporal resolution is greater and dynamic imaging to yield tracer kinetic data can be obtained. Absolute quantification of myocardial blood flow (MBF) (in mL/min/g of tissue) is possible.[10,26] The usefulness of flow quantification may be in defining balanced three-vessel disease or in assessing microvascular disease.[27] To date, however, studies have not clearly defined the added benefit of flow quantification to the imaging data.

In addition, the short $T_{1/2}$ of the commonly used PET tracer, [82]Rb, allows a short acquisition time with excellent count data. The short acquisition time is more comfortable for the patient and this may result in less patient motion. Rapid repeat studies are possible. As such, the study with acquisitions at rest then stress can be completed in less than 1 hour. This time frame is convenient for the patient and satisfaction is high. Laboratory efficiency can be high also.[4]

Detectors used in PET scanners are designed for optimal detection of the 511 keV coincidence gamma rays. An important consideration in PET detector design is the scintillation crystal material, whose characteristics directly affect the spatial resolution of the PET scanner and thus imaging performance. Recently, new crystal materials, such as lutetium oxyorthosilicate and gadolinium oxyorthosilicate, have become available along with others.[4,28] These newer crystals result in better spatial resolution and reduce partial volume effects. These materials are well suited to three-dimensional imaging mode (without septa) by increasing the sensitivity of the scanner and reducing noise from scattered and random coincidences.[10]

MPI with [82]Rb PET means ECG-gated studies can be obtained early after radiotracer injection, capturing ventricular function close to peak hyperemia with pharmacologic stress agents. Wall motion changes on PET MPI with vasodilator stress are thus more sensitive for ischemia, whereas wall motion changes on SPECT are post-stress and they reflect postischemic stunning. Ischemia-induced stress wall motion changes with PET MPI may enhance sensitivity for detecting more significant disease,[29–31] whereas post-stress wall motion changes with SPECT may be more specific for more severe disease.

Recent equipment developments have included the hybrid PET/CT cameras that not only can perform CT AC but also can acquire high-quality CT images, including coronary calcium scoring and CT coronary angiograms. This development combines the advantage of CT to assess anatomy and PET imaging to assess physiology. The potential exists to tailor the cardiac examination to the unique needs of the individual patient, in one setting. Evaluation of the potential advantage of hybrid imaging is the subject of ongoing investigation.

Disadvantages

The short $T_{1/2}$ of ^{82}Rb makes exercise imaging difficult. The studies are therefore done under pharmacologic stress.

The AC data are not acquired simultaneously with the PET data. As such, body motion or respiratory movement can lead to transmission–emission misalignment and potential AC-induced artifacts. Most PET/CT systems should include software tools to correct transmission–emission misalignments. Careful review of PET/CT data for quality control is still important and a required step before image interpretation. CT for AC is best obtained before the rest PET study and then again after the stress study.

Other potential sources of reconstruction artifacts include streak artifacts seen in large patients imaged with their arms down, artifacts secondary to metal implants, and residual radioactivity in

the IV line within the field of view.[4] Visceral uptake of ^{82}Rb in the stomach or ^{13}NH$_3$ in the liver can also lead to spill-over artifacts interfering with interpretation of the inferior wall.

Box 1 summarizes some the advantages and disadvantages of PET compared with SPECT MPI.

USE OF POSITRON EMISSION TOMOGRAPHY MYOCARDIAL PERFUSION IMAGING FOR THE DIAGNOSIS OF CORONARY ARTERY DISEASE

Indications for PET MPI have been reviewed in the ASNC/ACC/American Heart Association (AHA) clinical guidelines from 2003[32] and more recently in a joint position statement by the Canadian Cardiovascular Society and partnering Canadian imaging organizations from 2007.[1]

The diagnosis or risk stratification of patients for CAD with nondiagnostic or equivocal previous tests is an important indication for PET MPI (class I indication and evidence level B).[1,32] Patients who have had an inconclusive SPECT MPI study frequently undergo PET MPI as recommended in the AHA/ACC guidelines of nuclear cardiology.[32] Patients who have equivocal SPECT studies may have an increased risk for future cardiac events.

Box 1
Positron emission tomography myocardial perfusion imaging: advantages and disadvantages versus single photon emission computed tomography

Advantages

Higher extraction fraction of tracers

Linearity of uptake maintained at higher flow rates

Less gastrointestinal (GI) uptake of radiotracers

More accurate AC with CT

Absolute quantification of flow possible

Higher spatial, temporal, and contrast resolution

Reduced partial volume averaging effects

Shorter acquisition time

Gated images obtained during peak flow

Fewer equivocal reports

Higher quality images

Higher sensitivity, specificity

Disadvantages

Limited access to radiotracers, increased cost

Short physical half-life of ^{82}Rb

Some GI uptake occurs; liver uptake for ^{13}NH$_3$

AC data not acquired simultaneously with PET data

Greater attenuation

Reconstruction artifacts

Yoshinaga and colleagues[33] reported on a subgroup of 90 patients who had [82]Rb PET MPI following inconclusive SPECT MPI. The group with abnormal studies (n = 11) had an increase in their annual total cardiac event rate compared with those who had normal PET MPI (n = 79) (15.2% versus 1.3%) supporting the value of PET MPI for risk stratification in this group.

Patients who have left bundle branch block (LBBB) or ventricular pacing rhythm also benefit from MPI. PET MPI can be used for such patients (ACC/AHA/ASNC class IIa and Beanlands and colleagues: class I [level of evidence B]).[1,32]

Patients who are obese or those who have large body habitus prone to attenuation artifacts and thus to equivocal results could benefit from PET MPI (Beanlands and colleagues class I [level of evidence B]).[1]

It is also reasonable to consider PET MPI as the first test for detection of the extent and location of ischemia (ACC/AHA/ASNC 2003 class IIa and more recent evaluation by Beanlands and colleagues 2007: class I [level of evidence B]).[1,32]

In practice, the use of PET MPI as a first-line functional evaluation is generally reserved for those who may be prone to attenuation artifact (eg, obesity) or for those patients for whom the most definitive functional evaluation is required, as may be the case for a patient who has a moderate lesion on angiogram to determine hemodynamic significance before considering revascularization.

A recent review reported that the mean sensitivity and specificity of PET MPI for diagnosis of CAD were 89% and 90% with ranges from 83% to 100% and 73% to 100%, respectively (**Table 2**).[9,34–49]

Six studies comparing CAD diagnostic accuracy have demonstrated superiority of [82]Rb or [13]NH₃ PET MPI compared with ^{201}Tl SPECT imaging.[9,34,35,41,50,51] Recently, Bateman and colleagues[9] conducted a comparison of pharmacologically stress-gated [82]Rb PET MPI to gated SPECT MPI with ^{99m}Tc-sestamibi. They reported diagnostic accuracy of 89% for PET compared with 79% for SPECT (*P* = .03) supporting that PET MPI has advantages as a diagnostic tool compared with SPECT MPI.

More recently Sampson and colleagues[49] reported the sensitivity and specificity of [82]Rb PET/ CT MPI were 93% and 83%, respectively. Sampson also showed, however, that functional PET MPI findings and anatomic CAD findings demonstrated low agreement in patients who had multivessel disease (58%) suggesting that a given level of stenosis may have different degrees of functional significance. The SPARC trial (Study of

Perfusion versus Anatomy's Role in CAD) will help clarify the relative value of PET, SPECT, and CTA imaging.[52]

THE POTENTIAL ROLE OF POSITRON EMISSION TOMOGRAPHY ABSOLUTE BLOOD FLOW QUANTIFICATION IN THE CLINICAL SETTING: ADVANCED CORONARY ARTERY DISEASE

Relative perfusion imaging may underestimate the underlying extent of disease, which constitutes a current limitation. In recent years, considerable advances have been made in development of techniques aimed at noninvasive quantification of myocardial flow. PET is recognized as the most accurate noninvasive means by which to estimate MBF and myocardial flow reserve (MFR, ratio of stress MBF to rest MBF),[10,26] which are independent of relative perfusion measurements. MBF quantification provides additional information that may improve diagnostic accuracy in this setting.[10,26] The added value of quantification is currently the subject of intense interest and investigation. With relative perfusion, either by the use of SPECT or PET, an area of reduced flow is recognized by its reduced tracer uptake relative to a normal territory. Assessment is visual with semiquantitative analysis. With multivessel disease all territories may have reduced flow but only the territory with the lowest flow may be visually obvious when using relative perfusion methods. When all territories have reduced MFR, there can also be global reduction of flow in all territories without a discrete regional abnormality. This reliance on relative flow differences for the diagnosis of ischemia is a limitation of standard MPI with SPECT or PET. Quantification of flow with PET does not depend on the normal region and therefore may prove helpful in assessing multivessel disease as previously demonstrated.[27]

Yoshinaga and colleagues[13] compared PET MPI with ^{15}O-water to SPECT MPI with ^{99m}Tc-tetrofosmin in 27 patients who had known CAD and 11 normal subjects. Some 28% (16/58) of areas with a stenotic vessel showed ischemia on SPECT MPI. The remaining 72% of areas demonstrated a reduced MFR on PET MPI with no abnormalities seen on SPECT MPI. This reduction in flow was milder than that seen in the areas positive for ischemia on SPECT. PET flow measurements may be a sensitive means for detecting CAD.

The value of quantitative flow analysis with [82]Rb PET was further assessed by Parkash and colleagues.[27] They studied 13 patients who had three-vessel CAD who underwent [82]Rb PET MPI and 10 patients who had one-vessel disease for comparison. They quantified the retention of

Table 2
Diagnosis of coronary artery disease with positron emission tomography myocardial perfusion imaging

Author	Year	Number	Stress	Tracer	Reference CAG	Sensitivity			Specificity		
						Positive Test	Patient with CAD	%	Negative Test	Patient without CAD	%
Schelbert et al[34]	1982	45	Dipyridamole	$^{13}NH_3$	>50%	31	32	97	13	13	100
Tamaki et al[35]	1985	25	Exercise	$^{13}NH_3$	N/S	18	19	95	6	6	100
Yonekura et al[36]	1987	50	Exercise	$^{13}NH_3$	>75%	37	38	97	12	12	100
Tamaki et al[37]	1988	51	Exercise	$^{13}NH_3$	>50%	47	48	98	3	3	100
Gould et al[38,a]	1986	50	Dipyridamole	$^{82}Rb/^{13}NH_3$	QCA SFR <3	—	—	—	—	—	—
Demer et al[39,a]	1989	193	Dipyridamole	$^{82}Rb/^{13}NH_3$	QCA SFR <4	126	152	83	39	41	95
Go et al[40]	1990	202	Dipyridamole	^{82}Rb	>50%	142	152	93	39	50	78
Stewart et al[41]	1991	81	Dipyridamole	^{82}Rb	QCA >50%[b]	50	60	83	18	21	86
Marwick et al[42]	1992	74	Dipyridamole	^{82}Rb	>50%	63	70	90	4	4	100
Grover-McKay et al[43]	1992	31	Dipyridamole	^{82}Rb	>50%	16	16	100	11	15	73
Laubenbacher et al[44]	1993	34	Dipy/adenosine	$^{13}NH_3$	QCA >50%[b]	14	16	88	15	18	83
Wallhaus et al[45]	2001	45	Dipyridamole	^{64}Cu-PTSM	>50%	21	25	84	20	20	100
Bateman et al[9,c]	2006	112	Dipyridamole	^{82}Rb	>50%[b]	64	74	86	38	38	100
Walsh et al[46]	1988	33	Dipyridamole	^{15}O-H_2O	QCA	22	24	92	—	—	—
Williams et al[47,d]	1994	287	Dipyridamole	^{82}Rb	>67%	88	101	87	99	112	88
Simone et al[48,d]	1992	225	Dipyridamole	^{82}Rb	>67%	d	d	83	d	d	91
Sampson et al[49,e]	2007	102	Dipy/aden/dbt-CTAC	^{82}Rb	>70%	41	44	93	48	58	83
Husmann et al[50]	2007	70	Dipyridamole	$^{13}NH_3$	>50%	51	53	96	f	f	f
Totals + weighted mean	—	1660	—	—	—	831	924	90	365	411	89

Abbreviations: aden, adenosine; CAG, coronary angiogram; CTAC, CT attenuation correction; dbt, dobutamine; dipy, dipyridamole; N/S, not stated; QCA, quantitative coronary angiography; SFR, stenosis flow reserve based on QCA data.

[a] Study reported that 50 patients in Gould et al 1986 were included; thus Gould et al not included in mean calculations.

[b] Other cutoffs reported; >50% noted here.

[c] Electronic database, matched cohort design; values derived from reported population, sensitivity, and specificity.

[d] Retrospective study; MPI influenced CAG decision; mixed patient and region method for sensitivity/specificity; patients with/without disease could not be easily determined.

[e] Specificity was determined from combination of patients who had low likelihood of disease and those who had negative angiogram.

[f] Specificity reported for lesion only, not for patient diagnosis.

Data from Beanlands R, Chow BJ, Dick A, et al. CCS/CAR/CANM/CNCS/CanSCMR joint position statement on advanced non-invasive cardiac imaging using positron emission tomography, magnetic resonance imaging and multi-detector computed tomographic angiography in the diagnosis and evaluation of ischemic heart disease abbreviated report. Can J Cardiol 2007;23: 107–19.

[82]Rb and compared the retention between stress and rest. When the quantitative data were used to determine the size of a perfusion abnormality, in the patients who had three-vessel disease, the defects were larger using the regions with abnormal quantified stress-rest perfusion difference compared with the standard normalization using relative uptake method of assessment.

Absolute quantification of MFR and MFR with PET MPI seems promising particularly in the assessment of patients who have multivessel or diffuse CAD.

THE POTENTIAL ROLE OF POSITRON EMISSION TOMOGRAPHY ABSOLUTE BLOOD FLOW QUANTIFICATION IN THE CLINICAL SETTING: PRECLINICAL CORONARY ARTERY DISEASE AND NONISCHEMIC HEART DISEASES

Endothelial dysfunction has attracted much attention as an early marker of CAD. Many clinical states are known to be associated with endothelial dysfunction. PET perfusion imaging has the ability to assess diminished flow reserve before the development of clinical ischemia and this has made it a promising tool in this area. Detection of CAD at an earlier stage offers the hope of earlier and more aggressive medical and preventative interventions.

Impaired MFR has been observed in patients who have traditional cardiovascular risk factors for CAD, encompassing hypertension, diabetes mellitus, hyperlipidemia, smoking, gender, and age, before the development of overt CAD.[10,26] Furthermore, several nonischemic cardiomyopathies (dilated cardiomyopathy and hypertrophic cardiomyopathy) have been shown to have altered CFR. An impaired vasodilator response has been shown to predict long-term outcome in these conditions.[53,54] This approach may enable early detection of impaired endothelial or microvascular dysfunction. Such global impairment may also be confused with more serious multivessel atherosclerotic CAD, however. These questions are being addressed at several sites investigating the added value of PET MBF and MFR calculation. (Further discussion on flow quantification is presented in another section).

ASSESSMENT OF FUNCTION BY MEASUREMENT OF LEFT VENTRICULAR EJECTION FRACTION

Left ventricular ejection fraction (LVEF) is well recognized as a prognostic factor in CAD. With recent advances, PET images are now routinely gated and EF calculated at rest and during peak stress.[29,30] A delta increase in LVEF from rest to stress of 5% or more yielded a negative predictive value of 97% for ruling out left main or three-vessel CAD.[29] In addition, a recent study suggested that the magnitude of LVEF increase is determined in part by stress perfusion/reversible perfusion defects ($P = .009$).[30]

USE OF POSITRON EMISSION TOMOGRAPHY MYOCARDIAL PERFUSION IMAGING TO ASSESS PROGNOSIS IN CORONARY ARTERY DISEASE

Extent and severity of perfusion abnormalities as manifested by the summed stress score (SSS) on SPECT MPI has been well shown to correlate with increased risk for cardiac events.[55] Data are emerging on the prognostic value of PET MPI also. Marwick and colleagues[56] demonstrated incremental prognostic value in comparison with clinical and angiographic findings alone. Chow and colleagues[57] described a low hard event rate (0.09% per year) in a group of patients who had normal [82]Rb PET MPI scans. Unlike SPECT imaging, normal PET MPI was associated with a good prognosis, even with a positive dipyridamole ECG, likely because of the greater sensitivity of PET to detect CAD. **Fig. 1** shows an example of a normal PET MPI scan. Yoshinaga and colleagues[33] reported (N = 367 patients followed for 3.1 ± 0.9 years) that risk for adverse cardiac events is associated with the [82]Rb PET MPI SSS (**Fig. 2**) and SSS was an independent prognostic risk factor. The annual event rate for cardiac death and myocardial infarction (MI) was only 0.4% in the group with a normal SSS and was 7% in the moderate-severe group (SSS>8).

Fig. 3 shows an example of a high-risk PET perfusion study. Some of the SPECT MPI high-risk findings (ie, large myocardial perfusion defect, multiple myocardial perfusion defects in more than one coronary territory, and the presence of transient ischemic LV dilatation [TID], among others) are also noted with PET MPI. Recently, it has been shown that elevated TID index is a specific marker of single- and multiple-vessel CAD in pharmacologic stress [82]Rb PET MPI studies.[58]

Lertsburapa and colleagues[31] studied 1441 patients who had undergone [82]Rb PET MPI. Follow-up averaged 2.7 ± 0.8 years. Annualized mortality rates were lowest in those who had stress EF greater than 60% (2.1%) and highest in those who had stress EF less than 30% (9.9%). They concluded that LVEF has added prognostic value to [82]Rb PET MPI (**Fig. 4**A, B).

EFFECT OF POSITRON EMISSION TOMOGRAPHY MYOCARDIAL PERFUSION IMAGING ON COST

There have been previous conflicting assessments of cost using different cost models More recently,

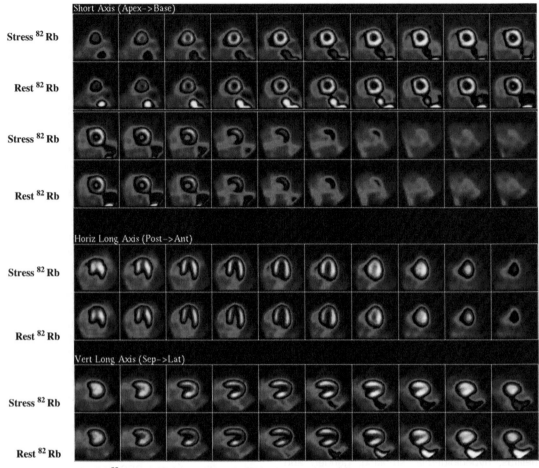

Fig. 1. 4DM display of ⁸²Rb PET MPI in a patient who had normal perfusion.

Merhige and colleagues[59] assessed cost saving with PET MPI. A total of 2159 actual patients who had an intermediate probability of CAD underwent PET MPI with ^{82}Rb and were compared with two control groups. The researchers concluded

that PET MPI led to cost savings because angiography rates were reduced. Revascularization rates were also reduced in the PET MPI group with no difference in cardiac death or MI. PET MPI thus seemed safe and cost effective. The reduced

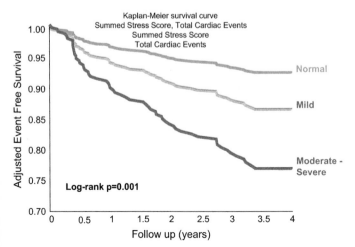

Fig. 2. Prognostic value of PET MPI. Risk-adjusted survival, free from any (total) cardiac events, as a function of summed stress score (SSS). (*From* Yoshinaga K, Chow BJ, Beanlands R, et al. What is the prognostic value of myocardial perfusion imaging using rubidium-82 positron emission tomography? J Am Coll Cardiol 2006;48:1029 –39; with permission). Color added to figure.

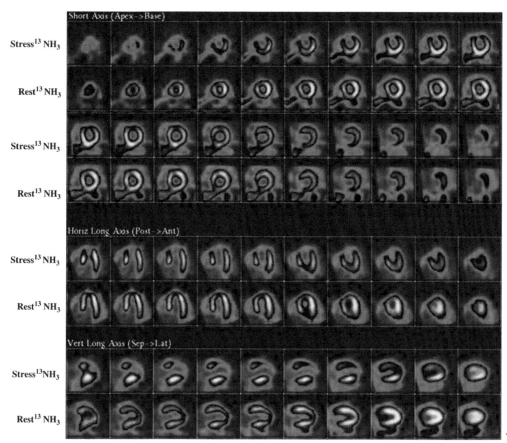

Fig. 3. 4DM display of $^{13}NH_3$ PET MPI in a patient who had reversible anterior, anteroseptal, and apical perfusion defect. There is transient ischemic dilatation (TID = 1.22). There was reversible wall motion on the gated images. High-risk scan.

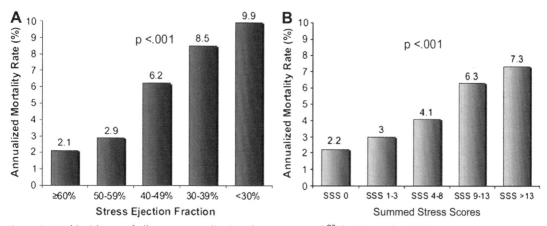

Fig. 4. Annual incidence of all-cause mortality in relation to gated ^{82}Rb PET results. (*A*) Event rates in relation to stress ejection fraction (EF). *P*<.001 across all groups. (*B*) Event rates in relation to perfusion (SSS). (*From* Lertsburapa K, Ahlberg A, Bateman T, et al. Independent and incremental prognostic value of left ventricular ejection fraction determined by stress gated rubidium 82 PET imaging in patients with known or suspected coronary artery disease. J Nuc Cardiol 2008;15:745–53; with permission.)

rate of invasive management was attributed to the increased accuracy of PET MPI. Improved image quality and fewer suboptimal images are seen with PET MPI and this may lead to greater confidence in the test result. Fewer false-positive MPI studies are reported with PET MPI, resulting in a higher specificity, which may be expected to reduce unnecessary diagnostic angiography.

ASSESSMENT OF MYOCARDIAL VIABILITY WITH POSITRON EMISSION TOMOGRAPHY

CHF is a leading cause of death and disability in North America, affecting more than 5 million individuals in the United States.[60] The morbidity of CHF includes recurrent hospitalizations, which also drive up health care costs. New therapies for CHF have improved outcomes, but mortality remains high. Because perioperative risk for revascularization is higher in patients who have reduced systolic dysfunction and the benefit may not always be certain, noninvasive risk stratification for patients who have viable myocardium becomes essential. Detection of myocardial viability in patients who have CAD and LV systolic dysfunction (with either MPI[32] or FDG imaging[1]) is generally regarded as a class I recommendation (level B evidence).

LV dysfunction in ischemic heart disease may be due to prior infarct and scar or viable tissue that can be stunned, hibernating, or normal remodeled myocardium. Approximately 70% of CHF is secondary to CAD and a significant number of these patients have myocardial hibernation.[61]

Stunning and Hibernation

Acute reduction in flow to myocardial tissue leads to ischemia with associated reduced contractile function in the region. Prolonged severe ischemia may result in infarction if flow is not restored. Following an episode of ischemia, contractile function may remain reduced for a period of time before eventually recovering even if there is no infarction. This phenomenon has been termed "stunning of the myocardium."[62] Prolonged or repetitive reductions in myocardial flow may lead to a state of chronically reduced contractility in viable myocardial tissue. Such viable tissue is still able to metabolize glucose but with impaired contractile function and associated reduction in perfusion represents a state often referred to as "hibernating myocardium."[63] Hibernating myocardium may recover function when flow is restored.

Viability assessment with ^{18}F-FDG assesses regional myocardial glucose metabolism in hypocontractile myocardial segments and compares it to perfusion imaging. Areas with maintained glucose metabolism, based on maintained FDG uptake, but with diminished perfusion, are so-called "perfusion-metabolism mismatch," a hallmark of hibernating myocardium (**Fig. 5**) indicating the potential for recovery of function after revascularization. The extent of mismatch is related to the degree of improvement with 18% or more of the LV predicting a significant change in CHF class after revascularization.[64] Conversely, regions with reduced perfusion and reduced glucose use based on reduced FDG uptake are considered a perfusion-metabolism match indicating scar and irreversible contractile dysfunction that will not improve after revascularization.[65] Other patterns, such as reverse mismatch pattern (normal perfusion, reduced metabolism relative to perfusion) can be observed in many patients who have LBBB,[66] in repetitive stunning, and in patients who have diabetes.[67] The significance of reverse mismatch is uncertain but preliminary work suggests that in patients who have LBBB, the presence of septal reverse mismatch may signal potential benefit from CRT.

Viability and Wall Motion Recovery

Recent meta-analyses demonstrate that dobutamine ECG is the most specific and least sensitive of all methods, whereas FDG PET is the most sensitive for predicting wall motion recovery (**Fig. 6**).[5]

Viability and Outcome

Patients who have CHF and extensive myocardial hibernation have higher rates of cardiac death and nonfatal MI if treated medically.[1,5] ^{18}F-FDG PET seems to provide the best incremental outcome benefit. The outcome data reported by the most recent meta-analysis study are shown (**Fig. 7**). This analysis addresses the importance of assessment of myocardial viability in patients who have systolic dysfunction secondary to CAD. Essentially, these predominantly retrospective observational studies have shown that when viability is present, such patients have better outcome with rather than without revascularization, particularly for FDG PET–defined viability. On the contrary, patients who do not have viability do not seem to gain benefit from revascularization (at least for FDG PET–defined viability [**Fig. 7**]). These data suggest great value for FDG PET to identify high-risk patients but until recently this was not supported by randomized controlled trial data.

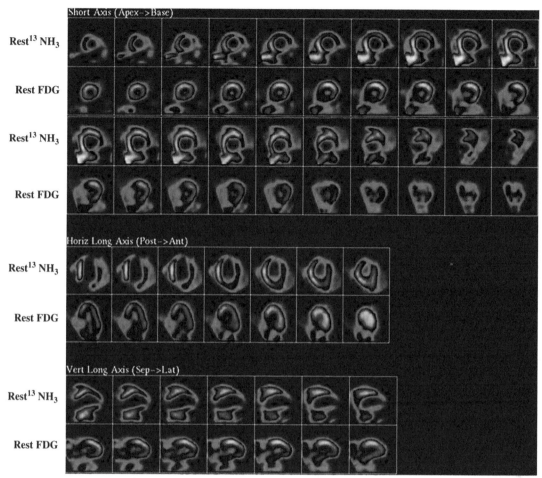

Fig. 5. PET $^{13}NH_3$ rest perfusion/^{18}FDG metabolism. PET perfusion images displayed on the top row, metabolic images displayed on second row. A large area of perfusion/metabolic mismatch involving the apex, mid to distal anterior, and anterolateral walls is noted. This finding is consistent with hibernating myocardium in the left anterior descending (LAD). In addition, a moderate region of perfusion/metabolic mismatch in the entire inferior and inferolateral walls is noted, consistent with hibernating myocardium in the left circumflex (LCX) territory.

Prospective Outcome Data on Viability Imaging in Severe Left Ventricular Dysfunction

The PARR-2 (Positron Emission Tomography And Recovery Following Revascularization–2) trial[68] represents the largest randomized study to evaluate viability imaging and the first to focus on patients who have severe LV dysfunction, the most relevant patient population for viability imaging. The results showed a trend for benefit in the arm that used ^{18}F-FDG PET to assist with management decisions. Although this did not reach statistical significance, when patients who adhered to PET recommendations were considered there was a significant outcome benefit (**Fig. 8**). Likewise, a predefined subgroup of high-risk patients who did not have recent angiography gained a significant

mortality benefit. Predictors of outcome included the following parameters: (a) renal function, (b) LV function (trend), and (c) interaction of hibernation with revascularization.[69] There was no such interaction with extent of scar, nor with other parameters. Parameters such as scar and LV function may have prognostic value but do not necessarily predict response to revascularization, whereas ischemia and hibernation identify the substrate for potential outcome benefit with revascularization. In patient evaluation, EF and scar are useful prognostic parameters predicting outcome regardless of therapy but it is degree of ischemia and hibernation that help identify those who will or will not gain benefit from revascularization.[54,69] Results from additional ongoing studies will help to better define those patients who would obtain the main benefit from various viability imaging.[70,71]

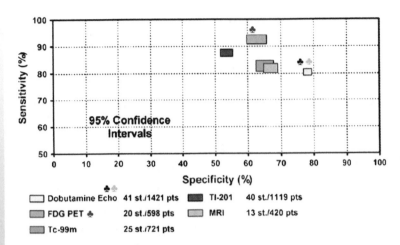

Fig. 6. Comparison of sensitivities and specificities with 95% confidence intervals of the various techniques for the prediction of recovery of regional LVEF after revascularization. Sensitivity: red clover, $P<.05$ better versus others; blue clover, $P<.05$ worse versus others. Specificity: green clover, $P<.05$ better versus others. (*From* Schinkel AFL, Ferrari R, Bax JJ, et al. Hibernating myocardium: diagnosis and patient outcomes. Curr Probl Cardiol 2007;32:375–410; with permission.)

USE OF FLUORODEOXYGLUCOSE POSITRON EMISSION TOMOGRAPHY IN INFLAMMATORY CARDIOVASCULAR DISORDERS

Cardiac Positron Emission Tomography to Detect Cardiac Sarcoidosis

Cardiac involvement with sarcoidosis is common but often silent. Cardiac PET has been evaluated as a diagnostic procedure in patients who have cardiac sarcoid with encouraging results. In one study, Okumura compared ^{18}F-FDG PET imaging, ^{99m}Tc-sestamibi SPECT, and ^{67}Ga scintigraphy in 22 patients according to the relevant Japanese Ministry of Health and Welfare guidelines for diagnosing cardiac sarcoidosis. ^{18}F-FDG PET imaging detected cardiac sarcoid with 100% sensitivity, whereas ^{99m}Tc-sestamibi SPECT had a sensitivity of 63.6% and ^{67}Ga scintigraphy of only 36.3%.[72]

In a head-to-head comparison with MRI, ^{18}F-FDG yielded a higher sensitivity for diagnosing cardiac sarcoidosis of 87.5% compared with

75% for MRI, but specificity was low at 38.5% compared with 76.9% for MRI.[73]

When patterns of ^{18}F-FDG uptake were compared between controls and patients known to have systemic sarcoidosis, focal uptake (or focal on diffuse uptake) of ^{18}F-FDG was seen only in patients who had sarcoidosis. A diffuse pattern of ^{18}F-FDG uptake was seen in about half of the control subjects, however, reducing the specificity of PET imaging.[74]

[13]NH$_3$/^{18}F-FDG imaging has also been used and the [13]NH$_3$ perfusion imaging had similar sensitivity as ^{18}F-FDG imaging, but the ^{18}F-FDG imaging abnormalities diminished on serial studies with steroid treatment and the [13]NH$_3$ images showed no change.[75] This finding suggests there may be a role for PET cardiac imaging in the assessment and follow-up of cardiac sarcoidosis.

PET imaging seems to be a promising diagnostic tool in cardiac sarcoidosis with particular value if the study is negative. Pulmonary FDG

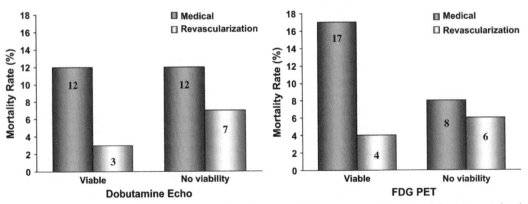

Fig. 7. Mortality rates. Revascularization or medical therapy—viable or nonviable using dobutamine echo (10 studies, 1645 patients) versus FDG PET (10 studies, 1002 patients). (*Adapted from* Schinkel AFL, Ferrari R, Bax JJ, et al. Hibernating myocardium: diagnosis and patient outcomes. Curr Probl Cardiol 2007;32:375–410; with permission.)

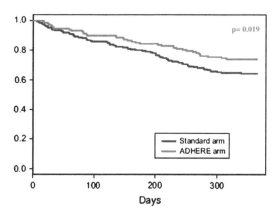

Fig. 8. PARR-2 trial. Survival curves (on the basis of time to first occurring outcome out of the composite event). The PET adherence group versus standard care arm. Mantel-Haenszel (log-rank) test for differences between two survival curves; adjusted hazard ratio = 0.62; 95% CI, 0.42 to 0.93; *P* = .019. (*From* Beanlands R, Ruddy T, deKemp R, et al. Positron emission tomography and recovery following revascularization (PARR-1): the importance of scar and the development of a prediction rule for the degree of recovery of left ventricular function. J Am Coll Cardiol 2002;40:1735–43; with permission.)

PET imaging has also been reported to be useful in tracking the response of pulmonary sarcoidosis to steroid therapy.[76]

CLINICAL APPLICATIONS OF FLUORODEOXYGLUCOSE POSITRON EMISSION TOMOGRAPHY UNDER INVESTIGATION
Applications of Positron Emission Tomography in Conditions with Vascular Inflammation

PET imaging has been explored as a tool to evaluate inflammatory processes in the vessel wall. In an animal model, Tawakol and colleagues[77] performed FDG PET imaging of inflamed vascular lesions and concluded that FDG accumulates in macrophage-rich atherosclerotic plaques and that vascular macrophage activity can be quantified with FDG PET.

In addition, Rudd and colleagues[78] performed serial FDG imaging of the carotid, iliac, and femoral arteries of 20 patients who had ^{18}F-FDG and concluded that results were reproducible. They suggested PET could be used to track response to therapy.

Meller performed ^{18}F-FDG PET imaging with a hybrid camera and MR imaging in five patients who had early Takayasu aortitis (TA). Abnormal FDG uptake in the wall of the aorta was noted in all patients and this group concluded that FDG PET was a useful screening method in early TA.[79]

Cardiac PET imaging has been used to evaluate patients who have Kawasaki disease. Hauser and colleagues[80] showed reduced MFR on ^{13}NH$_3$ PET MPI at rest and after vasodilatation in 10 asymptomatic children who had a history of Kawasaki arteritis suggesting residual damage. A second group studied 12 patients who had Kawasaki disease compared with 12 normal patients imaged using H$_2$^{15}O PET and showed reduced MBF in aneurysmal regions during the cold pressor test. They concluded that endothelial function was often impaired in these patients.[81]

Cardiac PET has been evaluated for its role in various syndromes with vasculitis. FDG PET imaging showed increased uptake in echocardiographically abnormal cardiac areas in six patients who had proven endocarditis/endocarteritis.[82] There are case reports demonstrating usefulness of PET imaging in cases of vasculitis. In one case, the FDG PET scan identified unsuspected active inflammation in the pulmonary artery that also responded to therapy. These examples demonstrate the potential usefulness of FDG PET (particularly when fused with CT imaging to detect and monitor active aortitis).[83] PET imaging has a promising future in the imaging of various vasculitis syndromes.

Other Potential Tracers for Clinical Application Under Investigation

Recent advances in molecular imaging with PET are promising. Among these, neurotransmitter and receptor imaging could facilitate our understanding of the pathophysiologic processes involved in several forms of heart disease, including CHF.[84] Carbon-11 (^{11}C)–meta-hydroxyephedrine in conjunction with FDG viability imaging may become useful to identify patients who have ischemic cardiomyopathy at risk for sudden cardiac death.[85]

Metabolic imaging represents another topic of growing interest. ^{11}C-acetate PET is used to measure oxidative metabolism, which is known to correlate with MVO$_2$.[86,87] The effects of multiple therapies on cardiac energetics have been and continue to be investigated.

SUMMARY

PET imaging has well-established clinical applications in the evaluation of patients who have actual or suspected cardiovascular disease. As the availability of PET continues to increase, its appropriate use and application will also grow. In CAD it has a role in diagnosis, risk stratification and prognosis, and assessment of function. New perfusion agents will expand capabilities to more sites and may expand PET MPI with pharmacologic stress testing to PET MPI with exercise stress. ^{18}F-FDG PET is a key element in the assessment of the difficult patient who has CAD and systolic dysfunction in assessment of viability. Cardiac PET is the most sensitive method for predicting recovery of function and has strong outcome data to support its clinical usefulness. PET can also be useful in the management of patients who have less common cardiac conditions, such as cardiac sarcoid, and inflammatory conditions, such as aortitis. Other applications of PET, including flow quantification, FDG use in other conditions such as cardiomyopathy and vascular disease, and the use of newer tracers in molecular imaging, are currently the subject of ongoing research. No doubt we have only begun to tap the potential uses of this imaging technology.

REFERENCES

1. Beanlands R, Chow BJ, Dick A, et al. CCS/CAR/ CANM/CNCS/CanSCMR joint position statement on advanced non-invasive cardiac imaging using positron emission tomography, magnetic resonance imaging and multi-detector computed tomographic angiography in the diagnosis and evaluation of ischemic heart disease abbreviated report. Can J Cardiol 2007;23:107–19.

2. Ziadi MC, Beanlands RSB, deKemp RA, et al. Diagnosis and prognosis in cardiac disease using cardiac PET perfusion imaging. In: Zaret BL, Beller GA (editors). Clinical nuclear cardiology: state of the art and future directions. Fourth edition, in press.

3. Machac J. Cardiac positron emission tomography imaging. Semin Nucl Med 2005;35:17–36.

4. Machac J, Bacharach S, Bateman T, et al. Positron emission tomography myocardial perfusion and glucose metabolism imaging. J Nucl Cardiol 2006; 13:121–51.

5. Schinkel AFL, Ferrari R, Bax JJ, et al. Hibernating myocardium: diagnosis and patient outcomes. Curr Probl Cardiol 2007;32:375–410.

6. Mullani NA, Goldstein RA, Gould KL, et al. Myocardial perfusion with rubidium-82. I. Measurement of extraction fraction and flow with external detectors. J Nucl Med 1983;24:898–906.

7. Wilson RA, Shea M, Landsheere CD, et al. Rubidium-82 myocardial uptake and extraction after transient ischemia: PET characteristics. J Comput Assist Tomogr 1987;11:60–6.

8. Chow BJ, Ananthasubramaniam K, deKemp RA, et al. Comparison of treadmill exercise versus dipyridamole stress with myocardial perfusion imaging using rubidium-82 positron emission tomography. J Am Coll Cardiol 2005;45:1227–34.

9. Bateman T, Heller G, McGhie A, et al. Diagnostic accuracy of rest/stress ECG-gated Rb-82 myocardial perfusion PET: comparison with ECG-gated Tc-99m sestamibi SPECT. J Nucl Cardiol 2006;13: 24–33.

10. deKemp R, Yoshinaga K, Beanlands R. Will 3-dimensional PET-CT enable the routine quantification of myocardial blood flow? J Nucl Cardiol 2007;14: 380–97.

11. Beanlands RS, Hutchins GD, Muzik O, et al. Heterogenicity of regional nitrogen 13-labeled ammonia tracer distribution in the normal human heart: comparison with rubidium 82 and copper 62-labeled PTSM. J Nucl Cardiol 1994;1:225–35.

12. Hickey R, Sciacca R, Bokhari S, et al. Assessment of cardiac wall motion and ejection fraction with gated PET using N-13 ammonia. Clin Nucl Med 2004;29: 243–8.

13. Yoshinaga K, Katoh C, Noriyasu K, et al. Reduction of coronary flow reserve in areas with and without ischemia on stress perfusion imaging in patients with coronary artery disease: a study using oxygen 15-labeled water PET. J Nucl Cardiol 2003;10: 275–83.

14. Sun KT, Yeatman LA, Buxton DB, et al. Simultaneous measurement of myocardial oxygen consumption and blood flow using 11-carbon acetate. J Nucl Med 1998;39:272–80.

15. Green MA, Mathias CJ, Welch MJ, et al. Copper-62-labeled pyruvaldehyde bis (N4-methylthiosemicarbazonato) copper (II): synthesis and evaluation as a positron emission tomography tracer for cerebral and myocardial perfusion. J Nucl Med 1990;31: 1989–96.

16. Lacy JL, Haynes NG, Nayak N, et al. PET myocardial perfusion imaging with generator produced radiopharmaceuticals. [62]Cu-PTSM and 62Cu-ETS. Clinical Nuclear Medicine 2000;25:396–402.

17. Madar I, Ravert H, DiPaula A, et al. Assessment of severity of coronary artery stenosis in a canine model using the PET agent ^{18}F-fluorobenzyl triphenyl phosphonium: comparison with 99mTc-tetrofosmin. J Nucl Med 2007;48:1021–30.

18. Yalamanchili P, Wexler E, Hayes M, et al. Mechanism of uptake and retention of F-18 BMS-747158-02 in cardiomyocytes: a novel PET myocardial imaging agent. J Nucl Cardiol 2007;14:782–8.

19. Chow BJ, Beanlands RS, Lee A, et al. Treadmill exercise produces larger perfusion defects than dipyridamole stress N-13 ammonia positron emission tomography. J Am Coll Cardiol 2006;47: 411–6.

20. Plössla K, Chandraa R, Qua W, et al. A novel gallium bisaminothiolate complex as a myocardial perfusion imaging agent. Nucl Med Biol 2008;35:83–90.

21. Sánchez-Crespo A, Andreo P, Larsson S. Positron flight in human tissues and its influence on PET

image spatial resolution. Eur J Nucl Med Mol Imaging 2004;31(1):44–51.

22. Ratib O, Phelps M, Huang S, et al. Positron tomography with deoxyglucose for estimating local myocardial glucose metabolism. J Nucl Med 1982; 23:577–86.

23. Hariharan R, Bray M, Ricky Ganim R, et al. Fundamental limitations of [^{18}F]2-deoxy-2-fluoro-D-glucose for assessing myocardial glucose uptake. Circulation 1995;91:2435–44.

24. Sabahat Bokhari S, Ficaro E, McCallister B, et al. Adenosine stress protocols for myocardial perfusion imaging. J Nucl Cardiol 2007;14:415–6.

25. Patlak CS, Blasberg RG. Graphical evaluation of blood-to-brain transfer constants from multiple-time uptake data: generalizations. J Cereb Blood Flow Metab 1985;5:584–90.

26. Kauffmann P, Camici P. Myocardial blood flow measurement by PET: technical aspects and clinical applications. J Nucl Med 2005;46:75–88.

27. Parkash R, deKemp R, Ruddy T, et al. Potential utility of rubidium 82 PET quantification in patients with 3-vessel disease. J Nucl Cardiol 2004;11(4):440–9.

28. Schwaiger M, Ziegler S, Nekolla S, et al. PET/CT: challenge for nuclear cardiology. J Nucl Med 2005; 46:1664–78.

29. Dorbala S, Kwong R, Di Carli MF, et al. Value of left ventricular ejection fraction reserve in assessment of severe left main/three-vessel coronary artery disease: a rubidium-82 PET-CT study. J Nucl Med 2007;48:349–58.

30. Brown TL, Merrill J, Bengel FM, et al. Determinants of the response of left ventricular ejection fraction to vasodilator stress in electrocardiographically gated 82-rubidium myocardial perfusion PET. Eur J Nucl Med Mol Imaging 2008;35:336–42.

31. Lertsburapa K, Ahlberg A, Bateman T, et al. Independent and incremental prognostic value of left ventricular ejection fraction determined by stress gated rubidium 82 PET imaging in patients with known or suspected coronary artery disease. J Nucl Cardiol 2008;15:745–53.

32. Klocke F, Baird M, Bateman T, et al. ACC/AHA/ASNC guidelines for the clinical use of cardiac radionuclide imaging. J Am Coll Cardiol 2003;42(7): 1318–33.

33. Yoshinaga K, Chow BJ, Beanlands R, et al. What is the prognostic value of myocardial perfusion imaging using rubidium-82 positron emission tomography? J Am Coll Cardiol 2006;48:1029–39.

34. Schelbert HR, Phelps ME, Wisenberg G, et al. Noninvasive assessment of coronary stenoses by myocardial imaging during pharmacologic coronary vasodilation. VI. Detection of coronary artery disease in human beings with intravenous N-13 ammonia and positron computed tomography. Am J Cardiol 1982;49:1197–207.

35. Tamaki N, Senda M, Yonekura Y, et al. Myocardial positron computed tomography with 13N-ammonia at rest and during exercise. Eur J Nucl Med 1985; 11:246–51.

36. Yonekura Y, Senda M, Tamaki N, et al. Detection of coronary artery disease with 13N ammonia and high resolution positron-emission computed tomography. Am Heart J 1987;113:645–54.

37. Tamaki N, Koide H, Saji H, et al. Value and limitation of stress thallium-201 single photon emission computed tomography: comparison with nitrogen-13 ammonia positron tomography. J Nucl Med 1988;29:1181–8.

38. Gould KL, Goldstein RA, Mullani NA, et al. Noninvasive assessment of coronary stenoses by myocardial perfusion imaging during pharmacologic coronary vasodilation. VIII. Clinical feasibility of positron cardiac imaging without a cyclotron using generator-produced rubidium-82. J Am Coll Cardiol 1986;7:775–89.

39. Demer LL, Gould KL, Goldstein RA, et al. Assessment of coronary artery disease severity by positron emission tomography. Comparison with quantitative arteriography in 193 patients. Circulation 1989;79: 825–35.

40. Go RT, Marwick TH, MacIntyre WJ, et al. A prospective comparison of rubidium-82 PET and thallium-201 SPECT myocardial perfusion imaging utilizing a single dipyridamole stress in the diagnosis of coronary artery disease. J Nucl Med 1990;31: 1899–905.

41. Stewart RE, Molina E, Popma J, et al. Comparison of rubidium-82 positron emission tomography and thallium-201 SPECT imaging for detection of coronary artery disease. Am J Cardiol 1991;67:1303–10.

42. Marwick TH, Nemec JJ, Salcedo EE, et al. Diagnosis of coronary artery disease using exercise echocardiography and positron emission tomography: comparison and analysis of discrepant results. J Am Soc Echocardiogr 1992;5:231–8.

43. Grover-McKay M, Ratib O, Schwaiger M, et al. Detection of coronary artery disease with positron emission tomography and rubidium 82. Am Heart J 1992;123:646–52.

44. Laubenbacher C, Rothley J, Sitomer J, et al. An automated analysis program for the evaluation of cardiac PET studies: initial results in the detection and localization of coronary artery disease using nitrogen-13-ammonia. J Nucl Med 1993;34:968–78.

45. Wallhaus TR, Lacy J, Stewart R, et al. Copper-62-pyruvaldehyde bis (N-methyl-thiosemicarbazone) PET imaging in the detection of coronary artery disease in humans. J Nucl Cardiol 2001;8:67–74.

46. Walsh MN, Bergmann SR, Kenzora JL, et al. Delineation of impaired regional myocardial perfusion by positron emission tomography with H2(15)O. Circulation 1988;78:612–20.

47. Williams BR, Jansen DE, Mullani NA, et al. A retrospective study of the diagnostic accuracy of a community hospital-based PET center for the detection of coronary artery disease using rubidium-82. J Nucl Med 1994;35:1586–92.

48. Simone GL, Mullani NA, Page DA, et al. Utilization statistics and diagnostic accuracy of a nonhospital-based positron emission tomography center for the detection of coronary artery disease using rubidium-82. Am J Physiol Imaging 1992;7:203–9.

49. Sampson UK, Di Carli MF, Dorbala S, et al. Diagnostic accuracy of rubidium-82 myocardial perfusion imaging with hybrid positron emission tomography/computed tomography in the detection of coronary artery disease. J Am Coll Cardiol 2007; 49:1052–8.

50. Husmann L, Kaufmann PA, Valenta L, et al. Diagnostic accuracy of myocardial perfusion imaging with single photon emission computed tomography and positron emission tomography: a comparison with coronary angiography. Int J Cardiovasc Imaging 2008;24(5):511–8.

51. Namdar M, Hany TF, Koepfli P, et al. Integrated PET/CT for the assessment of coronary artery disease: a feasibility study. J Nucl Med 2005;46:930–5.

52. Study of myocardial perfusion and coronary anatomy imaging roles in CAD (SPARC). Web page Available at: http://www.sparctrial.org. Accessed: September, 2008.

53. Neglia D, Michelassi C, Pratali L, et al. Prognostic role of myocardial blood flow impairment in idiopathic left ventricular dysfunction. Circulation 2002; 105:186–93.

54. Cecchi F, Olivotto I, Gistri R, et al. Coronary microvascular dysfunction and prognosis in hypertrophic cardiomyopathy. N Engl J Med 2003;349: 1027–35.

55. Hachamovitch R, Rozanski A, Hayes SW, et al. Predicting therapeutic benefit from myocardial revascularization procedures: are measurements of both resting left ventricular ejection fraction and stress-induced myocardial ischemia necessary? J Nucl Cardiol 2006;13:768–78.

56. Marwick T, Shan K, Sanjiv Patel S, et al. Incremental value of rubidium-82 positron emission tomography for prognostic assessment of known or suspected coronary artery disease. Am J Cardiol 1997;80: 865–70.

57. Chow BJ, Yoshinaga K, Williams K, et al. Prognostic significance of dypiridamole-induced ST depression in patients with normal 82Rb PET myocardial perfusion imaging. J Nucl Med 2005;46:1095–101.

58. Shi H, Santana CA, Rivero A, et al. Normal values and prospective validation of transient ischaemic dilation index in 82Rb PET myocardial perfusion imaging. Nucl Med Commun 2007;28:859–63.

59. Merhige M, Breen W, Shelton V, et al. Impact of myocardial perfusion imaging with PET and 82Rb on downstream invasive procedure utilization, costs, and outcomes in coronary disease management. J Nucl Med 2007;48:1069–76.

60. Rosamond W, Flegal K, Friday G, et al. Heart Disease and Stroke Statistics —2007 Update: A Report From the American Heart Association Statistics Committee and Stroke Statistics Subcommittee. Circulation 2007;115:e69–171.

61. Gheorghiade M, Bonow RO. Chronic heart failure in the United States: a manifestation of coronary artery disease. Circulation 1998;97:282–9.

62. Braunwald E, Kloner RA. The stunned myocardium: prolonged, postischemic ventricular dysfunction. Circulation 1982;66:1146–9.

63. Rahimtoola SH. From coronary artery disease to heart failure: role of the hibernating myocardium. Am J Cardiol 1995;75:16–22.

64. Di Carli MF, Asgazadie F, Schelbert HR, et al. Quantitative relation between myocardial viability and improvement in heart failure symptoms after revascularization in patients with ischemic cardiomyopathy. Circulation 1995;92:3436–44.

65. Beanlands R, Ruddy T, deKemp R, et al. Positron emission tomography and recovery following revascularization (PARR-1): the importance of scar and the development of a prediction rule for the degree of recovery of left ventricular function. J Am Coll Cardiol 2002;40:1735–43.

66. Thompson K, Saab G, Birnie D, et al. Is septal glucose metabolism altered in patients with left bundle branch block and ischemic cardiomyopathy? J Nucl Med 2006;47:1763–8.

67. Di Carli MF, Prcevski P, Singh TP, et al. Myocardial blood flow, function, and metabolism in repetitive stunning. J Nucl Med 2000;41: 1227–34.

68. Beanlands RSB, Ruddy T, et al. 18-Fluorodeoxyglucose positron emission tomography imaging-assisted management of patients with severe left ventricular dysfunction and suspected coronary disease a randomized controlled trial (PARR-2). J Am Coll Cardiol 2007;50:2002–12.

69. D'Egidio G, Nichol G, Williams K, et al. Hibernating myocardium identifies high risk patients with ischemic cardiomyopathy. Substudy of the PARR-2 trial. Can J of Card 2007;23(Supp c): 228C.

70. Joyce D, Loebe M, Noon GP, et al. Revascularization and ventricular restoration in patients with ischemic heart failure: the STICH trial. Curr Opin Cardiol 2003;18:454–7.

71. Cleland JG, Freemantle N, Ball SG, et al. The heart failure revascularization trial (HEART): rationale, design and methodology. Eur J Heart Fail 2003;5: 295–303.

72. Okumura W, Iwasaki T, Toyama T. Usefulness of fasting 18F-FDG PET in identification of cardiac sarcoidosis. J Nucl Med 2004;45(12):1989–98.

73. Ohira H, Tsujino I, Ishimaru S. Myocardial imaging with 18F-fluoro-2-deoxyglucose positron emission tomography and magnetic resonance imaging in sarcoidosis. Eur J Nucl Med Mol Imaging 2008;35:933–41.

74. Ishimaru H, Tsujino I, Takei T, et al. Focal uptake on 18F-fluoro-2-deoxyglucose positron emission tomography images indicates cardiac involvement of sarcoidosis. Eur Heart J 2005;26(15):1538–43.

75. Yamagishi H, Shirai N, Takagi M, et al. Identification of cardiac sarcoidosis with ^{13}NH$_3$/^{18}F-FDG PET. J Nucl Med 2003;44:1030–6.

76. Kaira K, Ishizuka T, Yanagitani N, et al. Value of FDG positron emission tomography in monitoring the effects of therapy in progressive pulmonary sarcoidosis. Clin Nucl Med 2007;32:114–6.

77. Tawakol A, Migrino R, Hoffmann U, et al. Noninvasive in vivo measurement of vascular inflammation with F-18 fluorodeoxyglucose positron emission tomography. J Nucl Cardiol 2005;12(3):294–301.

78. Rudd J, Myers K, Bansilal S, et al. Atherosclerosis inflammation imaging with 18F-FDG PET: carotid, iliac, and femoral uptake reproducibility, quantification methods, and recommendations. J Nucl Med 2008;49(6):871–8.

79. Meller J, Grabbe E, Becker W, et al. Value of F-18 FDG hybrid camera PET and MRI in early takayasu aortitis. Eur Radiol 2003;13:400–5.

80. Hauser M, Bengel F, Kuehn A, et al. Myocardial blood flow and coronary flow reserve in children with "normal" epicardial coronary arteries after the onset of Kawasaki disease assessed by positron emission tomography. Pediatr Cardiol 2004;25(2):108–12.

81. Furuyama H, Odagawa Y, Katoh C, et al. Assessment of coronary function in children with a history of Kawasaki disease using (15) O-water positron emission tomography. Circulation 2002;105(24):2878–84.

82. Yen RF, Chen YC, Wu YW, et al. Using 18-fluoro-2-deoxyglucose positron emission tomography in detecting infectious endocarditis/endoarteritis: a preliminary report. Acad Radiol 2004;11(3):316–21.

83. Mielniczuk L, DeKemp RA, Dennie C, et al. Images in cardiovascular medicine. Fluorine-18-labeled deoxyglucose positron emission tomography in the diagnosis and management of aortitis with pulmonary artery involvement. Circulation 2005;111:e375–6.

84. Valette H, Syrota A, Merlet P. Use of PET radiopharmaceuticals to probe cardiac receptors. In: Schwaiger M, editor. Cardiac positron emission tomography. Boston: Kluwer Academic Publishers; 1996. p. 331–51.

85. Fallavollita JA, Luisi AJ Jr, Michalek SM, et al. Prediction of arrhythmic events with positron emission tomography: PAREPET study design and methods. Contemp Clin Trials 2006;27:374–88.

86. Beanlands RS, Schwaiger M. Changes in myocardial oxygen consumption and efficiency with heart failure therapy measured by ^{11}C acetate PET. Can J Cardiol 1995;11:293–300.

87. Gropler RJ. Pet measurements of myocardial metabolism. In: Di Carli MF, Lipton MJ, editors. Cardiac PET and PET/CT imaging. Springer; 2007. p. 227–49.

Hybrid Imaging: Integration of Nuclear Imaging and Cardiac CT

Marcelo F. Di Carli, MD[a,b,*]

KEYWORDS

- PET • SPECT • Myocardial perfusion imaging
- Computed tomography • Atherosclerosis

The integration of nuclear medicine cameras with multidetector CT scanners (eg, positron emission tomography [PET]-CT and single photon emission CT [SPECT]-CT) provides a unique opportunity to delineate cardiac and vascular anatomic abnormalities and their physiologic consequences in a single setting. For the evaluation of patients with known or suspected coronary artery disease (CAD), it allows detection and quantification of the burden of the extent of calcified and noncalcified plaques (coronary artery calcium [CAC] and coronary angiography), quantification of vascular reactivity and endothelial health, identification of flow-limiting coronary stenoses, and assessment of myocardial viability. Consequently, by revealing the burden of anatomic CAD and its physiologic significance, hybrid imaging can provide unique information that may improve noninvasive diagnosis, risk assessment, and management of CAD. By integrating the detailed anatomic information from CT with the high sensitivity of radionuclide imaging to evaluate targeted molecular and cellular abnormalities, hybrid imaging may play a key role in shaping the future of molecular diagnostics and therapeutics. This article reviews potential clinical applications of hybrid imaging in cardiovascular disease.

RATIONALE FOR INTEGRATING NUCLEAR IMAGING AND CT

For many decades, CT and nuclear imaging have followed separate and distinct developmental pathways. Both modalities have their strengths; CT scanners image cardiac and coronary anatomy with high spatial resolution, whereas nuclear imaging can identify a functional abnormality in, for example, myocardial perfusion, metabolism, or receptors. Although it may seem that in many cases it would be equally effective to view separately acquired CT and nuclear images for a given patient on adjacent computer displays, with or without software registration, experience in the past 7 years with commercial PET/CT scanners has highlighted the superiority of the hybrid technology for improved detection and staging of cancer. The concept of applying dual-modality imaging to the evaluation of patients with known or suspected cardiovascular disease is relatively new and not without controversy, however. In thinking about the potentially complementary aspects of dual-modality imaging, one must necessarily begin by reviewing the strengths and limitations of single-modality approaches.

Myocardial Perfusion Imaging

It represents a robust approach to diagnosing obstructive CAD, quantifying the magnitude of myocardium at risk, assessing the extent of tissue viability, and guiding therapeutic management (ie, selection of patients for revascularization). The extensive published literature with SPECT suggests that its average sensitivity for detecting more than 50% angiographic stenosis is 87% (range, 71%–97%), whereas the average

[a] Noninvasive Cardiovascular Imaging Program, Departments of Medicine (Cardiology) and Radiology, Brigham and Women's Hospital, Harvard Medical School, Boston, MA 02115, USA
[b] Division of Nuclear Medicine and Molecular Imaging, Department of Radiology, Brigham and Women's Hospital, Harvard Medical School, 75 Francis St., Boston, MA 02115, USA
* Brigham and Women's Hospital, ASB L1-037C, Boston, MA 02115, USA.
E-mail address: mdicarli@partners.org

Cardiol Clin 27 (2009) 257–263
doi:10.1016/j.ccl.2008.12.001

specificity is 73% (range, 36%–100%).[1] With the use of attenuation correction methods, the specificity improves, especially among patients undergoing exercise stress testing.[1] With PET perfusion imaging, the reported average sensitivity for detecting more than 50% angiographic stenosis is 91% (range, 83%–100%), whereas the average specificity is 89% (range, 73%–100%).[2]

Despite its widespread use and acceptance, a recognized limitation of this approach is that it often uncovers only coronary territories supplied by the most severe stenosis and consequently is relatively insensitive to accurately delineate the extent of obstructive angiographic CAD, especially in the setting of multivessel CAD. For example, in a recent study of 101 patients with significant angiographic left main coronary stenosis, Berman and colleagues[3] reported that by perfusion assessment alone, high-risk disease with moderate to severe perfusion defects (involving > 10% myocardium at stress) was identified in only 59% by quantitative analysis. Conversely, absence of significant perfusion defect (> 5% myocardium) was seen in 15% of patients. Similar findings have been reported for PET imaging.[4]

Recent evidence suggests that two quantitative approaches (both unique to PET) may be able to help mitigate this limitation, at least in part. One of them relates to PET's unique ability to assess left ventricular function at rest and during peak stress (as opposed to poststress with SPECT).[4] The available evidence suggests that in normal subjects, left ventricular ejection fraction (LVEF) increases during peak vasodilator stress.[4] In patients with obstructive CAD, however, the delta change in LVEF (from baseline to peak stress) is inversely related to the extent of obstructive angiographic CAD. Patients with multivessel or left main disease show a frank drop in LVEF during peak stress, even in the absence of apparent perfusion defects (**Fig. 1**). In contrast, patients without significant CAD or with one-vessel disease show a normal increase in LVEF. Consequently, the diagnostic sensitivity of gated PET for correctly ascertaining the presence of multivessel disease increases from 50% to 79%.[4]

The second approach is based on the ability of PET to enable absolute measurements of myocardial blood flow (in mL/min/g) and coronary vasodilator reserve. In patients with so-called "balanced" ischemia or diffuse CAD,

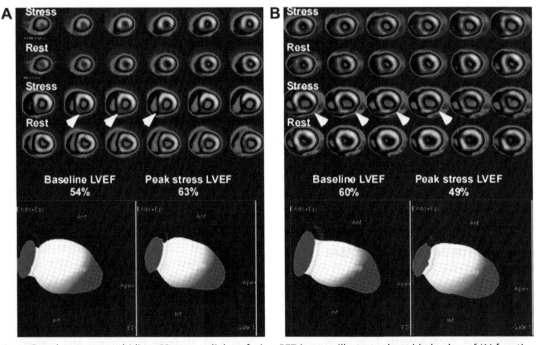

Fig. 1. Gated rest-stress rubidium-82 myocardial perfusion PET images illustrate the added value of LV function over the perfusion information. Panel A (*left*) demonstrates a normal rise in LVEF from rest to peak stress (*bottom*) in a patient with angiographic single vessel CAD, showing a single perfusion defect in the inferior wall on the PET images (*arrows*). Panel B (right) demonstrates an abnormal drop in LVEF from rest to peak stress in a patient with angiographic multivessel vessel CAD, also showing a single perfusion defect in the inferolateral wall on the PET images (*arrows*).(*From* Di Carli MF, Hachamovitch R. New technology for noninvasive evaluation of coronary artery disease. Circulation 2007;115:1464–80; with permission.)

measurements of coronary vasodilator reserve would uncover areas of myocardium at risk that would generally be missed by performing only relative assessments of myocardial perfusion.[5] It is important to point out, however, that neither of these approaches has been tested in prospective clinical trials. Another limitation of the myocardial perfusion imaging approach is that it fails to describe the presence and extent of subclinical atherosclerosis.[6,7] This is not unexpected because the myocardial perfusion imaging method is designed and targeted on the identification of flow-limiting stenoses. This is potentially important, especially in patient subgroups with intermediate-high clinical risk in whom there may be extensive subclinical CAD, and may partly explain the limitations of perfusion imaging alone to identify low-risk patients among those with high clinical risk (eg, diabetes, end-stage renal disease).[8]

Cardiac CT

Using state-of-the-art technology in carefully selected patients, it is possible to obtain high-quality images of the coronary arteries. The available evidence suggests that on a per-patient basis, the average weighted sensitivity for detecting at least one coronary artery with more than 50% stenosis is 94% (range, 75%–100%), whereas the average specificity is 77% (range, 49%–100%).[9] The corresponding average positive predictive values and negative predictive values are 84% (range, 50%–100%) and 87% (range, 35%–100%)respectively, and the overall diagnostic accuracy is 89% (range, 68%–100%).

Two multicenter, single vendor trials to evaluate the diagnostic accuracy of computed tomography angiography (CTA)-64 were completed and recently published.[10,11] The results of these two studies confirmed the robustness of CTA-64 for complete visualization of the coronary tree. The Assessment by Coronary Computed Tomographic Angiography of Individuals Undergoing Invasive Coronary Angiography (ACCURACY) trial enrolled 230 patients with a disease prevalence of 25%. On a patient-based model, the sensitivity, specificity, and positive predictive value and negative predictive value to detect 50% or more or 70% or more stenosis were 95%, 83%, 64%, and 99%, respectively, and 94%, 83%, 48%, 99%, respectively. The study reported no differences in sensitivity and specificity for nonobese patients compared with obese subjects, whereas calcium scores of 400 or more reduced specificity significantly. The Coronary Artery Evaluation Using 64-Row Multidetector Computed Tomography Angiography (CorE 64) trial[11] enrolled 291 patients

with a disease prevalence of 56% and provided additional evidence that is somewhat discordant to the ACCURACY trial and to initial results from single center studies. The CorE 64 study excluded patients with calcium scores of more than 600. On a per-patient basis, the sensitivity for detecting at least one coronary artery with 50% or more stenosis was 85%, considerably lower than in single-center studies and in the ACCURACY trial using similar technology, whereas the specificity was 90%, higher than previously reported. The corresponding average positive predictive value and negative predictive value were 91% and 83%, respectively, surprisingly different than most previous studies. On a per-vessel basis, the reported sensitivity rate for detecting coronary arteries with 50% or more stenosis was 75%, whereas the specificity rate was 93%. The corresponding positive predictive value and negative predictive value were 82% and 89%, respectively.

Except for the ACCURACY study, these reported accuracies of CTA to date should be interpreted in light of the relatively narrow range of CAD likelihood in patients examined (ie, high or intermediate-high), as evidenced by the high prevalence of obstructive CAD in these series (56%–62%).[9,11] Results are generally limited to relatively large vessel sizes ($\geq$ 1.5 mm), excluding the results of smaller or uninterpretable vessels (generally distal vessels and side branches), the inclusion of which lowers sensitivity. An ongoing problem with CT is that high-density objects, such as calcified coronary plaques and stent struts, limit its ability to accurately delineate the degree of coronary luminal narrowing.[12,13] Of note, the CorE 64 trial excluded patients with high calcium scores (> 600).[11] From a clinical perspective, a normal CTA is helpful because it effectively excludes the presence of obstructive CAD and the need for further testing, defines a low clinical risk, and makes management decisions straightforward. Because of its limited accuracy to define stenosis severity and predict flow-limiting disease,[14,15] however, abnormal CTA results are more problematic to interpret and use as the basis for defining the potential need of invasive coronary angiography and myocardial revascularization.

INTEGRATING NUCLEAR IMAGING AND CARDIAC CT FOR DIAGNOSIS AND MANAGEMENT
Diagnosing Obstructive Coronary Artery Disease

CTA provides excellent diagnostic sensitivity for stenoses in the proximal and mid segments (> 1.5 mm in diameter) of the main coronary arteries. Because of its relatively limited spatial resolution (compared with invasive angiography), the sensitivity of this approach is reduced substantially in more distal coronary segments and side branches.[9] This limitation can be offset by the scintigraphic information that is generally not affected by the location of coronary stenoses. More importantly, the stress perfusion information provides valuable clinical information regarding the physiologic significance of anatomic stenoses for identification of patients in need of potential revascularization. For example, Rispler and colleagues[16] reported a significant improvement in specificity (63%–95%) and positive predictive value (31%–77%) without a change in sensitivity or negative predictive value for detection of obstructive CAD as defined by quantitative coronary angiography in a cohort of 56 patients with known or suspected CAD undergoing hybrid SPECT/CTA imaging. On the other hand, CTA improves the detection of multivessel CAD, which is one of the main pitfalls of stress perfusion scintigraphy. The potential diagnostic appeal of a dual-modality approach needs to be weighed against the challenges that it poses, especially with regards to the added radiation dose to patients. It is unclear which patient subgroups may benefit from this hybrid imaging approach. Currently, nuclear imaging and CTA are more often used sequentially in selected patients. For example, nuclear imaging is often used as a follow-up of patients with abnormal CTA studies to define hemodynamic significance of coronary stenosis. Conversely, CTA can be used to follow patients with equivocal nuclear imaging studies or understand discrepancies in patients with markedly positive stress test results with normal nuclear imaging studies.

Assessing Prognosis

The potential to acquire and quantify rest and stress myocardial perfusion and CT information

from a single dual-modality study opens the door to expansion of the prognostic potential of stress nuclear imaging. For example, recent data from our laboratory suggest that quantification of CAC scores at the time of stress nuclear imaging using a hybrid approach with PET/CT can enhance risk predictions in patients with suspected CAD.[17] In a consecutive series of 621 patients undergoing stress PET imaging and CAC scoring in the same clinical setting, risk-adjusted analysis demonstrated a stepwise increase in adverse events (death and myocardial infarction) with increasing levels of CAC score for any level of perfusion abnormality. This finding was observed in patients with and without evidence of ischemia on PET myocardial perfusion imaging (MPI). The annualized event rate in patients with normal PET MPI and no CAC was substantially lower than among patients with normal PET MPI and a CAC level of 1000 or more (**Fig. 2**). Likewise, the annualized event rate in patients with ischemia on PET MPI and no CAC was lower than among patients with ischemia and a CAC value of 1000 or more. These findings suggest incremental risk stratification by incorporating information regarding the anatomic extent of atherosclerosis to conventional models using nuclear imaging alone, a finding that may serve as a more rational basis for personalizing the intensity and goals of medical therapy in a more cost-effective manner. Although CTA as an adjunct to perfusion imaging could expand the opportunities for identifying patients with non-calcified plaques at greater risk of adverse cardiovascular events, it is unclear how much added prognostic information there is in the contrast CT scan over the simple CAC scan.[18]

Guiding Patient Management

One of the most compelling arguments supporting a clinical role of dual-modality imaging is its potential ability for optimizing and personalizing management decisions. The importance of stress

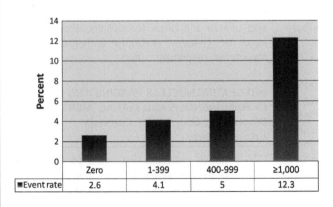

Fig. 2. Bar chart illustrates the stepwise increase of death or myocardial infarction with increasing coronary calcium scores in patients with intermediate likelihood of CAD undergoing evaluation for chest pain with PET/CT showing normal myocardial perfusion. (*Data from* Schenker MP, Dorbala S, Hong EC, et al. Interrelation of coronary calcification, myocardial ischemia, and outcomes in patients with intermediate likelihood of coronary artery disease. Circulation 2008;117:1693–700.)

perfusion imaging in the integrated strategy is the ability of noninvasive estimates of jeopardized myocardium to identify which patients may benefit from revascularization; that is, differentiating high-risk patients with extensive scar versus patients with extensive ischemia (**Fig. 3**). The advantages of this approach are clear—avoidance of unnecessary catheterizations that expose patients to risk and the potential for associated cost savings.[19] Multiple studies have shown the value of ischemia information for optimizing clinical decision making. The nonrandomized Coronary Artery Surgery Study (CASS) registry reported that surgical revascularization in patients with CAD improved survival only among patients with three-vessel disease with severe ischemia on exercise stress testing, whereas medical therapy was a superior initial strategy in patients without this finding.[20] Nonrandomized observational data using risk-adjustment techniques and propensity scores have demonstrated the ability of stress perfusion imaging to identify which patients may accrue a survival benefit from revascularization.[21]

The benefit of an ischemia-guided approach to management is further supported by invasive estimates of flow-limiting CAD (eg, fractional flow reserve).[22] In the setting of a fractional flow reserve of more than 0.75, revascularization can be safely deferred without increased patient risk, despite the presence of what visually appears to be a significant stenosis.[22] Cardiac event rates are low in these patients—even lower than predicted if treated with percutaneous coronary intervention,[23] and this differential risk seems to be sustained at the time of 5-year follow-up.[24] Importantly, in patients with visually defined left main coronary disease, a fractional flow reserve of more than 0.75 was associated with excellent 3-year survival and freedom from major adverse cardiovascular events.[23] Conversely, event rates are increased when lesions with fractional flow reserve of less than 0.75 are not revascularized.[25] By identifying which patients have sufficient ischemia to merit revascularization, it seems that stress perfusion imaging may play a significant role in the selection of patients for catheterization

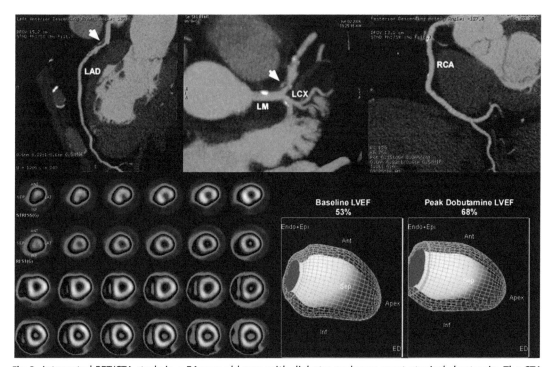

Fig. 3. Integrated PET/CTA study in a 54-year-old man with diabetes and new-onset atypical chest pain. The CTA images demonstrate a noncalcified plaque (*arrow*) in the proximal LAD with 50% to 70% stenosis. The rest and peak dobutamine stress myocardial perfusion PET study (*lower left panel*) demonstrates only minimal inferoapical ischemia, however. LVEF value was normal at rest and demonstrated a normal rise during peak dobutamine stress. In this patient, stress perfusion imaging clearly excluded the presence of severe ischemia despite the significant plaque on CTA, thereby excluding the need for revascularization at this time. (*From* Di Carli MF, Hachamovitch R. New technology for noninvasive evaluation of coronary artery disease. Circulation 2007;115:1464–80; with permission.)

within a strategy based on identification of patient benefit. These physiologic data may have greater clinical impact than visually defined coronary anatomy for revascularization decision making.

The dual-modality imaging approach also may facilitate identification of patients without flow-limiting disease (ie, normal perfusion) who have extensive, albeit subclinical, CAD. Recent data from multiple laboratories suggest that as many as 50% of patients with normal stress perfusion imaging may show extensive (non–flow limiting) coronary atherosclerosis (calcified and noncalcified plaques).[6,7] Although these patients do not require revascularization because of the absence of ischemia, patients with extensive atherosclerosis are a higher risk of adverse events[17,26,27] and probably warrant more aggressive medical therapy. Consequently, it may be possible to tailor antithrombotic, cholesterol reduction, and anti-inflammatory pharmacotherapy on the basis of CT findings. The major challenge for future developments is to identify which patients will benefit from a combined hybrid approach as opposed to a single-modality approach with stepwise testing. It is undefined whether all patients will require all pieces of information that can be acquired to optimize their care.

SUMMARY

Innovation in noninvasive cardiovascular imaging is rapidly advancing our ability to image in great detail the structure and function in the heart and vasculature, and hybrid PET/CT and SPECT/CT represent clear examples of this innovation. By providing concurrent quantitative information about myocardial perfusion and metabolism with coronary and cardiac anatomy, hybrid imaging offers the opportunity for a comprehensive noninvasive evaluation of the burden of atherosclerosis and its physiologic consequences in the coronary arteries and the myocardium. This integrated platform for assessing anatomy and biology offers a great potential for translating advances in molecularly targeted imaging into humans. The goals of future investigation are to refine these technologies, establish standard protocols for image acquisition and interpretation, address the issue of cost-effectiveness, and validate a range of clinical applications in large-scale clinical trials.

REFERENCES

1. Klocke FJ, Baird MG, Lorell BH, et al. ACC/AHA/ASNC guidelines for the clinical use of cardiac radionuclide imaging, executive summary: a report of the American College of Cardiology/American Heart Association Task Force on Practice Guidelines (ACC/AHA/ASNC Committee to Revise the 1995 Guidelines for the Clinical Use of Cardiac Radionuclide Imaging). J Am Coll Cardiol 2003;42(7):1318–33.
2. Di Carli MF, Dorbala S, Meserve J, et al. Clinical myocardial perfusion PET/CT. J Nucl Med 2007;48(5):783–93.
3. Berman DS, Kang X, Slomka PJ, et al. Underestimation of extent of ischemia by gated SPECT myocardial perfusion imaging in patients with left main coronary artery disease. J Nucl Cardiol 2007;14(4):521–8.
4. Dorbala S, Vangala D, Sampson U, et al. Value of vasodilator left ventricular ejection fraction reserve in evaluating the magnitude of myocardium at risk and the extent of angiographic coronary artery disease: a 82Rb PET/CT study. J Nucl Med 2007;48(3):349–58.
5. Parkash R, deKemp RA, Ruddy TD, et al. Potential utility of rubidium 82 PET quantification in patients with 3-vessel coronary artery disease. J Nucl Cardiol 2004;11(4):440–9.
6. Schuijf JD, Wijns W, Jukema JW, et al. Relationship between noninvasive coronary angiography with multi-slice computed tomography and myocardial perfusion imaging. J Am Coll Cardiol 2006;48(12):2508–14.
7. Di Carli MF, Dorbala S, Curillova Z, et al. Relationship between CT coronary angiography and stress perfusion imaging in patients with suspected ischemic heart disease assessed by integrated PET-CT imaging. J Nucl Cardiol 2007;14(6):799–809.
8. Shaw LJ, Iskandrian AE. Prognostic value of gated myocardial perfusion SPECT. J Nucl Cardiol 2004;11(2):171–85.
9. Di Carli MF, Hachamovitch R. New technology for noninvasive evaluation of coronary artery disease. Circulation 2007;115(11):1464–80.
10. Budoff MJ, Dowe D, Jollis JG, et al. Diagnostic performance of 64-multidetector row coronary computed tomographic angiography for evaluation of coronary artery stenosis in individuals without known coronary artery disease: results from the prospective multicenter ACCURACY (Assessment by Coronary Computed Tomographic Angiography of Individuals Undergoing Invasive Coronary Angiography) trial. J Am Coll Cardiol 2008;52(21):1724–32.
11. Miller JM, Rochitte CE, Dewey M, et al. Diagnostic performance of coronary angiography by 64-row CT. N Engl J Med 2008;359(22):2309–11.
12. Hoffmann U, Moselewski F, Cury RC, et al. Predictive value of 16-slice multidetector spiral computed tomography to detect significant obstructive coronary artery disease in patients at high risk for

coronary artery disease: patient-versus segment-based analysis. Circulation 2004;110(17):2638–43.

13. Mollet NR, Cademartiri F, van Mieghem CA, et al. High-resolution spiral computed tomography coronary angiography in patients referred for diagnostic conventional coronary angiography. Circulation 2005;112(15):2318–23.

14. Leber AW, Becker A, Knez A, et al. Accuracy of 64-slice computed tomography to classify and quantify plaque volumes in the proximal coronary system: a comparative study using intravascular ultrasound. J Am Coll Cardiol 2006;47(3):672–7.

15. Raff GL, Gallagher MJ, O'Neill WW, et al. Diagnostic accuracy of noninvasive coronary angiography using 64-slice spiral computed tomography. J Am Coll Cardiol 2005;46(3):552–7.

16. Rispler S, Keidar Z, Ghersin E, et al. Integrated single-photon emission computed tomography and computed tomography coronary angiography for the assessment of hemodynamically significant coronary artery lesions. J Am Coll Cardiol 2007; 49(10):1059–67.

17. Schenker MP, Dorbala S, Hong ECT, et al. Interrelation of coronary calcification, myocardial ischemia, and outcomes in patients with intermediate likelihood of coronary artery disease: a combined positron emission tomography/computed tomography study. Circulation 2008;117(13):1627–9.

18. Mahmarian JJ. Computed tomography coronary angiography as an anatomic basis for risk stratification: deja vu or something new? J Am Coll Cardiol 2007;50(12):1171–3.

19. Shaw LJ, Hachamovitch R, Berman DS, et al. The economic consequences of available diagnostic and prognostic strategies for the evaluation of stable angina patients: an observational assessment of the value of precatheterization ischemia. Economics of Noninvasive Diagnosis (END) Multicenter Study Group. J Am Coll Cardiol 1999;33(3): 661–9.

20. Weiner DA, Ryan TJ, McCabe CH, et al. The role of exercise testing in identifying patients with improved survival after coronary artery bypass surgery. J Am Coll Cardiol 1986;8(4):741–8.

21. Hachamovitch R, Hayes SW, Friedman JD, et al. Comparison of the short-term survival benefit associated with revascularization compared with medical therapy in patients with no prior coronary artery disease undergoing stress myocardial perfusion single photon emission computed tomography. Circulation 2003;107(23):2900–7.

22. Kern MJ, Lerman A, Bech JW, et al. Physiological assessment of coronary artery disease in the cardiac catheterization laboratory: a scientific statement from the American Heart Association Committee on Diagnostic and Interventional Cardiac Catheterization, Council on Clinical Cardiology. Circulation 2006;114:1321–41.

23. Bech GJ, De Bruyne B, Pijls NH, et al. Fractional flow reserve to determine the appropriateness of angioplasty in moderate coronary stenosis: a randomized trial. Circulation 2001;103:2928–34.

24. Pijls NH, van Schaardenburgh P, Manahoran G, et al. Percutaneous coronary intervention of functionally nonsignificant stenosis: 5-year follow-up of the DEFER study. J Am Coll Cardiol 2007;49:2105–11.

25. Chamuleau SAJ, Meuwissen M, Koch KT, et al. Usefulness of fractional flow reserve for risk stratification of patients with multivessel coronary artery disease and an intermediate stenosis. Am J Cardiol 2002;89:377–80.

26. Budoff MJ, Shaw LJ, Liu ST, et al. Long-term prognosis associated with coronary calcification: observations from a registry of 25,253 patients. J Am Coll Cardiol 2007;49(18):1860–70.

27. Greenland P, Bonow RO, Brundage BH, et al. ACCF/AHA 2007 clinical expert consensus document on coronary artery calcium scoring by computed tomography in global cardiovascular risk assessment and in evaluation of patients with chest pain: a report of the American College of Cardiology Foundation Clinical Expert Consensus Task Force (ACCF/AHA Writing Committee to Update the 2000 Expert Consensus Document on Electron Beam Computed Tomography) developed in collaboration with the Society of Atherosclerosis Imaging and Prevention and the Society of Cardiovascular Computed Tomography. J Am Coll Cardiol 2007;49(3):378–402.

Nuclear Imaging in Heart Failure

Jeroen J. Bax, MD, PhD*, Mark M. Boogers, MD,
Joanne D. Schuijf, PhD

KEYWORDS

- Heart failure • Nuclear imaging • Cardiac dyssynchrony
- Myocardial viability • Cardiac innervation
- Cardiac resynchronization therapy

Heart failure is becoming the main clinical challenge in cardiology in the twenty-first century and is associated with high morbidity and mortality. On a population level, congestive heart failure is associated with high morbidity and mortality. In the United States, hospital admissions for heart failure increased from 400,000 in 1979 to 1,084,000 in 2005. The number of visits to health care facilities for heart failure was 3.4 million in the year 2000.[1] The diagnostic and therapeutic costs involved are estimated to have exceeded $34 billion in 2008. Despite advances in therapies, the long-term prognosis for patients with heart failure remains poor: 80% of men and 70% of women greater than 65 years of age with heart failure die within 8 years.[1]

In almost 70% of patients, coronary artery disease is the underlying etiology.[2] Currently, several therapeutic options are available for heart failure patients including medical therapy; revascularization; advanced cardiac surgery (mitral valve surgery, left ventricular [LV] aneurysmectomy, LV restoration); device therapy (implantable cardioverter defibrillator [ICD] and cardiac resynchronization therapy [CRT]); and cardiac transplantation. Future therapies are directed at cell and gene therapy. In this article the role of nuclear imaging in the management of heart failure patients is discussed.

WHAT INFORMATION IS NEEDED TO TAILOR THERAPY?

To arrive at the optimal therapy for an individual heart failure patient, various information is needed. The underlying etiology of heart failure needs to be determined; most patients have coronary artery disease underlying heart failure (approximately 70%–80%). Nuclear imaging can help in the differentiation between patients with ischemic and nonischemic heart failure. In patients with ischemic cardiomyopathy, the precise coronary anatomy is also needed to determine if revascularization needs to be considered. At present, invasive angiography is performed to obtain the coronary anatomy, but multislice CT (MSCT) may also provide this information. Next, the presence of ischemia and viability needs to be determined to decide further if revascularization is indicated. Nuclear imaging is considered the first choice technique for assessment of ischemia and viability; both single-photon emission CT (SPECT) and positron emission tomography (PET) can provide this information. It is anticipated that the newer hybrid imaging systems (SPECT-PET CT scanners) can provide the integrated information on coronary anatomy (with CT) and ischemia-viability (with SPECT-PET).

In addition, information on the LV size (volumes) and shape (aneurysms) is needed to decide

Jeroen J. Bax has research grants from Medtronic (Tolochenaz, Switzerland); Boston Scientific (Maastricht, The Netherlands); BMS Medical Imaging (North Billerica, Massachusetts); St. Jude Medical (Veenendaal, The Netherlands); Biotronik (Berlin, Germany); GE Healthcare (St. Giles, United Kingdom); and Edwards Lifesciences (Saint-Prex, Switzerland). M.M. Boogers is supported by the Dutch Heart Foundation grant number 2008R004.
Department of Cardiology, Leiden University Medical Center, Albinusdreef 2, PO Box 9600, 2300 RC Leiden, The Netherlands
* Corresponding author.
E-mail address: j.j.bax@lumc.nl (J.J. Bax).

Cardiol Clin 27 (2009) 265–276
doi:10.1016/j.ccl.2009.01.001
0733-8651/09/$ – see front matter © 2009 Elsevier Inc. All rights reserved.

whether LV surgery is needed in addition to revascularization. Gated SPECT or PET imaging can provide information on LV volumes and ejection fraction, but MRI is probably the most accurate technique for this purpose, whereas echocardiography may be the most practical approach in daily clinical management.

Next, many patients with severely dilated left ventricles develop so-called "functional mitral regurgitation;" this valvular insufficiency is related to mitral annular dilatation, with systolic retraction of the mitral leaflets, resulting in poor leaflet coaptation. This is mainly evaluated with echocardiography, and can also be assessed by MRI. Nuclear imaging does not play a role in assessment of mitral regurgitation.

The final clinical question that comes up is: does the patient need an ICD or biventricular pacemaker? Current guidelines mainly focus on LV ejection fraction for ICD selection (<30%–40%).[3] Also for CRT selection, LV ejection fraction (<35%) is a criterion, in addition to New York Heart Association class III to IV and wide QRS complex (>120 millisecond).[4] LV ejection fraction can be assessed by gated SPECT-PET imaging but in practice is most often assessed by echocardiography or MRI. Nuclear imaging, however, may provide unique information in the selection of candidates for ICD and CRT. It has been shown that cardiac denervation-innervation is related to ventricular arrhythmias, and can be used in selection for ICD therapy; SPECT imaging with 123-iodine metaiodobenzylguanidine (MIBG) and PET imaging with carbon-11 metahydroxyephedrine can provide information on cardiac innervation. Moreover, cardiac dyssynchrony is considered important for the response to CRT, and this can be evaluated with phase analysis derived from gated SPECT imaging.

The next paragraphs address the specific use of nuclear imaging in differentiation between ischemic and nonischemic cardiomyopathy, assessment of ischemia, assessment of viability, assessment of cardiac innervation, and assessment of cardiac dyssynchrony.

DIFFERENTIATION BETWEEN ISCHEMIC AND NONISCHEMIC CARDIOMYOPATHY

Nuclear imaging can provide some indirect evidence in the differentiation between ischemic and nonischemic cardiomyopathy. With stress-rest SPECT imaging, reversible defects indicate ischemia and fixed defects indicate scar tissue; both these findings are markers of coronary artery disease. Based on these markers, SPECT myocardial perfusion imaging has been shown to have a high accuracy for the diagnosis of coronary artery disease with an average sensitivity and specificity of 86% and 74% based on pooled analysis of 79 studies with 8964 patients included (**Fig. 1**).[5] The lower specificity can be attributed to the posttest referral bias; a better parameter may be the normalcy rate, which was 89% in pooled data from 10 studies with 549 patients.[5]

Moreover, earlier studies with nuclear perfusion imaging demonstrated that patients with ischemic cardiomyopathy had extensive and diffuse perfusion defects, whereas tracer uptake was mostly homogenous in patients with nonischemic cardiomyopathy. Danias and colleagues[6] evaluated 37 heart failure patients with technetium-99 m sestamibi SPECT and demonstrated a significant difference in summed stress, rest, and reversibility scores (reflecting both reversible and irreversible defects) between the patients with ischemic and nonischemic cardiomyopathy. In particular, much higher summed stress scores were observed in patients with ischemic cardiomyopathy (32.9 ± 7.7 as compared with 6.9 ± 3.8 in nonischemic cardiomyopathy; P<.001).

In a second study, the same authors evaluated 164 heart failure patients and indicated that the summed stress score had a sensitivity of 87% with a specificity of 63% to detect coronary artery disease.[7]

Similarly, PET studies also demonstrated that patients with nonischemic cardiomyopathy had more homogeneous tracer uptake, whereas patients with ischemic cardiomyopathy had areas

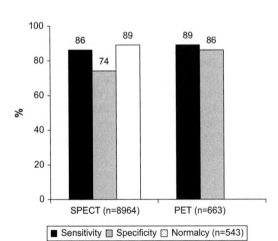

Fig. 1. Pooled diagnostic accuracy of nuclear imaging techniques (SPECT and PET) to detect coronary artery disease. (*From* Schuijf JD, Poldermans D, Shaw LJ, et al. Diagnostic and prognostic value of non-invasive imaging in known or suspected coronary artery disease. Eur J Nucl Med Mol Imaging 2006;33:93–104; with permission.)

of severely reduced tracer uptake (reflecting scar formation). For example, Eisenberg and coworkers[8] evaluated 20 patients with C11-palmitate PET; patients with ischemic cardiomyopathy had extensive areas of reduced accumulation of C11-palmitate, whereas patients with nonischemic cardiomyopathy had homogeneous tracer uptake. Accordingly, nuclear imaging can help in the differentiation between ischemic and nonischemic cardiomyopathy, but for the diagnosis of underlying coronary artery disease, visualization of the coronary arteries is needed. Invasive angiography is the technique of choice, but recently MSCT has been introduced for noninvasive angiography. With the older generations of MSCT scanners, a substantial number of segments were of insufficient image quality, resulting in suboptimal diagnostic accuracy. With 64-slice MSCT and dual-source slice MSCT, however, more consistent image quality is obtained with improved visualization of the coronary artery tree. With 64-slice MSCT, a sensitivity and specificity of 92% and 96% on average are observed.[9] What is most important is that the negative predictive value approaches 100%, indicating perfect rule out of coronary artery disease. MSCT should not be used to rule out significant stenoses, but rather complete exclusion of coronary artery disease (ie, complete absence of coronary artery calcium, and absence of any noncalcified lesions). An example of a patient with normal coronary arteries on MSCT is shown in **Fig. 2**.

Currently, not much experience has been obtained in heart failure patients with MSCT. Ghostine and colleagues[10] evaluated the accuracy of 64-slice MSCT to identify coronary artery disease in 93 heart failure patients (LV ejection fraction 31% $\pm$ 7%) and demonstrated a high diagnostic accuracy. Once coronary anatomy is known, however, additional information on ischemia and viability is needed to decide on coronary revascularization.

ASSESSMENT OF ISCHEMIA

In the presence of a flow-limiting stenosis, resting myocardial perfusion is preserved, but once an increased myocardial oxygen demand occurs, a perfusion demand-supply mismatch follows, resulting in myocardial ischemia. Then, a sequence of events is initiated, which is referred to as the "ischemic cascade" (**Fig. 3**).[11,12] Perfusion abnormalities occur at an early stage, whereas diastolic and systolic LV dysfunction occur later. ECG changes and angina are only induced at the end of the cascade. Accordingly, such techniques as nuclear imaging that detect perfusion abnormalities should have a high sensitivity for detection of ischemia, because these abnormalities occur early in the cascade. Different radionuclides have been used for assessment of perfusion with SPECT, including thallium-201, technetium-99 m sestamibi, and technetium-99 m tetrofosmin. Average sensitivity and specificity, based on a pooled analysis of 79 studies with 8964 patients included, are 86% and 74% (see **Fig. 1**).[5] With the introduction of ECG gated SPECT, assessment of LV volumes and ejection fraction, and wall motion, can simultaneously be performed, which has significantly increased diagnostic accuracy of the technique.

Smanio and colleagues[13] compared ungated SPECT (only using perfusion) and gated SPECT (using integrated perfusion and wall motion) and demonstrated an increase in normalcy rate from 74% to 93%, whereas the number of inconclusive tests decreased from 31% to 10% through addition of systolic function data to the original perfusion data.

PET is also increasingly used for perfusion imaging. The main advantages of PET over SPECT are the possibility to perform attenuation correction and absolute quantification of perfusion. Nitrogen-13 ammonia and rubidium-82 are the most commonly used tracers, but O15-labeled water can also be used. Pooled analysis of seven PET perfusion studies (with 663 patients) yielded a sensitivity of 89% with a specificity of 86% to detect coronary artery disease (see **Fig. 1**).[14] Because of the aforementioned advantages over SPECT, PET has a higher specificity for the detection of coronary artery disease; moreover, the high spatial resolution of PET permits differentiation between epicardial and endocardial perfusion.

In heart failure patients, the combination between the coronary anatomy (stenoses) and the presence of ischemia in the territories of the stenotic vessels determines the need for revascularization. In the absence of ischemia, the presence of viability needs to be evaluated.

ASSESSMENT OF MYOCARDIAL VIABILITY

From the observational studies by Rahimtoola[15] it became clear that many patients with chronic LV dysfunction can improve in function after revascularization. This observation was the basis for the concept of myocardial viability: some dysfunctional myocardium in patients with chronic coronary artery disease may not be irreversibly damaged but may still be viable, although not functioning properly, and may recover in function following adequate restoration of blood flow. From further studies it became clear that patients

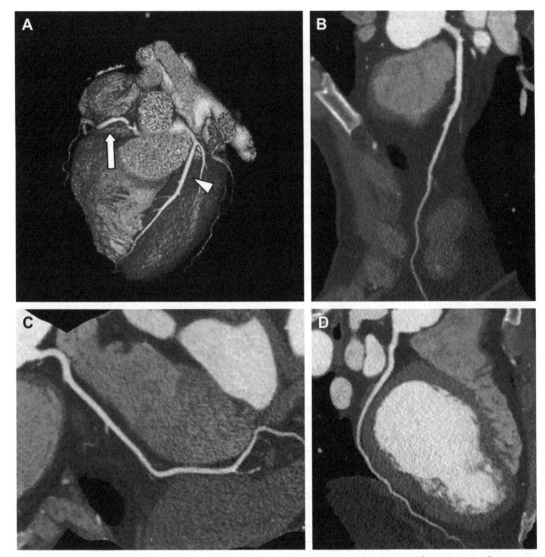

Fig. 2. A 320-slice MSCT to rule out coronary artery disease in a 43-year-old patient with an intermediate pretest likelihood of CAD. (*A*) On the three-dimensional volume-rendered reconstruction, a normal left anterior descending coronary artery (LAD, *arrowhead*) and right coronary artery (RCA, *arrow*) can be observed. (*B–D*) Curved multiplanar reconstructions of, respectively, the LAD, RCA, and left circumflex coronary artery showing normal coronary arteries.

with viable myocardium may have chronically hypoperfused myocardium at rest (referred to as "hibernation") or preserved resting perfusion with reduced flow reserve (referred to as "repetitive stunning"); probably, these two entities represent the ends of a spectrum, with repetitive stunning representing less damaged myocardium and hibernation representing severely damaged myocardium. In the clinical setting these different situations may coexist in the same patient; for both conditions, revascularization is needed, and the term "jeopardized but viable myocardium" may include the entire spectrum from (repetitive)

stunning to chronic stunning to hibernation. The fact that revascularization is warranted is underlined by the fact that jeopardized but viable myocardium (and particularly hibernation) is an unstable substrate, which can easily progress to cell death and scar formation if revascularization is delayed.[16]

Observational imaging studies have demonstrated that jeopardized but viable myocardium occurs often in patients with chronic LV dysfunction and there should be a systematic evaluation for viability in these patients to decide whether or not revascularization is needed. Schinkel and

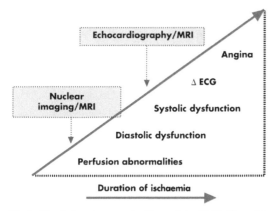

Fig. 3. The ischemic cascade. (*From* Schuijf JD, Shaw LJ, Wijns W, et al. Cardiac imaging in coronary artery disease: differing modalities. Heart 2005;91:1110–7; with permission.)

colleagues[17] demonstrated that the prevalence of myocardial viability as evaluated by nuclear imaging (with combined perfusion/glucose use assessment) was 61%. Even in patients with a previous myocardial infarction with Q-waves on the ECG, a clinically significant amount of residual myocardial viability may be present.[18]

Jeopardized, viable myocardium has certain features and these form the basis for the different imaging techniques that are available for viability assessment (**Table 1**). These features include preserved glucose and (possibly) fatty acid metabolism; cell membrane integrity; intact mitochondria; and inotropic reserve. It has been demonstrated that the presence or absence of these different features may be related to the severity of ultrastructural damage at the myocyte level. All the features can be evaluated by nuclear imaging with PET or SPECT using different radionuclides. Glucose use can be evaluated with F18-fluorodeoxyglucose (FDG) and PET or SPECT; free fatty acid metabolism can be assessed by beta-methyl-iodophenyl-pentadecanoic acid and SPECT; cell membrane integrity can be evaluated by thallium-201 with SPECT; intact mitochondria can be assessed by technetium-99 m sestamibi or technetium-99 m tetrofosmin with SPECT; and contractile reserve has been assessed most often by low-dose dobutamine echocardiography (or MRI). Contractile reserve can also be evaluated, however, using gated SPECT imaging with technetium-99 m labeled tracers or thallium-201. Finally, contrast-enhanced MRI is frequently used for viability assessment, but one needs to realize that this technique is excellent for assessment of scar tissue (because of the high spatial resolution) but does not provide information on the remaining viable myocardium (whether that is jeopardized, viable myocardium, which needs revascularization or normal, viable myocardium, which does not need revascularization).

In clinical studies, viability techniques have been used to predict outcome after revascularization, focusing on improvement of regional function, improvement of global function, improvement of heart failure symptoms and exercise capacity, and improvement of long-term prognosis.

Pooled analysis of the different techniques was performed recently, using the end point of improvement of regional function postrevascularization (**Fig. 4**).[19] For FDG-PET imaging, 24 studies were available (756 patients), and the weighted mean sensitivity and specificity were 92% and 63%, respectively. For thallium-201 imaging, 40 studies were available (1119 patients) and the

Table 1
Viability techniques, based on viability features and their viability criteria

Technique	Feature	Viability Criteria
FDG imaging with PET or SPECT	Glucose use	Normal perfusion/FDG uptake Perfusion-FDG mismatch
BMIPP imaging with SPECT	Free fatty acid use	Tracer activity >50%
Thallium-201 imaging with SPECT	Intact cell membrane	Redistribution Tracer activity >50%
Tc-99 m sestamibi imaging with SPECT	Intact mitochondria	Tracer activity >50% Improved tracer uptake postnitrates
Dobutamine echo/MRI	Contractile reserve	Improved contraction during low-dose dobutamine infusion
Contrast-enhanced MRI	Scar tissue	Transmurality of hyperenhancement

Abbreviations: BMIPP, Beta-methyl-iodophenyl-pentadecanoic acid; FDG, F18-Fluorodeoxyglucose; MRI, Magnetic resonance imaging; PET, Positron emission tomography; SPECT, Single photon emission computed tomography; Tc-99 m, Technetium-99 m.

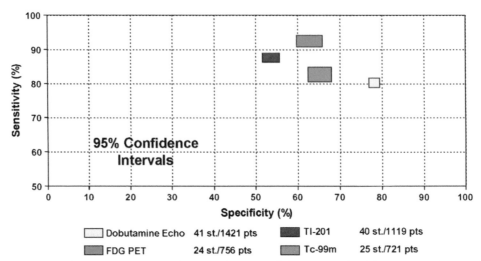

Fig. 4. Comparison of sensitivities and specificities with 95% confidence intervals of the various techniques for the prediction of recovery of regional function after revascularization. TI-201, thallium-201; Tc-99 m, technetium-99 m labeled tracers; FDG-PET, F18-fluorodeoxyglucose and positron emission tomography. (*From* Schinkel AF, Bax JJ, Poldermans D, et al. Hibernating myocardium: diagnosis and patient outcomes. Curr Probl Cardiol 2007;32: 375–410; with permission.)

weighted mean sensitivity and specificity were 87% and 54%. Nuclear imaging with technetium-99 m labeled agents was used in 25 studies (721 patients), yielding a weighted mean sensitivity and specificity of 83% and 65%, respectively. With dobutamine stress echocardiography, 41 studies (1421 patients) were available, yielding a weighted mean sensitivity and specificity of 80% and 78%.

Comparison of the techniques revealed the following. FDG-PET had the highest sensitivity (P<.05 versus other techniques), followed by nuclear imaging using thallium-201, and technetium-99 m labeled agents. In general, the nuclear imaging techniques had a higher sensitivity (P<.05) than dobutamine stress echocardiography. Specificity was highest, however, for dobutamine echocardiography (P<.05 versus other techniques).

Pooled analysis (13 studies, 641 patients) was also performed for the different techniques to predict improvement of global LV function after revascularization (**Fig. 5**). The results are summarized in **Table 2**. It is clear that not many studies are available for the prediction of improvement of global LV function after revascularization. The nuclear imaging techniques had a fairly high sensitivity, whereas dobutamine stress echocardiography had a lower sensitivity (P<.05). Conversely, the specificity of dobutamine stress echocardiography was higher than for the nuclear imaging techniques (P<.05). The lower specificity indicates that some segments (or patients) are classified as

viable according to the imaging techniques, but do not improve in function postrevascularization. Improvement of function may not be the ideal end point, however, and revascularization of viable segments may still be important, because this may prevent ventricular arrhythmias (sudden death) or LV remodeling (dilatation), and may thereby still result in improved survival, although functional recovery was not achieved.

Prognostic data were also pooled from the available viability studies (29 studies, 3640 patients). The annualized mortality rates obtained from the pooled analysis are summarized in **Table 3**. Patients with viable myocardium who underwent revascularization had the best survival, whereas the highest annualized mortality rate was noted in viable patients receiving medical therapy. Intermediate mortality rates were noted in nonviable patients who were treated medically or underwent revascularization. These trends were observed with all different viability techniques.

Accordingly, viability assessment is useful in the therapeutic decision-making process, and patients with viability should be considered for revascularization.

ASSESSMENT OF CARDIAC INNERVATION, IMPLICATIONS FOR IMPLANTABLE CARDIOVERTER DEFIBRILLATOR

Hyperactivity of the sympathetic nervous system with an increase in plasma norepinephrine plays a major role in the pathophysiology of heart failure.

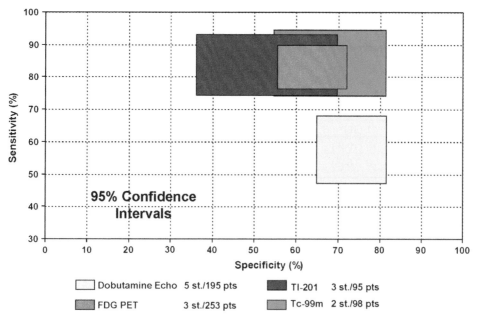

Fig. 5. Comparison of sensitivities and specificities with 95% confidence intervals of the various techniques for the prediction of recovery of global LV function after revascularization. The number of available studies and patients are indicated per technique. TI-201, thallium-201; Tc-99 m, technetium-99 m labeled tracers; FDG-PET, F18-fluorodeoxyglucose and positron emission tomography. (*From* Schinkel AF, Bax JJ, Poldermans D, et al. Hibernating myocardium: diagnosis and patient outcomes. Curr Probl Cardiol 2007;32:375–410; with permission.)

At first this increased activity is supporting the cardiovascular system by increasing heart rate, contractility, and venous return. In chronic heart failure, however, this hyperactivity of the sympathetic nervous system is unfavorable and can cause myocardial β-adrenoceptor down-regulation. Cardiac innervation can be evaluated with PET and carbon-11 metahydroxyephedrine, but in the clinical setting, SPECT imaging with MIBG is most often used. MIBG is a norepinephrine analog and is labeled with 123-iodine to visualize uptake and storage of MIBG in the presynaptic nerve endings. MIBG uptake is primarily performed by the presynaptic norepinephrine transporter (uptake 1), but uptake can also be performed by nonneuronal mechanisms, consisting of uptake 2 (carrier-facilitated process) and metabolic diffusion.

In heart failure patients, cardiac innervation is reduced and MIBG uptake is globally reduced (in contrast to patients with ischemic heart disease, in whom MIBG uptake is mainly reduced in the ischemic or infarcted areas). MIBG is used with both planar and SPECT imaging. Images are acquired at two different phases; early planar and SPECT imaging are performed 10 to 20 minutes after tracer administration, whereas late planar and SPECT imaging are performed 3 to 4 hours after MIBG injection. From the planar images, global myocardial MIBG uptake can be

Table 2
Pooled data from the available studies (13,641 patients) using the different viability techniques to predict improvement of global LV function after revascularization

Technique	N Studies	N Patients	Sens (%)	Spec (%)
Thallium-201	3	95	84	53
Technetium-99 m	2	98	84	68
FDG-PET	3	253	83	64
DSE	5	195	57	73

Abbreviations: DSE, Dobutamine stress echocardiography; FDG, F18-Fluorodeoxyglucose; PET, Positron emission tomography.

Table 3
Pooled data from the available studies (29 studies, 3640 patients) using the different viability techniques focusing on long-term outcome

Technique	N Studies (N Patients)	Mortality Rate % (Patients)			
		V+/Rev	V+/Med	V−/Rev	V−/Med
Thallium-201	8 (893)	4	7	14	7
Technetium-99 m	1 (56)	3	9	—	—
FDG-PET	10 (1046)	4	17	6	8
DSE	10 (1645)	3	12	7	12

The mortality rates for the patients are categorized according to the presence (V+) or absence (V-) of viability, and therapy.
Abbreviations: DSE, Dobutamine stress echocardiography; FDG, F18-Fluorodeoxyglucose; MED, Medical therapy; PET, Positron emission tomography; REV, Revascularization.

assessed using the heart-to-mediastinum (H/M) ratio (**Fig. 6**). In addition to global myocardial MIBG uptake, regional cardiac MIBG uptake can be appreciated from the SPECT images.

Extensive evidence is available on the prognostic value of global MIBG uptake in heart failure patients. Merlet and colleagues[20] evaluated the predictive value of innervation imaging using MIBG scintigraphy in 90 patients with heart failure. Only H/M ratio on delayed planar imaging was used to semiquantify cardiac sympathetic nerve innervation. Besides MIBG scintigraphy, patients underwent radionuclide angiography, chest radiograph, and M-mode echocardiography and among all baseline variables, H/M ratio on late planar imaging was the most powerful independent predictor of adverse cardiovascular events over a mean follow-up of 27 months. Moreover, a cutoff value of 120% of late H/M ratio was able to predict adverse outcome with sensitivity and specificity values of 95% and 93%, respectively. Similarly, Manrique and coworkers[21] recently evaluated 94 patients with nonischemic cardiomyopathy, and demonstrated that global cardiac MIBG uptake on delayed planar imaging was the only independent predictor for primary (cardiac death or heart transplantation) and secondary (cardiac death, heart transplantation, or recurrent heart failure) study end points over a mean follow-up of 37 ± 16 months.

The occurrence of ventricular arrhythmias has also been related to a dysfunctional state of the cardiac autonomic nervous system. Some studies have suggested that viable myocardium with reduced innervation may be hyperresponsive to catecholamines, leading to enhanced automaticity and triggering. In this respect, the border zone of myocardial infarction may be prone to develop re-entrant circuits and ventricular arrhythmias because these areas are viable but may have damaged autonomic innervation.

Accordingly, some studies have evaluated the use of MIBG imaging for the prediction of ventricular arrhythmias and sudden cardiac death (SCD).[22–24] Nagahara and colleagues[22] have reported some interesting findings on the use of MIBG scintigraphy for selection of patients at risk for SCD. Based on the presence of an appropriate ICD discharge or SCD, patients were divided into two groups: patients with an appropriate ICD discharge or SCD showed significantly lower values of late H/M ratio (indication of cardiac denervation) than patients without appropriate ICD therapy or SCD, over a mean follow-up of 15 months (**Fig. 7**). Univariate predictors for lethal arrhythmic events were brain natriuretic peptide, pharmacologic treatment, and delayed H/M ratio on MIBG imaging; multivariate model identified late H/M ratio as an independent predictor for appropriate ICD therapy or SCD. Arora and

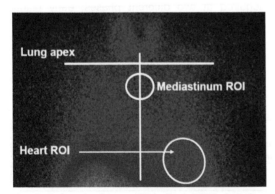

Fig. 6. Delayed planar 123-iodine MIBG imaging. Global cardiac sympathetic innervation is expressed by the heart-to-mediastinum (H/M) ratio on planar imaging. Regions of interest are manually drawn over the heart and upper mediastinum and the mean cardiac counts per pixel are divided by the mean mediastinum counts per pixel. ROI, region of interest.

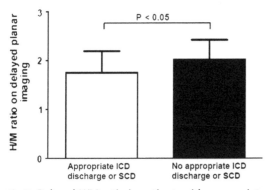

Fig. 7. Delayed H/M ratio in patients with appropriate ICD discharge or SCD and in patients without appropriate ICD discharge or SCD (1.75 ± 0.44 versus 2.02 ± 0.40; P<.05). (*Data from* Arora R, Ferrick KJ, Nakata T, et al. I-123 MIBG imaging and heart rate variability analysis to predict the need for an implantable cardioverter defibrillator. J Nucl Cardiol 2003;10:121–31.)

colleagues[23] evaluated 17 patients with a previously implanted ICD with MIBG imaging; 10 patients received an appropriate ICD discharge during a follow-up of 14 ± 11 months, and these patients had significantly lower values of early H/M ratio than patients without an appropriate ICD discharge. Few studies have evaluated regional cardiac MIBG uptake with SPECT. Bax and colleagues[24] evaluated 50 patients (depressed LV function, previous infarction) with MIBG-SPECT aiming to predict inducibility of ventricular arrhythmias on electrophysiologic examination. Patients with a positive electrophysiologic test

had significantly larger defects on MIBG-SPECT as compared with patients with a negative electrophysiologic test. Moreover, the MIBG defect score was the only independent predictor for inducibility during electrophysiologic testing and a summed defect score of 37 was able to predict a positive electrophysiologic test with a sensitivity and specificity of 77% and 75%, respectively.

Accordingly, the available studies have provided evidence that cardiac sympathetic innervation imaging is useful for risk stratification and prognostication in heart failure patients. Patients with larger MIBG defects may have a higher likelihood of ventricular arrhythmias and SCD (**Fig. 8**), and may play an important role in selection of patients who may benefit from ICD therapy. Despite encouraging results, larger trials are needed to establish the actual role of innervation imaging in risk stratification in patients with heart failure.

ASSESSMENT OF CARDIAC DYSSYNCHRONY, IMPLICATIONS FOR CARDIAC RESYNCHRONIZATION THERAPY

Selection of patients with high likelihood of response to CRT remains difficult. In addition to the classical selection criteria, the presence and extent of cardiac dyssynchrony have been demonstrated to be of use in the prediction of response to CRT.

The presence of a dyssynchronous contraction pattern within the left ventricle can be assessed with several nuclear imaging modalities, including gated blood-pool ventriculography, gated

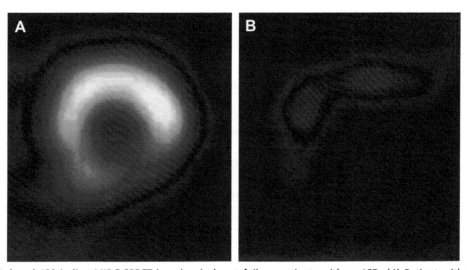

Fig. 8. Delayed 123-iodine MIBG-SPECT imaging in heart failure patients with an ICD. (*A*) Patient with normal cardiac MIBG uptake on SPECT imaging. This patient did not receive appropriate ICD discharges during follow-up. (*B*) Patient example with severe defects in cardiac MIBG uptake on SPECT imaging. This patient received an appropriate ICD discharge 6 months after implantation.

blood-pool SPECT, and gated myocardial perfusion SPECT (GMPS).

A novel count-based approach for the assessment of LV dyssynchrony from GMPS has been developed by Chen and colleagues.[25] From gated short-axis images, location and intensity (number of counts) of each myocardial segment is determined during the cardiac cycle (8 frames or 16 frames per cardiac cycle). Differences in segmental location indicate segmental wall motion, whereas an increase in segmental intensity reflects wall thickening because of the partial-volume effect. For each myocardial short-axis segment, the count-based curve is generated by approximation of first Fourier harmonic function and provides amplitude (end-systolic wall thickness) and phase (onset of mechanical contraction). Next, phase distribution of the entire LV can be displayed in polar map and histogram format. The most important parameters derived from phase analysis include histogram bandwidth and phase SD.

Comparative studies between phase analysis with GMPS and echocardiographic techniques to assess LV dyssynchrony were published. In 75 heart failure patients, phase analysis from GMPS correlated well with tissue Doppler echocardiography for assessment of LV dyssynchrony.[26] Henneman and coworkers[27] evaluated 42 heart failure patients who underwent CRT, and 6 months follow-up was obtained. All baseline characteristics were similar between responders (N = 30) and nonresponders (N = 12) to CRT, except for more extensive LV dyssynchrony in responders as compared with nonresponders, reflected in a significantly larger histogram bandwidth (175 degrees ± 63 degrees versus 117 degrees ± 51 degrees; $P<.01$) and phase SD (56.3 degrees ± 19.9 degrees versus 37.1 degrees ± 14.4 degrees; $P<.01$). Receiver-operator characteristic curve analysis demonstrated that the optimal value for prediction of response to CRT was 135 degrees for histogram bandwidth (providing a sensitivity and specificity of 70%) and 43 degrees for phase SD (providing a sensitivity and specificity of 74%). An example of a patient with extensive cardiac dyssynchrony on GMPS is shown in **Fig. 9**.

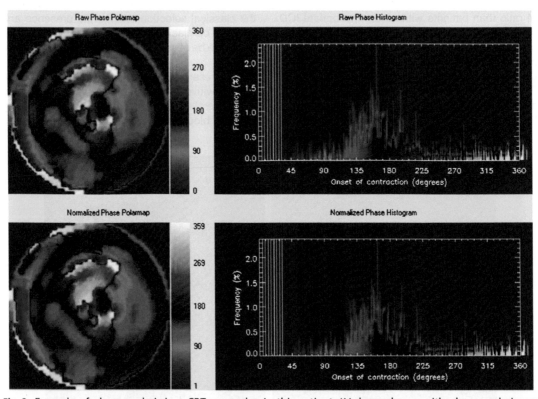

Fig. 9. Example of phase analysis in a CRT responder. In this patient, LV dyssynchrony with phase analysis was present at baseline (evidenced by the wide phase histogram), and clinical and echocardiographic improvement at 6 months follow-up was observed. (*From* Henneman MM, Chen J, Dibbets-Schneider P, et al. Can LV dyssynchrony as assessed with phase analysis on gated myocardial perfusion SPECT predict response to CRT? J Nucl Med 2007;48:1104–11; reprinted by permission of the Society for Nuclear Medicine.)

Besides cardiac dyssynchrony, nuclear imaging can also provide information on viability and scar tissue, which are also important for CRT response. Ypenburg and coworkers[28] evaluated 51 heart failure patients before CRT implantation with GMPS using technetium-99 m tetrofosmin. After 6 months, clinical and echocardiographic follow-up was obtained, and it was demonstrated that the extent of viable myocardium was positively related to the extent of reverse LV remodeling and the increase in LV ejection fraction; the extent of scar tissue, however, was inversely related to the changes in volumes and ejection fraction. These findings highlight the potential use of nuclear imaging in the improved selection for CRT patients.

SUMMARY

This article provides an overview of the merits of nuclear imaging in heart failure patients. Nuclear imaging provides integrated assessment of ischemia, viability, innervation, and dyssynchrony. The assessment of ischemia and viability are accepted approaches, whereas innervation imaging and assessment of cardiac dyssynchrony with nuclear imaging are relatively new. This information provides the framework for therapeutic decision-making in the individual heart failure patient.

REFERENCES

1. Rosamond W, Flegal K, Furie K, et al, for the American Heart Association Statistics Committee and Stroke Statistics Heart disease and stroke statistics—2008 update. A Report from the American Heart Association Statistics Committee and Stroke Statistics Subcommittee. Circulation 2008;117: e25–146.

2. Gheorgiade M, Bonow RO. Chronic heart failure in the Unites States: a manifestation of coronary artery disease. Circulation 1998;97:282–9.

3. Goldberger JJ, Cain ME, Hohnloser SH, et al. American Heart Association/American College of Cardiology Foundation/Heart Rhythm Society Scientific Statement on Noninvasive Risk Stratification. Techniques for Identifying Patients at Risk for Sudden Cardiac Death. A scientific statement from the American Heart Association Council on Clinical Cardiology Committee on Electrocardiography and Arrhythmias and Council on Epidemiology and Prevention. J Am Coll Cardiol 2008;52:1179–99.

4. Vardas PE, Auricchio A, Blanc JJ, et al. Guidelines for cardiac pacing and cardiac resynchronization therapy. Task Force for Cardiac Pacing and Cardiac Resynchronization Therapy of the European Society of Cardiology. Europace 2007;9:959–98.

5. Underwood SR, Anagnostopoulos C, Cerqueira M, et al. Myocardial perfusion scintigraphy: the evidence. Eur J Nucl Med Mol Imaging 2004;31: 261–91.

6. Danias PG, Ahlberg AW, Clark BA III, et al. Combined assessment of myocardial perfusion and left ventricular function with exercise technetium-99m sestamibi gated single-photon emission computed tomography can differentiate between ischemic and nonischemic dilated cardiomyopathy. Am J Cardiol 1998;82:1253–8.

7. Danias PG, Papaioannou GI, Ahlberg AW, et al. Usefulness of electrocardiographic-gated stress technetium-99m sestamibi single-photon emission computed tomography to differentiate ischemic from nonischemic cardiomyopathy. Am J Cardiol 2004;94:14–9.

8. Eisenberg JD, Sobel BE, Geltman EM. Differentiation of ischemic from nonischemic cardiomyopathy with positron emission tomography. Am J Cardiol 1987; 59:1410–4.

9. Schuijf JD, Jukema JW, van der Wall EE, et al. The current status of multislice computed tomography in the diagnosis and prognosis of coronary artery disease. J Nucl Cardiol 2007;14:604–12.

10. Ghostine S, Caussin C, Habis M, et al. Non-invasive diagnosis of ischaemic heart failure using 64-slice computed tomography. Eur Heart J 2008;29(17): 2133–40.

11. Nesto RW, Kowalchuk GJ. The ischemic cascade: temporal sequence of hemodynamic, electrocardiographic and symptomatic expressions of ischemia. Am J Cardiol 1987;59:23C–30C.

12. Schuijf JD, Shaw LJ, Wijns W, et al. Cardiac imaging in coronary artery disease: differing modalities. Heart 2005;91:1110–7.

13. Smanio PE, Watson DD, Segalla DL, et al. Value of gating of technetium-99m sestamibi single-photon emission computed tomographic imaging. J Am Coll Cardiol 1997;30:1687–92.

14. Schuijf JD, Poldermans D, Shaw LJ, et al. Diagnostic and prognostic value of non-invasive imaging in known or suspected coronary artery disease. Eur J Nucl Med Mol Imaging 2006;33:93–104.

15. Rahimtoola SH. The hibernating myocardium. Am Heart J 1989;117:211–21.

16. Bax JJ, Schinkel AFL, Boersma E, et al. Early versus delayed revascularization in patients with ischemic cardiomyopathy and substantial viability: impact on outcome. Circulation 2003;108(Suppl 1):II39–42.

17. Schinkel AFL, Bax JJ, Sozzi FB, et al. Prevalence of myocardial viability assessed by single photon emission computed tomography in patients with chronic ischaemic left ventricular dysfunction. Heart 2002;88:125–30.

18. Schinkel AFL, Bax JJ, Elhendy A, et al. Assessment of viable tissue in Q-wave regions by metabolic imaging using single-photon emission computed

tomography in ischemic cardiomyopathy. Am J Cardiol 2002;89:1171–5.

19. Schinkel AF, Bax JJ, Poldermans D, et al. Hibernating myocardium: diagnosis and patient outcomes. Curr Probl Cardiol 2007;32:375–410.

20. Merlet P, Valette H, Dubois-Rande JL, et al. Prognostic value of cardiac metaiodobenzylguanidine imaging in patients with heart failure. J Nucl Med 1992;33:471–7.

21. Manrique A, Bernard M, Hitzel A, et al. Prognostic value of sympathetic innervation and cardiac asynchrony in dilated cardiomyopathy. Eur J Nucl Med Mol Imaging 2008;35:2074–81.

22. Nagahara D, Nakata T, Hashimoto A, et al. Predicting the need for an implantable cardioverter defibrillator using cardiac metaiodobenzylguanidine activity together with plasma natriuretic peptide concentration or left ventricular function. J Nucl Med 2008;49:225–33.

23. Arora R, Ferrick KJ, Nakata T, et al. I-123 MIBG imaging and heart rate variability analysis to predict the need for an implantable cardioverter defibrillator. J Nucl Cardiol 2003;10:121–31.

24. Bax JJ, Kraft O, Buxton AE, et al. [123]-I-MIBG scintigraphy to predict inducibility of ventricular arrhythmias on cardiac electrophysiology testing. Circ Cardiovasc Imaging 2008;1:131–40.

25. Chen J, Garcia EV, Folks RD, et al. Onset of left ventricular mechanical contraction as determined by phase analysis of ECG-gated myocardial perfusion SPECT imaging: development of a diagnostic tool for assessment of cardiac mechanical dyssynchrony. J Nucl Cardiol 2005;12:687–95.

26. Henneman MM, Chen J, Ypenburg C, et al. Phase analysis of gated myocardial perfusion single-photon emission computed tomography compared with tissue Doppler imaging for the assessment of left ventricular dyssynchrony. J Am Coll Cardiol 2007;49:1708–14.

27. Henneman MM, Chen J, Dibbets-Schneider P, et al. Can LV dyssynchrony as assessed with phase analysis on gated myocardial perfusion SPECT predict response to CRT? J Nucl Med 2007;48:1104–11.

28. Ypenburg C, Schalij MJ, Bleeker GB, et al. Extent of viability to predict response to cardiac resynchronization therapy in ischemic heart failure patients. J Nucl Med 2006;47:1565–70.

Quantification of Myocardial Blood Flow: What is the Clinical Role?

Heinrich R. Schelbert, MD, PhD

KEYWORDS

- PET • Coronary artery disease • Myocardial blood flow
- Microvascular disease • Endothelial function

The ability to measure myocardial blood flow in absolute units adds an important new dimension to standard myocardial perfusion imaging. As a widely applied diagnostic test, standard perfusion imaging evaluates the relative distribution of myocardial blood flow at rest and in response to physiologic or pharmacologic stress. It accurately predicts presence or absence of flow-limiting coronary artery disease, delineates the extent and severity of such disease, and is of considerable prognostic value. However, there are distinct limitations to standard perfusion imaging. For example, it cannot identify disease-related disturbances of the coronary circulation that do not lead to regional blood flow heterogeneities but that affect blood flow homogeneously throughout the left ventricular myocardium. Therefore, disease at the microvascular level—and also of the coronary arteries—may remain unrecognized. In these instances where measurements of myocardial blood flow and its responses to targeted pharmacologic and physiologic stresses, positron emission tomography (PET) can provide important clinical information. This article presents technical aspects of PET-based measurements of myocardial blood flow, examines major determinants of blood flow regulation, and explores how quantification of myocardial blood flow can contribute to diagnosis, risk assessment, and treatment of cardiovascular disease.

TECHNICAL CONSIDERATIONS OF MYOCARDIAL BLOOD FLOW MEASUREMENTS

PET measures regional myocardial blood flow in absolute units. Positron-emitting radiotracers of blood flow, which are currently in use for investigational and, importantly, clinical studies, include: oxygen-15–labeled (O-15) water; nitrogen-13 (N-13) ammonia; and rubidium-82 (Rb-82). Each agent possesses unique physical and tracer kinetic properties with distinct advantages and limitations.[1–6]

O-15– labeled water exhibits tracer kinetic properties that very closely approach those of the ideal tracer of blood flow. The myocardial radiotracer tissue concentration follows in strict linear proportion changes in myocardial blood flow, ie, O-15–labeled water linearly tracks changes of myocardial blood flow. Yet, the physical half-life of O-15 is only 124 seconds; as a result, measurements of myocardial blood flow require close coordination with the cyclotron O-15 production. Additionally, O-15–labeled water not only exchanges from blood into myocardium but equilibrates with the water spaces in blood, requiring corrections for tracer activity in the left ventricular blood pool and the vascular space of the myocardium. Correction routines include subtraction of blood pool activity after labeling the blood pool with inhalation of O-15 or C-11 carbon monoxide (binding to hemoglobin) or through image-based algorithms.[1,4,7]

N-13 ammonia, also cyclotron produced, is logistically less demanding because of its 10-minute physical half-life. Administered intravenously, it rapidly exchanges into the myocardium and clears from blood so that high contrast myocardial perfusion images are obtained within 5–15 minutes after the N-13 ammonia administration. Because the physical half-life is longer for N-13 than O-15, more counts are recorded with N-13

Department of Molecular and Medical Pharmacology, David Geffen School of Medicine at UCLA, University of California at Los Angeles, B2-085J; Box 95648, 650 Charles E. Young Drive South, Los Angeles, CA 90095-6948, USA

E-mail address: hschelbert@mednet.ucla.edu

Cardiol Clin 27 (2009) 277–289
doi:10.1016/j.ccl.2008.12.009

ammonia, typically resulting in high-count density myocardial perfusion images of good diagnostic quality. Unlike when using O-15 water, however, N-13 ammonia activity concentrations do not linearly increase with changes in myocardial blood flow. The first-pass radiotracer extraction (or retention) fraction (ie, the fraction of tracer that exchanges across the capillary wall [or is retained in myocardium] during a single passage through the coronary circulation) though high at resting flows, gradually and nonlinearly declines with higher flows.[8] Accordingly, the radiotracer net uptake (as the product of flow and first-pass extraction fraction) in myocardium increases with higher flows but in a nonlinear fashion until reaching a "plateau" (approximately at flows of 2.5–3.0 mL/min/gm) when further flow increases are associated with progressively smaller increases in myocardial N-13 ammonia concentrations.

Rb-82 exhibits tracer kinetic properties that are similar to those of N-13 ammonia, ie, a nonlinear relationship between blood flow and myocardial activity concentrations. Its first-pass extraction fraction is lower than that of N-13 ammonia and, consequently, reaches the "plateau phase" at somewhat lower flows (ie, 2.0–2.5 mL/min/gm). Nevertheless, Rb-82 offers distinct logistical advantages. It is available through a generator that typically is operated by a semi-automated intravenous infusion system that facilitates close coordination between pharmacologic or other stress interventions and the tracer administration. Radiotracer activity doses are preselected and delivered by the push-button operated infusion system. Because of its ultrashort physical half-life of only 78 seconds, image acquisition typically commences between 90–120 seconds after tracer administration and continues for 5–7 minutes. The high kinetic energy of Rb-82 positrons (associated with longer distances of travel in tissue before losing their energy, combining with an electron and annihilation) together with the ultra-short physical half-life, produces myocardial perfusion images of lower count density and spatial resolution—although the images are usually of good diagnostic quality.

Fundamental to measurements of myocardial blood flow is the high spatial and temporal resolution of PET capability, together with its quantitative imaging capability. Rapidly acquired serial images (typically with 5–10 second frame rates) track the initial transit of the radiotracer bolus through the central circulation and its exchange from blood into the myocardium. The serially acquired images are corrected for photon-attenuation either via prerecorded transmission images obtained with a rotating external positron-emitting rod source or,

more recently, for integrated PET/CT systems, with a pre-recorded CT image of the mediastinum. These images, therefore, quantitatively depict the true regional radiotracer activity concentrations. Through regions or volumes of interest assigned to the arterial blood of the left ventricular cavity and to the left ventricular myocardium, time–activity curves of the arterial radiotracer input function and the myocardial tissue response are obtained (**Fig. 1**). Fitted with operational equations derived from tracer kinetic models, which relate the externally observed tissue kinetics to absolute values of myocardial blood flow, estimates of myocardial blood flow in units of ml/blood/min/gm are obtained. It is also possible to apply graphical analysis approaches to the serially acquired images and to display regional estimates of myocardial blood flow in the form of color-coded parametric images (**Fig. 2**).[9]

The noninvasive flow estimates accurately reflect regional myocardial blood flows as validated by the arterial reference microsphere technique in animal experiments. In these comparison studies, the noninvasive PET blood flow estimates closely and linearly correlated with microsphere flows as high as 5.0 mL/min/gm. Flow estimates as verified with the microsphere approach were equally accurate for O-15 water and N-13 ammonia studies.[10–13] More recently, a similar linear correlation with microsphere blood flows has been reported for Rb-82.[14]

Importantly, measurements of regional myocardial blood flows with PET at rest, as well as during pharmacologically stimulated hyperemia or with cold pressor testing, are highly reproducible as confirmed by repeat blood flow measurements during the same study session or by repeat measurements several days later.[15–21]

REGULATION OF CORONARY BLOOD FLOW

The coronary circulation can be viewed as consisting of two functionally distinct but closely interconnected compartments: the coronary resistance and the coronary conduit vessels. Flow through the coronary circulation depends on the pressure gradient between the aorta and the right atrium. Under normal circumstances, the epicardial coronary conduit vessels exert little if any resistance to flow. Accordingly, intracoronary pressures approach those in the aorta and are fully maintained along the conduit artery. In contrast, in the resistance vessel, intracoronary pressure gradually declines with decreasing vessel diameter (from 500 μm–100 μm at the pre-arteriolar level and to less than 100 μm at the arteriolar level).[22] Control of vascular resistance and, thus,

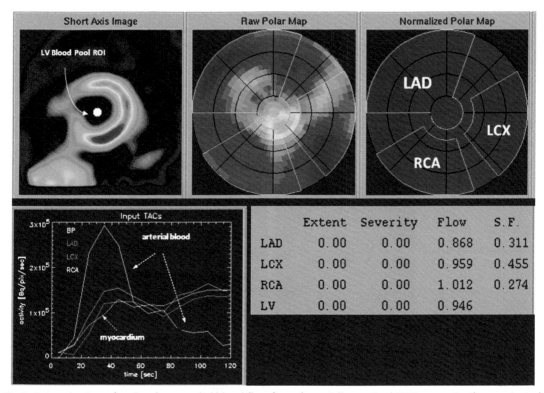

Fig.1. Determination of regional myocardial blood flow from the serially acquired PET images. On the re-oriented short-axis image of the left ventricular myocardium (*upper left panel*), a region of interest is assigned to the left ventricular blood pool. The polar map displays the relative distribution of the flow tracer throughout the left ventricular myocardium. Based on a comparison to a database of normal, no regional reductions in radiotracer activity are identified. Regions of interest are assigned to the territories of the left anterior descending (LAD), the left circumflex (LCX) and the right coronary artery (RCA). The corresponding time–activity curves for arterial blood and the myocardial regions are shown in the left lower panel. The final read out is shown in the lower left panel; extent and severity of regional flow defects are indicated but listed as zero because of the normal homogenous radiotracer distribution. Values of flow in ml/min/g are indicated for each of the vascular territories as well as the entire left ventricular myocardium. *Abbreviations*: SF, spillover fraction, for cross contamination of activity from blood into myocardium.

of coronary blood flow resides mostly at the level of the pre-arterioles and arterioles.[23]

Rates of blood flow and, thus, of substrate delivery are constantly adjusted to match energy demand, mostly dictated by myocardial work with heart rate, pressure development, and contractility as major determinants. Hence, metabolism-dependent regulatory mechanisms, presumably mediated by adenosine, adjust the diameter of the pre-arteriolar and arteriolar vessels and, thus, their resistance to flow. A predominantly vascular smooth muscle–mediated change in coronary blood flow is further modulated by the endothelium. For example, increases in flow velocity lead to a shear-stress–mediated increased availability of vasodilator substances, especially of nitric oxide (or at the level of the microvasculature, of hyperpolarizing substances), which amplify the vasodilator effect and further

lower the resistance to flow. This modulatory shear-stress–mediated and endothelium-dependent dilator effect adjusts the conduit vessel diameter to reduce the resistance to higher velocity flows. Resistance to flow depends on its velocity, the coronary pressure and, importantly, on the fourth power of the vessel diameter; the latter determinant emphasizes the importance of the flow-related conduit vessel dilation for maintaining resistance to flow at the minimum.

In addition to these more intrinsic coronary regulatory mechanisms, neurohumeral factors integrate the coronary vascular function into the overall function of the circulatory system. Neuronal regulation includes the sympathetic system with stimulation of local α- and β-adrenoreceptors.[23] Under normal conditions, α-adrenergically mediated vasoconstrictor effects on the vascular smooth muscle are opposed by shear-stress as

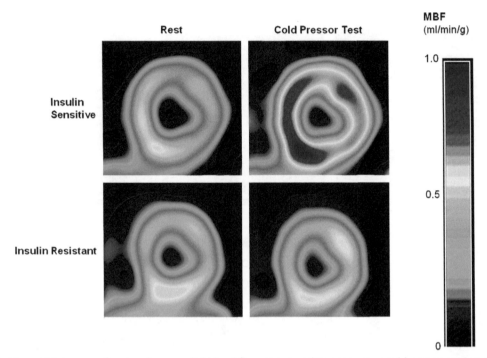

Fig. 2. Parametric images of regional myocardial blood flow at rest and in response to cold pressor testing. Examples are shown for a normal, insulin-sensitive volunteer (*upper panel*) and an insulin-resistant individual (*lower panel*). Regional myocardial blood flows are color coded as shown on the color scale on the right. Note the increase in regional myocardial blood flows from rest to cold pressor testing in the insulin-sensitive individual as compared with a markedly attenuated flow response in the insulin-resistant individual.

well as endothelial, α-adrenergically mediated vasodilator effects. Decreases in the bioavailability of vasodilator substances and, in particular, of nitric oxide in diseased states diminish the opposing vasodilator effect such that vasoconstrictor effects may prevail. Vasodilator responses to increased flow demand are then attenuated, absent, or paradoxical, that is, flow actually declines. Hence, hyperemic responses to exercise or to vasodilator stimulation may be diminished. Moreover, at the level of the conduit vessels, inadequately opposed vasoconstrictor effects may attenuate or even abolish the flow-related diameter increase. Accordingly, resistance to high velocity flow increases, associated with a gradual decline in intracoronary pressure over the length of the epicardial conduit vessel.

Disturbances of the coronary circulatory function originate with functional or structural alterations of the vascular resistance, which reside either at the level of the conduit vessel (eg, a flow-limiting coronary stenosis) or at the level of the microvasculature (eg, because of microangiopathies) or both.[22] Because of the considerable vasodilator reserve of the coronary circulation, functional or structural alterations early in the course of coronary vascular disease can be adequately compensated for so

that coronary blood flow at rest is fully maintained. However, when this compensatory mechanism and, thus, the residual vasodilator reserve are progressively exhausted, flow at rest ultimately declines. Use of the compensatory reserve is associated with a reduction in vasoreactivity, which can be demonstrated with invasive and noninvasive study techniques. Invasive probes of the coronary circulatory function include intracoronary flow velocity measurements and quantitative coronary angiography at baseline and during pharmacologic stimulation of vascular smooth muscle and endothelium.[24–26]

TARGETS OF CORONARY CIRCULATORY FUNCTION

Among the noninvasive approaches for the study of the coronary circulatory function in humans, the foremost approach entails PET measurement of myocardial blood flow, including of its responses to target-specific physiologic and pharmacologic challenges (**Fig. 3**). Targets of PET blood flow measurements include: (a) integrated vasodilator capacity; (b) endothelium-related vasomotion; and (c) epicardial conduit vessel function.

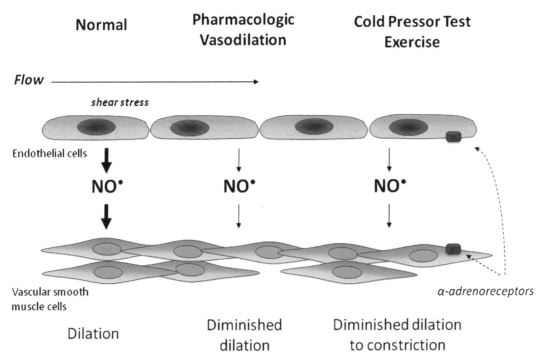

Fig. 3. Highly schematic depiction of the interplay between the endothelium related vasodilator and vascular smooth muscle–mediated vasoconstrictor effects at baseline, during pharmacologic vasodilation and during cold pressor testing. Under normal condition, increases in coronary flow velocity lead to a shear-stress–mediated release of vasodilator substances, especially of nitric oxide (NO) from the endothelium. In instances of diminished bioavailability of vasodilator substances and especially of NO, the vasodilator response to pharmacologically induced hyperemia is attenuated or absent. During sympathetic stimulation (*on the right*) norepinephrine–mediated stimulation of α-adrenoreceptors prompts a vasoconstrictor effect that under normal conditions is offset by flow-related and adrenergically stimulated endothelial release of vasodilator substances. In endothelial dysfunction however, this opposing vasodilator effect is diminished so that flow responses are diminished or vasoconstriction may prevail.

Integrated Vasodilator Capacity

Its assessment entails intravenous administration of vascular smooth muscle–relaxing agents like dipyridamole, adenosine, and adenosine-triphosphate or, more recently, adenosine receptor agonists.[27–29] These agents maximally reduce resistance of flow and initiate an increase in flow that is augmented by shear-stress–mediated and endothelium-dependent vasodilation. Endothelium-related factors may contribute as much as 26% to the total vasodilator response or as much as 19% of the total hyperemic flow according to PET flow measurements during pharmacologically induced hyperemia after pharmacologic inhibition of the nitric oxide synthase in young normal volunteers.[30]

The total hyperemic response to pharmacologic stress reflects the combined vasodilator effect of vascular smooth muscle and endothelium and is, therefore, defined as the "total integrated vasodilator capacity." It typically is expressed in units of ml/min/gm. This measurement can be further related to the coronary driving pressure and be described as "minimal coronary resistance" or the ratio of mean arterial blood pressure and myocardial blood flow. Coronary—or preferably, myocardial—flow reserve serves as another, more conventional measure of the vasodilator capacity. The term "coronary flow reserve" has gained wide acceptance in the past, especially because initial invasive approaches measured only changes in flow velocity but not absolute rates of myocardial blood flow. As the ratio of hyperemic to baseline flows, coronary flow reserve depends also on the baseline flows so that it does not fully and consistently reflect the true vasodilator capacity.

Endothelium-Related Coronary Vasomotion

Assessment of endothelium-related vasomotion targets the response of myocardial blood flow to sympathetic stimulation with cold pressor testing. The validity of this response measurement as an indicator of endothelial function has been established through invasive measurements where sympathetic stimulation induced changes in coronary blood flow and in conduit vessel diameter that closely correlate with changes induced by pharmacologic stimulation of the endothelium as well as of the vascular smooth muscle cells.[24–26]

Assessment of endothelium-dependent coronary vasomotion entails PET measurements of myocardial blood flow at baseline and, then again, during the peak hemodynamic response (heart rate and systolic blood pressure) to cold exposure (typically 30–60 seconds after immersion of a hand in a slush of ice water).[31,32] The difference between rest and cold pressor flows constitutes the cold pressor flow response, which is expressed in absolute flow units or as a percentage of baseline flow. Again, as in the case of the myocardial flow reserve, flow responses given in percent of baseline flow depend also on baseline flows, which may limit the value when flows are elevated at baseline, for example, in arterial hypertension. In contrast, when expressed in absolute units of flow, the response to cold pressor stress is less dependent on baseline hemodynamic conditions.[33]

Epicardial Conduit Vessel Function

The concept underlying the assessment of epicardial coronary artery function relates to the importance of the conduit vessel diameter for the resistance to high velocity flows. As mentioned, shear-stress–related and endothelium-mediated regulatory mechanisms adjust the vessel diameter to changes in flow velocity such that resistance to high velocity flows remains low and intracoronary pressures remain constant over the length of the epicardial conduit vessel. If, however, as pointed out by Gould and colleagues,[34] and subsequently confirmed by de Bruyne and colleagues,[35] such dilatory response is impaired, either due to diffuse luminal narrowing, increased vessel wall stiffness or diminished bioavailability of vasodilator substances, then the resistance to high velocity flow increases and leads, as de Bruyne and colleagues[35] have demonstrated, to a gradual loss of intracoronary pressure along the conduit vessel. As a consequence, downstream perfusion progressively declines, leading to a progressive, longitudinal, base-to-apex perfusion gradient. In patients who have coronary artery disease, for example, distal intracoronary pressures during pharmacologic hyperemia in nonstenosed coronary vessels were on average 10 ± 8 mmHg lower than in the aorta as compared with statistically nonsignificant pressure differences in normal volunteers.[35] In some patients, the aorta to distal coronary artery pressure gradient was as high as

that seen in vessels with obstructive coronary stenosis and may be associated with ischemia. Moreover, relative values of perfusion or of myocardial blood flows during dipyridamole-induced hyperemia were on average 11% lower in the apical than in the more basal portions of the left ventricular myocardium.[34,36] In contrast, in normal human healthy volunteers, values for hyperemic blood flows were similar in apical and midleft ventricular myocardial regions. A longitudinal perfusion gradient may also develop even when myocardial blood flow remains constant, but when the conduit vessel diameter declines (eg, in response to sympathetic stimulation with cold pressor testing).[37]

It is possible to probe with PET flow measurements different aspects of coronary circulatory function. When used together, they offer a more comprehensive assessment of the functional state of the coronary circulation as well as the extent and severity of functional disturbances, that is, whether disease-related alterations are confined to the endothelium or encroach upon vascular smooth muscle function. Moreover, flow responses to pharmacologic stimuli (eg, smooth muscle relaxing agents) considerably vary between individuals.[27] Combined use of the different functional probes may then allow clinicians to more definitively distinguish between normal and abnormal states of coronary vasomotor function. Conversely, use of only one functional probe may suffice when only mild alterations are anticipated or for repeat studies when the effect of specific therapeutic interventions are to be monitored.

CLINICAL APPLICATIONS OF FLOW MEASUREMENTS

Numerous investigations with PET measurements of myocardial blood flow have explored the human coronary circulation. These studies examined: (1) functional consequences of macrovascular as well as microvascular coronary artery disease; (2) the effects of structural and functional manifestations of metabolism disorders like type 2 diabetes and insulin resistance; and (3) conventional coronary risk factors on circulatory function and potentially beneficial responses to coronary risk reduction strategies. These investigations have also demonstrated the prognostic value of measurements of myocardial blood flow for long-term cardiovascular events. From these observations, several clinical conditions emerged in which measurements of myocardial blood flow can aid in diagnosis, risk assessment, and patient management. Specifically, PET flow measurements may prove clinically useful for: (a) determining the "total ischemic burden of the myocardium;" (b) assessing coronary risk and for risk stratification; and (c) monitoring the effectiveness of risk reducing therapeutic strategies.

Assessment of the "Total Ischemic Burden"

The potential of flow measurements for assessing the myocardium's "total ischemic burden" extends beyond macrovascular manifestations of coronary atherosclerosis to disease manifestations at the microcirculatory level. As recently emphasized by Neglia,[38] impairments of microcirculatory flow at rest or of the microvascular reserve in coronary and noncoronary artery disease may limit tissue perfusion and, similar to fluid dynamically significant coronary stenosis, lead to contractile dysfunction. In this change of paradigm, microvascular disease represents as much as macrovascular disease an "ischemic burden" to the myocardium.

Macrovascular Disease

Standard stress-rest SPECT myocardial perfusion imaging with Tc-99 m labeled flow agents identifies the presence and extent of coronary artery disease and has proved clinically important for risk stratification of patients who have coronary artery disease. Perfusion imaging either with SPECT or PET delineates the relative distribution of myocardial blood flow. Regional reductions in radiotracer activity on the perfusion images reflect the presence of an upstream fluid dynamically significant coronary stenosis or of myocardial tissue injury. In contrast, regions with the highest radiotracer activity are considered to be subtended by nonstenosed coronary vessels. Yet, these regions might also be subtended by diseased coronary arteries; their disease severity is less than that of vessels with downstream regional tracer uptake defects. Imaging only the relative distribution of myocardial blood flow during stress and rest therefore limits the assessment of the full extent of coronary artery disease, especially in instances of multivessel disease, balanced coronary lesions, and left main disease.

In these conditions, especially, regional flow responses to vasodilator stress, measured in absolute units, will more accurately reveal the full extent of coronary artery disease. For example, in a study of 23 coronary artery disease patients (10 with single vessel and 13 with triple vessel disease), standard myocardial perfusion imaging correctly identified only 6 of the 13 patients (46%) as having triple vessel disease as compared with 12 of 13 patients (92%) by the quantitative imaging approach.[39] Quantitative flow estimates correctly identified 37 of the 39 stenosed vessels (95%) in triple vessel disease patients as compared with only 31 (80%) with standard imaging. The study approach used the quantitative radiotracer retention as a measure of absolute flow and a threshold value for distinguishing between normal and diminished hyperemic blood flows.

Clinical investigations in support of quantitative flow measurements for determining the extent of coronary artery disease are still limited in number. Importantly, however, the finding of a stenosis-related reduction in hyperemic flow in these studies is consistent with PET flow observations of an inverse correlation between stenosis severity and downstream hyperemic blood flow.[40,41] In one study for example, 70% to 90% area stenosis were associated with an average 48% reduction in hyperemic flows, which is comparable to an average 58% reduction in hyperemic flows for 60% to 79% diameter stenosis measured in the second study.

Microvascular Disease

Impairments in myocardial perfusion, even in noncoronary disease, either at rest or as more frequently observed, during pharmacologically stimulated hyperemia similarly reflect the "ischemic burden of the heart." **Fig. 4** illustrates an example of diffuse vasodilator impairment with apparently normal stress rest perfusion images in a 16-year-old female who had an orthotopic heart transplant two years earlier and who presented with intermittent chest pain with ST-segment changes, elevated troponin levels, and a left ventricular ejection fraction of only 30%. The perfusion images were normal during stress and at rest. However, measurements of myocardial blood flow revealed severely reduced adenosine-stimulated hyperemic flows and a markedly reduced flow reserve. The patient was subsequently re-transplanted; histopathology of the explanted cardiac allograft revealed extensive concentric narrowing of the epicardial and intramyocardial arteries, which most likely accounted for the reduced vasodilator capacity.

Similar to this patient's example of advanced transplant vasculopathy, myocardial blood flow at rest in patients with ischemic cardiomyopathy, with idiopathic dilated cardiomyopathy, with hypertrophic cardiomyopathy or with diabetic cardiomyopathy is almost invariably normal, while hyperemic flow responses or the myocardial flow reserve are markedly diminished.[42–44] The impairment in vasodilator capacity in patients who have noncoronary cardiac disease or in "remote myocardium" in patients who have coronary disease has been attributed to functional and/or structural alterations of the coronary microvasculature.

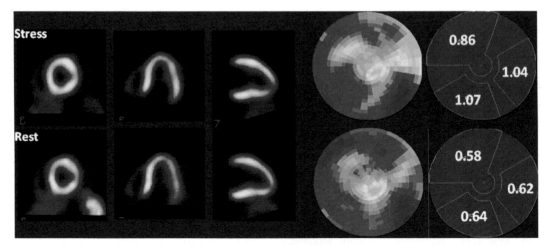

Fig. 4. An example of diffusely impaired vasodilator reserve in an orthotopic heart transplant patient. This 16-year-old female had received an orthotopic heart transplant 2 years earlier and currently presents with intermittent chest pain associated with ST-segment abnormalities, elevated troponin levels, and progressive deterioration of left ventricular function. The N-13 ammonia stress and rest myocardial perfusion images show normal homogeneous perfusion (panel on the left). However, the adenosine stimulated myocardial blood flows are severely reduced so that the myocardial flow reserve was only 1.62 and thus, markedly diminished. (The values in each of the coronary artery territories represent the actual flow values in ml/min/gm).

The severity of impairment in microvascular vasodilator function contains prognostic information. In patients who have hypertrophic cardiomyopathy or who have mild idiopathic left ventricular systolic dysfunction, severely reduced dipyridamole flows were —on multivariate analysis— highly predictive of cardiac death and of left ventricular remodeling and progressive deterioration of left ventricular function.[42,43] In these studies, dipyridamole flows of 0.89 mL/min/gm in hypertrophic cardiomyopathy[42] and of 1.27 mL/min/gm in idiopathic dilated cardiomyopathy[43] (or flow reserves of 1.47 and 1.29, respectively) predicted an unfavorable outcome whereas dipyridamole flows of 2.28 mL/min/gm and of 1.67 mL/min/gm (or flow reserves of 2.18 and 2.4, respectively) were associated with a more favorable outcome. Even in patients with normal left ventricular dimensions and function did the severe reductions of dipyridamole predict the progressive left ventricular remodeling and worsening of contractile function.[45] The predictive value of the diminished dipyridamole flows exceeded that of the left ventricular ejection fraction. In ischemic cardiomyopathy patients, global hyperemic myocardial blood flows similarly contained important prognostic information, as recently reported.[46] In 344 consecutive coronary artery disease patients who had at least one prior myocardial infarction, the global myocardial flow reserve proved to be more predictive than the left ventricular ejection fraction of subsequent cardiac death or major cardiovascular events. Dipyridamole flows of less than 1.49 mL/min/g or flow reserves of less than 1.49 in that study were associated with a significantly lower cardiac event free survival than higher hyperemic flow or flow reserves. In contrast to prior investigations in ischemic cardiomyopathy patients, the presence and extent of perfusion metabolism matches or mismatches were not associated in this study population with future cardiac events.

Mechanisms that account for the predictive value of low hyperemic flows remain uncertain. It is also unclear whether the flow reduction is secondary to other disease related alterations or is causative. Possible explanations include: the increased wall stress of the enlarged left ventricle with elevated extravascular resistive forces, apoptosis and replacement fibrosis as reported for idiopathic left ventricular systolic dysfunction;[43] and structural alterations of the microvessels as observed in hypertrophic cardiomyopathy.[42] Some evidence suggests that the impairment in microcirculatory reactivity may be associated with repetitive ischemic episodes, which, in turn, might account for the progressive left ventricular remodeling.[45] Structural alterations of the microvasculature, apart from functional disturbances, likely account for the diminished vasodilator capacity, for example, shown in hypertrophic cardiomyopathy or type 2 diabetic patients who have diabetic retinopathy or coronary microangiopathies.[47,48]

Importantly, functional alterations that are potentially reversible also contribute to the impairment in microcirculatory reactivity. In type 2 diabetic patients, for example, glycemic control was associated with significant improvements in total vasodilator capacity as well as, as shown in another study, in endothelium-related vasomotion, possibly related to a reduction in hyperglycemia-related oxidative stress.[49,50] Furthermore, improvements in microcirculatory reactivity have also been observed after treatment with verapamil or with ACE inhibitors and diuretics,[51,52] further implicating potentially reversible endothelial dysfunction as a significant contributor or cause of the diminished vasodilator reserve.

Quantitation of regional flow responses to vasodilator stress allows a more comprehensive assessment of the severity and extent of coronary artery disease. Importantly, these measurements contain predictive information that appears to exceed that available through other measures of left ventricular function or that is not available with other techniques. The flow measurement can thus aid in patient risk assessment as well as contribute to patient management especially because impairments of microcirculatory function may be partially reversible.

CORONARY RISK ASSESSMENT

Measurements of myocardial blood flow may also prove useful for assessing the coronary risk in individuals without clinical coronary artery disease and for monitoring the efficacy of therapeutic strategies for risk reduction. Conventional coronary risk factors may affect the total vasodilator capacity as reported by some investigations,[53–59] but may involve only the endothelial function.[25,26,31,32,60–62] For example, in individuals who have insulin resistance of increasing severity, the total vasodilator capacity remained fully preserved in milder insulin-resistant states and declined only with type 2 diabetes.[63] However, endothelial function, determined by PET measured flow responses to cold pressor testing, were already attenuated in even the mildest forms of insulin resistance and progressively worsened with more severe states of insulin resistance.

Reductions in endothelium-related coronary vasomotion have also been observed in young individuals with angiographically normal coronary arteries but with conventional coronary risk factors.[32] In these individuals, the flow responses to cold correlated closely with flow-related changes in conduit vessel diameter by quantitative coronary angiography, lending further support to the validity of the noninvasively measured flow responses to cold pressor testing as indicators of endothelial function. Other PET investigations demonstrated coronary vasomotor abnormalities

in postmenopausal women;[60] the vasomotor abnormalities involved both the total vasodilator capacity and endothelial function in women with coronary risk factors but were confined to the endothelium-related coronary vasomotion in the absence of coronary risk factors. Obesity similarly was associated with functional alterations of the coronary circulation that paralleled in severity the body weight or BMI.[61] The severity of coronary vasomotor disturbances appeared to correspond to the number of risk factors. Insulin resistance alone in normoglycemic individuals was associated only with disturbances of endothelium-related vasomotion whereas the diminished vasodilator capacity in type 2 diabetes patients was associated with a cluster of risk factors that included hyperlipidemia, hypertriglyceridemia and, most importantly, hyperglycemia and related oxidative stress.[63]

The degree of coronary circulatory dysfunction thus appears to parallel the severity of underlying disease and, possibly, the level of the cardiovascular risk. More severe states of dysfunction involve both the total coronary vasodilator capacity as reflected by the hyperemic flow response to pharmacologic vasodilators and the endothelium-related vasomotion as reflected by the flow response to cold pressor stimulation. Milder and presumably earlier states of disease appear to affect only the endothelium-dependent vasoreactivity. Delineation of the endothelium-related vasomotor function is therefore important; Rask-Madsen and King have appropriately referred to endothelial dysfunction as the "link between complex phenomena at the molecular level and vascular pathogenesis like atherosclerosis."[64]

Dysfunction of the endothelium may reflect loss of anti-atherogenic and anti-thrombotic properties as a pivotal step in the development of atherosclerosis. It may thus indicate an increase in coronary risk as also demonstrated previously with highly invasive[65] and more recently with noninvasive PET measurements.[62] In 72 individuals with angiographically normal coronary arteries but with risk factors for coronary artery disease, cold pressor flow responses proved to be predictive of future cardiovascular events.[62] Over an average 60-month follow-up period, the incidence of cardiovascular events including sudden cardiac death, acute coronary syndrome, nonfatal myocardial infarction, coronary revascularization, and ischemic stroke was strongly associated with an attenuated, absent or paradoxical flow response to cold pressor testing. Quantitation of myocardial blood flow response to sympathetic stimulation with cold pressor testing may indeed be clinically useful for identifying the risk for future coronary events.

Moreover, flow measurements may also contribute to elucidating underlying mechanisms and, at the same time, guide therapeutic interventions. In one study, acute antioxidant treatment with vitamin C restored the flow response to cold pressor stress, which was fully maintained with chronic vitamin C administration when re-examined several months later.[66] In hypercholesteremic patients in contrast, acute vitamin C administration failed to improve the flow response to cold, which accurately predicted the failure of chronic vitamin C treatment. These findings implicate reactive oxygen species as a main contributor to the endothelium-related coronary vasomotor dysfunction in chronic smokers; other factors accounted for the endothelial dysfunction in hypercholesterolemia. Acute challenges in these studies were predictive of long-term responses and thus may aid in target-specific therapeutic strategies.

Other studies have shown the possibility of demonstrating improvements in the coronary vasoreactivity in response to lifestyle modification,[67] lipid lowering,[68–71] glycemic control in type 2 diabetes[49,50] or PPARγ agonists in insulin resistance.[72] Of course, whether such improvements in coronary vasoreactivity translate into a coronary risk reduction awaits further confirmation. Such improvement appears possible because improvements in coronary vasoreactivity in postinfarction patients[73] or in brachial artery flow-related dilation in hypertensive women[74] were associated with significant improvements in long-term event free survival.

SUMMARY AND FUTURE DEVELOPMENTS

Quantification of myocardial blood flow and of its responses to specifically targeted stimuli with PET offers new investigative and clinical possibilities. Flow measurements may prove to be especially important when standard imaging of the relative distribution of myocardial blood flow remains of limited diagnostic value, for example. in multi-vessel coronary artery disease or, even more importantly, in noncoronary cardiovascular diseases with microvascular dysfunction. In these instances, quantitative flow measurements offer unique and clinically relevant prognostic information. In addition, flow measurements can also be used for coronary risk assessments and for monitoring the effectiveness of risk-lowering strategies.

However, several aspects of quantitative flow measurements with PET have limited PET's more widespread clinical use. Although radiotracer administration and serial image acquisition are relatively straightforward but require careful quality control, widely available, reliable, and robust software applications for routine clinical use are still under development. Further, use of N-13 ammonia and of O-15 water as tracers of myocardial blood flow depend on on-site cyclotrons and require close coordination with radiopharmaceutical production. The commercial availability of the generator-produced Rb-82 has largely alleviated this problem, yet the initial, high purchase cost of the generator needs to be offset by high patient volumes to be cost-effective. This situation, in turn, limits the use of Rb-82 in PET facilities with high-volume oncologic studies and occasional cardiac studies. However, the current development and evaluation of F-18 labeled flow tracers with a 2-hour physical half-life promise to overcome this limitation.[75–78] Individual patient doses will then become available through regional PET distribution centers. Based on initial findings in animal experiments and in human investigations, these novel F-18–labeled radiotracers are avidly extracted by the myocardium and they exhibit an exceedingly high first-pass extraction fraction that, in addition, is flow-independent and yields high contrast and high diagnostic quality myocardial perfusion images.[79,80] If the myocardial uptake of these novel radiotracers closely tracks changes in myocardial blood flow, it should markedly facilitate the quantitation of myocardial blood flow and its implementation for routine clinical use.

ACKNOWLEDGMENT

The author wishes to thank Mary Allene Smith for her skillful assistance in preparing this manuscript.

REFERENCES

1. Bergmann SR, Herrero P, Markham J, et al. Noninvasive quantitation of myocardial blood flow in human subjects with oxygen-15-labeled water and positron emission tomography. J Am Coll Cardiol 1989;14: 639–52.
2. El Fakhri G, Sitek A, Guerin B, et al. Quantitative dynamic cardiac 82Rb PET using generalized factor and compartment analyses. J Nucl Med 2005;46: 1264–71.
3. Hutchins GD, Schwaiger M, Rosenspire KC, et al. Noninvasive quantification of regional blood flow in the human heart using N-13 ammonia and dynamic positron emission tomographic imaging. J Am Coll Cardiol 1990;15:1032–42.
4. Iida H, Kanno I, Takahashi A, et al. Measurement of absolute myocardial blood flow with H2150 and dynamic positron-emission tomography. Strategy

for quantification in relation to the partial-volume effect. Circulation 1988;78:104–15.

5. Krivokapich J, Smith GT, Huang SC, et al. 13N ammonia myocardial imaging at rest and with exercise in normal volunteers. Quantification of absolute myocardial perfusion with dynamic positron emission tomography. Circulation 1989;80:1328–37.

6. Lortie M, Beanlands RS, Yoshinaga K, et al. Quantification of myocardial blood flow with 82Rb dynamic PET imaging. Eur J Nucl Med Mol Imaging 2007;34:1765–74.

7. Hermansen F, Ashburner J, Spinks TJ, et al. Generation of myocardial factor images directly from the dynamic oxygen-15-water scan without use of an oxygen-15-carbon monoxide blood-pool scan. J Nucl Med 1998;39:1696–702.

8. Schelbert HR, Phelps ME, Huang SC, et al. N-13 ammonia as an indicator of myocardial blood flow. Circulation 1981;63:1259–72.

9. Choi Y, Huang SC, Hawkins RA, et al. Quantification of myocardial blood flow using 13N-ammonia and PET: comparison of tracer models. J Nucl Med 1999;40:1045–55.

10. Bergmann SR, Fox KA, Rand AL, et al. Quantification of regional myocardial blood flow in vivo with H215O. Circulation 1984;70:724–33.

11. Bol A, Melin JA, Vanoverschelde JL, et al. Direct comparison of [13N]ammonia and [15O]water estimates of perfusion with quantification of regional myocardial blood flow by microspheres. Circulation 1993;87:512–25.

12. Kuhle WG, Porenta G, Huang SC, et al. Quantification of regional myocardial blood flow using 13N-ammonia and reoriented dynamic positron emission tomographic imaging. Circulation 1992;86:1004–17.

13. Muzik O, Beanlands RS, Hutchins GD, et al. Validation of nitrogen-13-ammonia tracer kinetic model for quantification of myocardial blood flow using PET. J Nucl Med 1993;34:83–91.

14. Lautamaki R, George RT, Kitagawa K, et al. Rubidium-82 PET-CT for quantitative assessment of myocardial blood flow: validation in a canine model of coronary artery stenosis. Eur J Nucl Med Mol Imaging 2008.

15. Jagathesan R, Kaufmann PA, Rosen SD, et al. Assessment of the long-term reproducibility of baseline and dobutamine-induced myocardial blood flow in patients with stable coronary artery disease. J Nucl Med 2005;46:212–9.

16. Kaufmann PA, Gnecchi-Ruscone T, Yap JT, et al. Assessment of the reproducibility of baseline and hyperemic myocardial blood flow measurements with 15O-labeled water and PET. J Nucl Med 1999; 40:1848–56.

17. Nagamachi S, Czernin J, Kim AS, et al. Reproducibility of measurements of regional resting and hyperemic myocardial blood flow assessed with PET. J Nucl Med 1996;37:1626–31.

18. Sawada S, Muzik O, Beanlands RS, et al. Interobserver and interstudy variability of myocardial blood flow and flow-reserve measurements with nitrogen 13 ammonia-labeled positron emission tomography. J Nucl Cardiol 1995;2:413–22.

19. Schindler TH, Zhang XL, Prior JO, et al. Assessment of intra- and interobserver reproducibility of rest and cold pressor test-stimulated myocardial blood flow with (13)N-ammonia and PET. Eur J Nucl Med Mol Imaging 2007;34:1178–88.

20. Siegrist PT, Gaemperli O, Koepfli P, et al. Repeatability of cold pressor test-induced flow increase assessed with H(2)(15)O and PET. J Nucl Med 2006; 47:1420–6.

21. Wyss CA, Koepfli P, Namdar M, et al. Tetrahydrobiopterin restores impaired coronary microvascular dysfunction in hypercholesterolaemia. Eur J Nucl Med Mol Imaging 2005;32:84–91.

22. Camici PG, Crea F. Coronary microvascular dysfunction. N Engl J Med 2007;356:830–40.

23. Heusch G, Baumgart D, Camici P, et al. alpha-adrenergic coronary vasoconstriction and myocardial ischemia in humans. Circulation 2000;101: 689–94.

24. Zeiher AM, Drexler H, Wollschlaeger H, et al. Coronary vasomotion in response to sympathetic stimulation in humans: importance of the functional integrity of the endothelium. J Am Coll Cardiol 1989;14: 1181–90.

25. Zeiher AM, Drexler H, Wollschlager H, et al. Modulation of coronary vasomotor tone in humans. Progressive endothelial dysfunction with different early stages of coronary atherosclerosis. Circulation 1991;83:391–401.

26. Zeiher AM, Drexler H, Wollschlager H, et al. Endothelial dysfunction of the coronary microvasculature is associated with coronary blood flow regulation in patients with early atherosclerosis. Circulation 1991;84:1984–92.

27. Chan SY, Brunken RC, Czernin J, et al. Comparison of maximal myocardial blood flow during adenosine infusion with that of intravenous dipyridamole in normal men. J Am Coll Cardiol 1992;20:979–85.

28. Heinonen I, Nesterov SV, Liukko K, et al. Myocardial blood flow and adenosine A2A receptor density in endurance athletes and untrained men. J Physiol 2008;586:5193–202.

29. Kubo S, Tadamura E, Toyoda H, et al. Effect of caffeine intake on myocardial hyperemic flow induced by adenosine triphosphate and dipyridamole. J Nucl Med 2004;45:730–8.

30. Buus NH, Bottcher M, Hermansen F, et al. Influence of nitric oxide synthase and adrenergic inhibition on adenosine-induced myocardial hyperemia. Circulation 2001;104:2305–10.

31. Campisi R, Czernin J, Schoder H, et al. Effects of long-term smoking on myocardial blood flow,

coronary vasomotion, and vasodilator capacity. Circulation 1998;98:119–25.

32. Schindler TH, Nitzsche EU, Olschewski M, et al. PET-measured responses of MBF to cold pressor testing correlate with indices of coronary vasomotion on quantitative coronary angiography. J Nucl Med 2004;45:419–28.

33. Prior JO, Schindler TH, Facta AD, et al. Determinants of myocardial blood flow response to cold pressor testing and pharmacologic vasodilation in healthy humans. Eur J Nucl Med Mol Imaging 2007;34:20–7.

34. Gould KL, Nakagawa Y, Nakagawa K, et al. Frequency and clinical implications of fluid dynamically significant diffuse coronary artery disease manifest as graded, longitudinal, base-to-apex myocardial perfusion abnormalities by noninvasive positron emission tomography. Circulation 2000; 101:1931–9.

35. De Bruyne B, Hersbach F, Pijls NH, et al. Abnormal epicardial coronary resistance in patients with diffuse atherosclerosis but "Normal" coronary angiography. Circulation 2001;104:2401–6.

36. Hernandez-Pampaloni M, Keng FY, Kudo T, et al. Abnormal longitudinal, base-to-apex myocardial perfusion gradient by quantitative blood flow measurements in patients with coronary risk factors. Circulation 2001;104:527–32.

37. Schindler TH, Facta AD, Prior JO, et al. PET-measured heterogeneity in longitudinal myocardial blood flow in response to sympathetic and pharmacologic stress as a non-invasive probe of epicardial vasomotor dysfunction. Eur J Nucl Med Mol Imaging 2006;33:1140–9.

38. Neglia D, L'Abbate A. Myocardial perfusion reserve in ischemic heart disease. J Nucl Med 2009;50:175–7.

39. Parkash R, deKemp RA, Ruddy TD, et al. Potential utility of rubidium 82 PET quantification in patients with 3-vessel coronary artery disease. J Nucl Cardiol 2004;11:440–9.

40. Di Carli M, Czernin J, Hoh CK, et al. Relation among stenosis severity, myocardial blood flow, and flow reserve in patients with coronary artery disease. Circulation 1995;91:1944–51.

41. Uren NG, Melin JA, De Bruyne B, et al. Relation between myocardial blood flow and the severity of coronary-artery stenosis. N Engl J Med 1994;330:1782–8.

42. Cecchi F, Olivotto I, Gistri R, et al. Coronary microvascular dysfunction and prognosis in hypertrophic cardiomyopathy. N Engl J Med 2003;349:1027–35.

43. Neglia D, Michelassi C, Trivieri MG, et al. Prognostic role of myocardial blood flow impairment in idiopathic left ventricular dysfunction. Circulation 2002; 105:186–93.

44. Stolen KQ, Kemppainen J, Kalliokoski KK, et al. Myocardial perfusion reserve and peripheral endothelial function in patients with idiopathic dilated cardiomyopathy. Am J Cardiol 2004;93:64–8.

45. Olivotto I, Cecchi F, Gistri R, et al. Relevance of coronary microvascular flow impairment to long-term remodeling and systolic dysfunction in hypertrophic cardiomyopathy. J Am Coll Cardiol 2006;47:1043–8.

46. Tio RA, Dabeshlim A, Siebelink H-MJ, et al. Comparison between the prognostic value of left ventricular function and myocardial perfusion reserve in patients with ischemic heart disease. J Nucl Med 2009;50(2):214–9.

47. Maron BJ, Wolfson JK, Epstein SE, et al. Intramural ("small vessel") coronary artery disease in hypertrophic cardiomyopathy. J Am Coll Cardiol 1986;8:545–57.

48. Yokoyama I, Yonekura K, Ohtake T, et al. Coronary microangiopathy in type 2 diabetic patients: relation to glycemic control, sex, and microvascular angina rather than to coronary artery disease. J Nucl Med 2000;41:978–85.

49. Schindler TH, Facta AD, Prior JO, et al. Improvement in coronary vascular dysfunction produced with euglycaemic control in patients with type 2 diabetes. Heart 2007;93:345–9.

50. Yokoyama I, Ohtake T, Momomura S, et al. Hyperglycemia rather than insulin resistance is related to reduced coronary flow reserve in NIDDM. Diabetes 1998;47:119–24.

51. Gistri R, Cecchi F, Choudhury L, et al. Effect of verapamil on absolute myocardial blood flow in hypertrophic cardiomyopathy. Am J Cardiol 1994; 74:363–8.

52. Mourad JJ, Hanon O, Deverre JR, et al. Improvement of impaired coronary vasodilator reserve in hypertensive patients by low-dose ACE inhibitor/ diuretic therapy: a pilot PET study. J Renin Angiotensin Aldosterone Syst 2003;4:94–5.

53. Dayanikli F, Grambow D, Muzik O, et al. Early detection of abnormal coronary flow reserve in asymptomatic men at high risk for coronary artery disease using positron emission tomography. Circulation 1994;90:808–17.

54. Pitkanen OP, Nuutila P, Raitakari OT, et al. Coronary flow reserve in young men with familial combined hyperlipidemia. Circulation 1999;99:1678–84.

55. Sundell J, Laine H, Raitakari OT, et al. Positive family history of coronary artery disease is associated with reduced myocardial vasoreactivity in healthy men. Int J Cardiol 2006;112:289–94.

56. Yokoyama I, Murakami T, Ohtake T, et al. Reduced coronary flow reserve in familial hypercholesterolemia. J Nucl Med 1996;37:1937–42.

57. Yokoyama I, Ohtake T, Momomura S, et al. Reduced coronary flow reserve in hypercholesterolemic patients without overt coronary stenosis. Circulation 1996;94:3232–8.

58. Yokoyama I, Ohtake T, Momomura S, et al. Altered myocardial vasodilatation in patients with

hypertriglyceridemia in anatomically normal coronary arteries. Arterioscler Thromb Vasc Biol 1998; 18:294–9.

59. Yokoyama I, Ohtake T, Momomura S, et al. Impaired myocardial vasodilation during hyperemic stress with dipyridamole in hypertriglyceridemia. J Am Coll Cardiol 1998;31:1568–74.

60. Campisi R, Nathan L, Pampaloni MH, et al. Noninvasive assessment of coronary microcirculatory function in postmenopausal women and effects of short-term and long-term estrogen administration. Circulation 2002;105:425–30.

61. Schindler TH, Cardenas J, Prior JO, et al. Relationship between increasing body weight, insulin resistance, inflammation, adipocytokine leptin, and coronary circulatory function. J Am Coll Cardiol 2006;47:1188–95.

62. Schindler TH, Nitzsche EU, Schelbert HR, et al. Positron emission tomography-measured abnormal responses of myocardial blood flow to sympathetic stimulation are associated with the risk of developing cardiovascular events. J Am Coll Cardiol 2005;45:1505–12.

63. Prior JO, Quinones MJ, Hernandez-Pampaloni M, et al. Coronary circulatory dysfunction in insulin resistance, impaired glucose tolerance, and type 2 diabetes mellitus. Circulation 2005;111:2291–8.

64. Rask-Madsen C, King GL. Mechanisms of Disease: endothelial dysfunction in insulin resistance and diabetes. Nat Clin Pract Endocrinol Metab 2007;3: 46–56.

65. Schachinger V, Britten MB, Zeiher AM. Prognostic impact of coronary vasodilator dysfunction on adverse long-term outcome of coronary heart disease. Circulation 2000;101:1899–906.

66. Schindler TH, Nitzsche EU, Munzel T, et al. Coronary vasoregulation in patients with various risk factors in response to cold pressor testing: contrasting myocardial blood flow responses to short- and long-term vitamin C administration. J Am Coll Cardiol 2003;42:814–22.

67. Czernin J, Barnard RJ, Sun KT, et al. Effect of short-term cardiovascular conditioning and low-fat diet on myocardial blood flow and flow reserve. Circulation 1995;92:197–204.

68. Baller D, Notohamiprodjo G, Gleichmann U, et al. Improvement in coronary flow reserve determined by positron emission tomography after 6 months of cholesterol-lowering therapy in patients with early stages of coronary atherosclerosis. Circulation 1999;99:2871–5.

69. Guethlin M, Kasel AM, Coppenrath K, et al. Delayed response of myocardial flow reserve to lipid-lowering therapy with fluvastatin. Circulation 1999; 99:475–81.

70. Huggins GS, Pasternak RC, Alpert NM, et al. Effects of short-term treatment of hyperlipidemia on coronary vasodilator function and myocardial perfusion in regions having substantial impairment of baseline dilator reverse. Circulation 1998;98:1291–6.

71. Yokoyama I, Momomura S, Ohtake T, et al. Improvement of impaired myocardial vasodilatation due to diffuse coronary atherosclerosis in hypercholesterolemics after lipid-lowering therapy. Circulation 1999; 100:117–22.

72. Quinones MJ, Hernandez-Pampaloni M, Schelbert H, et al. Coronary vasomotor abnormalities in insulin-resistant individuals. Ann Intern Med 2004;140:700–8.

73. Fichtlscherer S, Breuer S, Zeiher AM. Prognostic value of systemic endothelial dysfunction in patients with acute coronary syndromes: further evidence for the existence of the "vulnerable" patient. Circulation 2004;110:1926–32.

74. Modena MG, Bonetti L, Coppi F, et al. Prognostic role of reversible endothelial dysfunction in hypertensive postmenopausal women. J Am Coll Cardiol 2002;40:505–10.

75. Madar I, Ravert H, Dipaula A, et al. Assessment of severity of coronary artery stenosis in a canine model using the PET agent 18F-fluorobenzyl triphenyl phosphonium: comparison with 99mTc-tetrofosmin. J Nucl Med 2007;48:1021–30.

76. Madar I, Ravert HT, Du Y, et al. Characterization of uptake of the new PET imaging compound 18F-fluorobenzyl triphenyl phosphonium in dog myocardium. J Nucl Med 2006;47:1359–66.

77. Yu M, Guaraldi M, Kagan M, et al. Assessment of (18)F-labeled mitochondrial complex I inhibitors as PET myocardial perfusion imaging agents in rats, rabbits, and primates. Eur J Nucl Med Mol Imaging 2009;36:63–72.

78. Yu M, Guaraldi MT, Mistry M, et al. BMS-747158-02: a novel PET myocardial perfusion imaging agent. J Nucl Cardiol 2007;14:789–98.

79. Higuchi T, Nekolla SG, Huisman MM, et al. A new 18F-labeled myocardial PET tracer: myocardial uptake after permanent and transient coronary occlusion in rats. J Nucl Med 2008;49:1715–22.

80. Maddahi J, Schiepers C, Czernin J, et al. First human study of BMS747158, a novel F-18 labeled tracer for myocardial perfusion imaging. J Nucl Med 2008;49:70P.

Translation of Myocardial Metabolic Imaging Concepts into the Clinics

Adil Bashir, PhD[a], Robert J. Gropler, MD[a,b],*

KEYWORDS

• Heart • Metabolism • Tomography • Glucose • Fatty acids

Flexibility in myocardial substrate metabolism for energy production is fundamental to cardiac health. This loss in plasticity or flexibility leads to an overdependence on the metabolism of an individual category of substrates, with the predominance in fatty acid metabolism characteristic of diabetic heart disease and the accelerated glucose use associated with pressure-overload left ventricular hypertrophy being prime examples. Important unresolved questions include the extent to which these metabolic patterns are adaptive and have the propensity to become maladaptive, what the key determinants of these metabolic perturbations are, do they alter prognosis, and do they represent robust targets for novel therapeutics. Accelerating our understanding of the role of alterations in myocardial substrate metabolism in cardiac disease is the development of transgenic models targeting key aspects of myocardial substrate use. The relevance of the metabolic phenotype of these models to the corresponding human condition is frequently unclear, however. In addition, applied genomics have identified numerous gene variants intimately involved in the regulation of myocardial substrate use. Yet, identifying the clinically significant genetic variants remains elusive. For all these reasons, there is a strong demand for accurate noninvasive imaging approaches of myocardial substrate metabolism that can facilitate the crosstalk between the bench and the bedside leading to improved patient management paradigms. Currently the most successful example is the detection of ischemic but viable myocardium with PET and ^{18}F-fluorodexoglucose (FDG) for the management of patients who have ischemic cardiomyopathy. In this article potential future applications of metabolic imaging, particularly radionuclide approaches, for assessment of cardiovascular disease are discussed.

OVERVIEW OF MYOCARDIAL METABOLISM—THE NEED FOR FLEXIBILITY

The heart is an omnivore capable of switching from one substrate to another for energy production. This flexibility in substrate use occurs in response to numerous stimuli, including substrate availability, the hormonal environment, the level of tissue perfusion, and the level of workload by the heart (**Fig. 1**).[1,2] The control of substrate switching can represent an acute or chronic adaptation in response to either short or prolonged alterations in the physiologic environment. Examples of acute or short-term adaptations would include inhibitory effects of fatty acid oxidation on glucose oxidation and the converse, and the increasing oxidation of glycogen, lactate, and glucose in response to

Supported by grants POI-HL15851, ROI-HLE9100 and AG15644.

[a] Division of Radiological Sciences, Cardiovascular Imaging Laboratory, Edward Mallinckrodt Institute of Radiology, 510 South Kingshighway, St. Louis, MO 63110, USA
[b] Cardiovascular Division, Department of Medicine, Washington University School of Medicine, St. Louis, MO, USA
* Corresponding author. Division of Radiological Sciences, Cardiovascular Imaging Laboratory, Edward Mallinckrodt Institute of Radiology, 510 South Kingshighway, St. Louis, MO 63110, USA.
E-mail address: groplerr@mir.wustl.edu (R. Gropler).

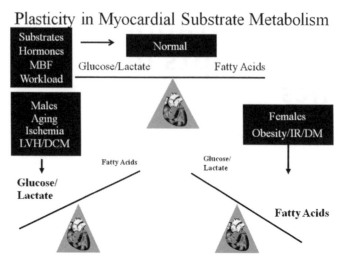

Fig. 1. Summary of myocardial substrate metabolism demonstrating the need for flexibility in myocardial substrate use to maintain myocardial health. DCM, dilated cardiomyopathy; DM, diabetes mellitus; IR, insulin resistance (*Reproduced from* Herrero P, Gropler RJ. Imaging of myocardial metabolism. J Nucl Cardiol 2005;12(3):345–58; with permission).

increasing workload. Regulating these rapid changes is a host of enzymes, such as pyruvate dehydrogenase complex and enzyme carnitine palmityl transferase 1, which is regulated by the concentration of malonyl-CoA.[3–7]

In contrast, chronic metabolic adaptations reflect alterations in the metabolic machinery of the heart. These changes occur primarily at the transcriptional level through the coordinated up-regulation of enzymes and proteins in key metabolic pathways. A prominent example in this case is the nuclear receptor peroxisome proliferator-activated receptor alpha (PPARα), which is a key regulator of myocardial fatty acid uptake, oxidation, and storage.[8] For example, in diabetes mellitus, PPARα activity is increased leading to an up-regulation in genes controlling fatty acid uptake and oxidation.[9] In contrast, in pressure-overload hypertrophy PPARα activity is reduced leading to a down-regulation of genes controlling fat metabolism and in turn leading to an up-regulation of glucose use.[10] These chronic adaptations can induce numerous detrimental effects that extend beyond alterations in energy production and may include increases in oxygen free radical production, impaired energetics, increases in apoptosis, and the induction of left ventricular dysfunction. Subsequent sections discuss how metabolic imaging has helped characterize this loss of metabolic flexibility due to these chronic adaptations in various disease processes.

METHODS TO IMAGE MYOCARDIAL METABOLISM

There are currently three methods to image myocardial metabolism noninvasively: magnetic resonance spectroscopy (MRS), single photon emission computed tomography (SPECT) and positron emission tomography (PET). A summary of each technique is provided here.

Magnetic Resonance Spectroscopy

This technology offers numerous advantages for the measurement of myocardial metabolism. They include the ability to measure multiple metabolic pathways simultaneously, relative ease in performing serial measurements, and the lack of ionizing radiation. When combined with MRI, near-simultaneous measurements of myocardial perfusion and mechanical function are possible. MRS allows direct measurement of biochemical information about in vivo processes. These biochemical data can be acquired repeatedly with minimal interference to tissue function. Several biologically important nuclei can be measured, including phosphorous (^{31}P), hydrogen (^{1}H), carbon (^{13}C), sodium (^{23}Na), nitrogen (^{15}N), and fluorine (^{19}F). The basic principle of MRS is that the chemical environment of a nucleus induces local magnetic fields that shift its resonance frequency. The different frequency shift for different metabolites results in an NMR signal consisting of one or more discrete resonance frequencies. The Fourier transform of the acquired signal produces a spectrum with peaks at distinct frequencies. The MRS spectrum displays the signal intensity as a function of frequency measured in parts per million (ppm) relative to the frequency of a reference compound. The signal intensity at a given frequency is proportional to the amount of the respective metabolite and can be used to determine the absolute concentration of the metabolite using appropriate calibrating reference signal.[11,12]

MRS is limited by inherent low signal to noise, concomitant limited spatial resolution, intravoxel signal contamination, and long acquisition times. Compared with nuclear imaging methods, MRS has a much lower sensitivity (detecting millimolar as opposed to nanomolar concentrations). Although recent studies suggest imaging of cardiac metabolism using C-13 labeled agents is possible in intact animals, studies in humans are still not possible.[13] Cardiac applications for MRS become more limited as one moves from rodent to man as opposed to nuclear methods wherein the reverse occurs. This difference seems to be a function of the higher field strength in the small bore systems and the use of radiofrequency coils that are in closer proximity to the entire heart used in small animal imaging. These advantages overcome the need for markedly improved spatial resolution. Indeed, as opposed to rodent hearts wherein the measurements of the left ventricular myocardium are obtained, measurements in human myocardium are typically limited to the anterior myocardium. Currently, only ^{31}P and ^{1}H have been widely used for in vivo clinical cardiac examinations focusing on myocardial energetics (^{31}P) and lipid accumulation (^{1}H).[11,13,14]

Single Photon Emission Computed Tomography

An advantage of SPECT is the inherent high sensitivity of the radionuclide method to measure metabolic processes. The technology is widely available in the clinical and research settings. With ECG gating, measurements of myocardial function can be obtained simultaneously. Because of the long physical half-life of SPECT radionuclides radiopharmaceutical delivery to multiple sites is possible, facilitating the performance of multicenter studies that incorporate measurements of myocardial substrate metabolism. Theoretically, assessing more than one metabolic process simultaneously is possible if the heart is imaged after the administration of radiopharmaceuticals labeled with radionuclides with different primary photon energies. Finally, small animal SPECT and SPECT/CT systems are rapidly advancing, facilitating the performance of myocardial metabolic studies in rodent models of cardiac disease. The major disadvantage of SPECT is the inability to quantify cellular metabolic processes primarily because of the technical limitations of SPECT (relatively poor temporal and spatial resolution and inaccurate correction for photon attenuation).

Metabolic Processes that can be Measured by SPECT Include:

Glucose metabolism: No specific SPECT radiotracers are currently available to measure myocardial glucose metabolism. When combined with the appropriate detection scheme or collimator design, however, myocardial glucose metabolism can be measured with SPECT and FDG.[15]

Fatty acid metabolism: Over the past 20 years numerous radiotracers have been developed to assess myocardial fatty acid metabolism with SPECT. The earliest and most promising was 15-(p-iodophenyl)-pentadecanoic acid (IPPA).[16–18] This radiotracer demonstrated rapid accumulation in the heart and exhibited clearance kinetics that followed a biexponential function characteristic for ^{11}C-palmitate. Moreover, the clearance rates correlated directly with beta oxidation. Initial studies in humans who had coronary atherosclerosis demonstrated reduced uptake and washout in regions subtended by occluded arteries.[19] The kinetics of IPPA thus made it attractive as a radiotracer of fatty acid metabolism. Unfortunately, SPECT systems did not have the temporal resolution to take advantage of the rapid turnover of IPPA. As a consequence quantification of myocardial fatty acid metabolism was not possible and image quality was reduced; this led to the development of branched-chain analogs of IPPA, such as ^{123}I-beta-methyl-P-iodophenylpentadecanoic acid (BMIPP) (**Fig. 2**).[18–21] Alkyl branching inhibits beta oxidation and shunting radiolabel to the triglyceride pool thereby increasing radiotracer retention. The metabolic stability of BMIPP affords retention of radioactivity in the heart long enough to allow sufficient blood clearance such that high-quality SPECT imaging can be performed.

Positron Emission Tomography

The two major advantages of PET are its intrinsic quantitative capability and the use of radiopharmaceuticals labeled with the positron-emitting radionuclides. The PET detection scheme permits accurate quantification of activity in the field of view. The positron-emitting radionuclides of the

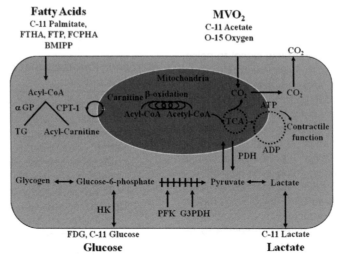

Fig. 2. Summary of the various PET and SPECT radiopharmaceuticals to assess myocardial substrate metabolism. ADP, adenosine diphosphate; BMIPP, ^{123}I-beta-methyl-P iodophenylpentadecanoic acid; FCPHA, trans-9(*RS*)-^{18}F-fluoro-3,4(*RS,RS*) methyleneheptadecanoic acid; FTHA, F-18 fluoro-6-thia-heptadecanoic acid; G3PDH, glyceraldehyde 3-phosphate dehydrogenase; HK, hexokinase; PDH, pyruvate dehydrogenase; PFK, phosphofructokinase; TCA; tricarboxylic acid cycle; TG, triglyceride; αGP, alpha-glycerol phosphate (*Reproduced from* Herrero P, Gropler RJ. Imaging of myocardial metabolism. J Nucl Cardiol 2005;12(3):345–58; with permission).

biologically ubiquitous elements oxygen (^{15}O), carbon (^{11}C), and nitrogen (^{13}N), and fluorine (^{18}F) substituting for hydrogen, can be incorporated into a wide variety of substrates or substrate analogs that participate in diverse biochemical pathways without altering the biochemical properties of the substrate of interest (see **Fig. 2**). By combining the knowledge of the metabolic pathways of interest with kinetic models that faithfully describe the fate of the tracer in tissue, an accurate interpretation of the tracer kinetics as they relate to the metabolic process of interest can be achieved. The major disadvantages of PET are its complexity in radiotracer design and image quantification schemes and its expense. Metabolic processes that are typically measured with PET are:

Myocardial Oxygen Consumption (MVO₂)

[15]O-oxygen: Because oxygen is the final electron acceptor in all pathways of aerobic myocardial metabolism, PET with ^{15}O-oxygen has also been used to measure MVO₂. The major advantage of the approach is that it provides a measure of myocardial oxygen extraction and measures MVO₂ directly. Because of the short half-life of this tracer, ^{15}O-oxygen is readily applicable in studies requiring repetitive assessments, such as those with an acute pharmacologic intervention. Its major disadvantages are the need for

a multiple-tracer study (to account for myocardial blood flow and blood volume) and fairly complex compartmental modeling to obtain the measurements.[22–24]

[11]C-acetate: PET using ^{11}C-acetate is the preferred method of measuring MVO₂ non-invasively. Once taken up by the heart, acetate, a two–carbon chain free fatty acid, is rapidly converted to acetyl-CoA. The primary metabolic fate of acetyl-CoA is metabolism through the tricarboxylic acid cycle. Because of the tight coupling of the tricarboxylic acid cycle and oxidative phosphorylation, the myocardial turnover of ^{11}C-acetate reflects overall flux in the tricarboxylic acid cycle and, thus, overall oxidative metabolism or MVO₂. Either exponential curve fitting or compartmental modeling is used to calculate MVO₂. The latter is typically preferable in situations of low cardiac output wherein marked splaying of the input function and spill-over of activity from the lungs to the myocardium can decrease the accuracy of the curve-fitting method.[25–29]

Carbohydrate Metabolism

FDG: Most studies of myocardial glucose metabolism with PET have used FDG. This radiotracer competes with glucose for facilitated transport into the sarcolemma then for hexokinase-mediated phosphorylation. The resultant F-FDG-6-phosphate is trapped in the cytosol and the myocardial uptake of FDG is believed to reflect overall anaerobic and aerobic myocardial glycolytic flux.[30–33] Regional myocardial glucose use can be assessed in either relative or in absolute terms (ie, in $nmol \cdot g^{-1} \cdot min^{-1}$). In the latter case, a mathematical correction for the kinetic differences between FDG and glucose called the lumped constant must be used calculate rates of glucose. This value may vary, however, depending on the prevailing plasma substrate and hormonal conditions decreasing the accuracy of the measurement.[32,34–36] Other disadvantages of FDG include the limited metabolic fate of FDG in tissue, precluding determination of the metabolic fate (ie, glycogen formation versus glycolysis) of the extracted tracer and glucose, and limitations on the performance of serial measurements of myocardial glucose use because of the relatively long physical half-life of [18]F. On the other hand, the myocardial kinetics of FDG have been well characterized, the acquisition scheme is relatively straightforward, and its production has become routine owing in part to the rapid growth of its clinical use in oncology; as such, it remains the most widely used tracer for determination of myocardial glucose metabolism.

Carbon-11 glucose: More recently, quantification of myocardial glucose use has been performed with PET using glucose radiolabeled in the 1-carbon position with [11]C (^{11}C-glucose). Because ^{11}C-glucose is chemically identical to unlabeled glucose it has the same metabolic fate as glucose, thus obviating the need for the lumped constant correction. It has been demonstrated that measurements of myocardial glucose use based on compartmental modeling of tracer kinetics are more accurate with ^{11}C-glucose than with FDG.[37,38] Moreover, it has been recently demonstrated that PET with ^{11}C-glucose permits the estimation of glycogen synthesis, glycolysis, and glucose oxidation (**Fig. 3** and **4**).[39] Disadvantages of this method include compartmental modeling that is more demanding with ^{11}C-glucose than it is with FDG, the need to correct the arterial input function for the production of [11]CO_2 and ^{11}C-lactate,

a fairly complex synthesis of the tracer, and the short physical half-life of ^{11}C requiring an on-site cyclotron.

[11]C-lactate: Lactate metabolism in the heart correlates with serum lactate level at rest but this relationship may vary with exercise or ischemia. Recently, a multicompartmental model was developed for the assessment of myocardial lactate metabolism using PET and L-3 [^{11}C] lactic acid. Under a wide variety of conditions, PET-derived extraction of lactate correlated well with lactate oxidation measured by arterial and coronary sinus sampling (**Fig. 5**).[40] This model may help delineate the clinical role of lactate metabolism in various pathologic conditions, such as diabetes mellitus and myocardial ischemia. Moreover, when combined with either FDG or ^{11}C-glucose it permits a more comprehensive measurement of myocardial carbohydrate metabolism.

Fatty Acid Metabolism

[11]C-palmitate: The major advantage of ^{11}C-palmitate is that its myocardial kinetics are identical to labeled palmitate. With appropriate mathematical modeling techniques its use permits the assessment of various aspects of myocardial fatty acid metabolism, such as uptake, oxidation, and storage.[41–44] This attribute is important because exactly which component of myocardial fatty acid metabolism is the contributor to a pathologic process is frequently not fully elucidated. This approach does suffer from several disadvantages, however, including reduced image quality and biologic specificity, a more complex analysis, and the need for an on-site cyclotron and radiopharmaceutical production capability.

Fatty acid tracers that are trapped: Most of the PET tracers in this category have been designed to reflect myocardial beta oxidation. 14-(R,S)-^{18}F-fluoro-6-thiaheptadecanoic acid (FTHA) was one of the first radiotracers developed using this approach. Initial results were promising with uptake and retention in the myocardium accordingly with changes in substrate delivery, blood flow, and workload in animal models.[45,46] As a consequence, PET with FTHA was used to evaluate the effects of various diseases,

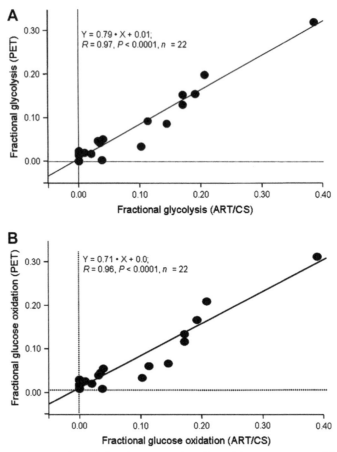

Fig. 3. Correlation between PET and arterial and coronary sinus (ART/CS) measurement of fractional glycolysis (*A*) and glucose oxidation (*B*) (*Reproduced from* Herrero P, Kisrieva-Ware Z, Dence CS, et al. PET measurements of myocardial glucose metabolism with 1-^{11}C-glucose and kinetic modeling. J Nucl Med 2007;48(6):955–64; reprinted by permission of the Society for Nuclear Medicine.)

such as coronary artery disease and cardiomyopathy, on myocardial fatty acid metabolism.[47,48] Enthusiasm for FTHA has waned somewhat primarily because its uptake and retention have been shown to be insensitive to the inhibition of beta oxidation by hypoxia.[49] Subsequently, 16-^{18}F-fluoro-4-thia-palmitate (FTP) has been developed. This modification retains the metabolic trapping function of the tracer, which is proportional to fatty acid oxidation under normal oxygenation and hypoxic conditions.[49,50] The lumped constant for FTP is relatively independent of the substrate environment but is sensitive to the presence of ischemia. The ability to quantify fatty acid oxidation with this radiotracer is still unclear. Currently, FTP is undergoing commercialization and entering early phase 1 evaluation. Recently, a new F-18–labeled fatty acid radiotracer,

trans-9(*RS*)-^{18}F-fluoro-3,4(*RS,RS*) methyleneheptadecanoic acid (FCPHA), has been developed.[51] Results of initial studies show that uptake of FCPHA into rat myocardium was approximately 1.5% injected dose per gram tissue at 5 minutes with little change over a period of 60 minutes and low blood activity over the same period. The impact of alterations in plasma substrates, workload, and blood flow on myocardial kinetics is unknown. This radiotracer is also undergoing commercialization.

GENDER AND AGING

Both gender and aging impact the myocardial metabolic phenotype. Results of studies in animal models show that there are sex differences in myocardial substrate metabolism, with female rats exhibiting less myocardial glucose and more

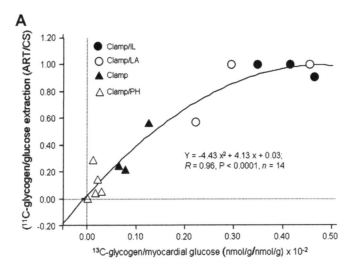

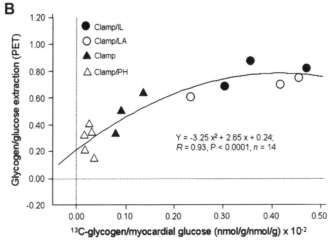

Fig. 4. Correlation between glycogen formation expressed as fraction of myocardial glucose obtained from ART/CS ^{11}C measurements (y-axis) and heart ^{13}C-glycogen content (x-axis) (A). Corresponding correlation between PET ^{11}C and heart ^{13}C-glycogen measurements (B). Fasted group was excluded from analysis because of negligible glucose extraction (*Reproduced from* Herrero P, Kisrieva-Ware Z, Dence CS, et al. PET measurements of myocardial glucose metabolism with 1-^{11}C-glucose and kinetic modeling. J Nucl Med 2007;48(6):955–64; reprinted by permission of the Society for Nuclear Medicine.)

fatty acid metabolism.[52,53] Recently, using PET with ^{11}C-glucose and ^{11}C-plamitate, these observations were confirmed in young healthy volunteers.[54] Women exhibited lower levels of glucose metabolism compared with men (**Fig. 6**). Although no differences in myocardial fatty acid metabolism were noted, women also exhibited higher MVO$_2$ compared with men as measured by PET with ^{11}C-acetate. These gender differences in substrate metabolism become more pronounced as one transitions to more pathologic conditions. For example, in addition to the changes in glucose metabolism and MVO$_2$, obese women exhibited higher fatty acid uptake and oxidation compared with obese men.[55] In both these studies, the

differences in myocardial metabolism could not be explained by differences in myocardial blood flow, insulin sensitivity, hemodynamics, myocardial work, or the plasma substrate environment.

In various experimental models of aging, the contribution of fatty acid oxidation to overall myocardial substrate metabolism declines with age.[56,57] It seems the cause for the decrease in fatty acid oxidation is multifactorial, including changes in mitochondrial lipid content, lipid composition, and protein interactions, along with oxygen free radical injury, a decline in carnitine palmitoyltransferase-1 activity, and an age-related decline in myocardial PPARα activity.[58–60] Using the PET approaches described previously, it has

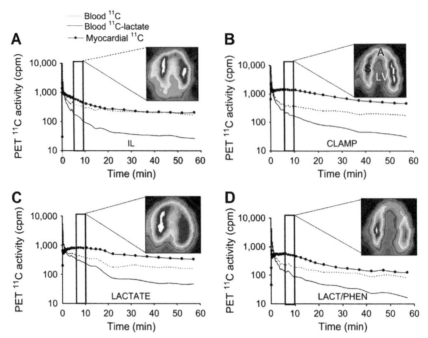

Fig. 5. Representative PET time–activity curves of L-3-^{11}C-lactate obtained from intralipid (IL), insulin clamp (CLAMP), lactate infusion (LACTATE), or lactate and phenylephedrine (LAC/PHEN) studies and corresponding myocardial images obtained 5 to 10 minutes after tracer injection and depicting primarily early tracer uptake. Images are displayed on horizontal long axis. Blood ^{11}C indicates ^{11}C time–activity curves obtained from region of interest (ROI) placed on left atrium; blood ^{11}C-lactate indicates blood ^{11}C time–activity curves after removing [11]CO_2, ^{11}C-neutral, and ^{11}C-basic metabolites; myocardial ^{11}C indicates ^{11}C time–activity curves obtained from ROI placed on lateral wall. A, apical wall; L, lateral wall; LV, left ventricle; S, septal wall (*Reproduced from* Herrero P, Dence CS, Coggan AR, et al. L-3-^{11}C-lactate as a PET tracer of myocardial lactate metabolism: a feasibility study. J Nucl Med 2007;48(12):2046–55; reprinted by permission of the Society for Nuclear Medicine.)

been shown that a similar metabolic shift occurs in healthy older humans.[61] Moreover, older individuals are not able to increase glucose use in response to β-adrenergic stimulation with dobutamine to the same extent as younger individuals. This impaired metabolic response may represent a stress-related energy deprivation state in the aging heart or potentially indicate that the heart is more susceptible to injury during periods of ischemia.[62] Recently it has been shown that this impairment in metabolic reserve can be ameliorated by endurance exercise training in older subjects.[63] It seems the myocardial metabolic response to dobutamine following endurance exercise training is gender specific with men demonstrating an increase in myocardial glucose metabolism and women exhibiting an increase in both glucose and fatty acid metabolism. Although requiring further study, these gender and age differences in metabolism may provide a partial explanation for the gender- and age-related outcome differences for various cardiovascular diseases in which altered myocardial metabolism plays a role.

ISCHEMIA

Under conditions of mild to moderate myocardial ischemia, fatty acid oxidation ceases and anaerobic metabolism supervenes. Glucose becomes the primary substrate for increased anaerobic glycolysis and for continued, albeit diminished, oxidative metabolism.[64] This metabolic switch is prerequisite for continued energy production and cell survival. When the ischemic insult is reversed, oxygen availability increases and oxidative metabolism resumes. It seems that these abnormalities in myocardial substrate metabolism may persist well after the resolution of ischemia, so-called "ischemic memory." Demonstration of either accelerated myocardial glucose metabolism or reduced fatty acid metabolism using FDG and BMIPP, respectively, has been used to document this phenomenon. For example, more than 20 years ago it was shown that PET myocardial FDG uptake was increased in patients who had unstable angina during pain-free episodes.[65] Moreover, in patients who had stable angina, increased FDG uptake was demonstrated

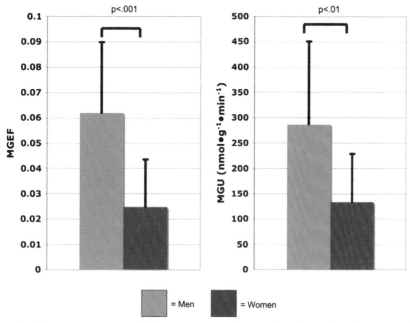

Fig. 6. Sex-related differences in myocardial glucose extraction fraction (MGEF) and myocardial glucose use (MGU) (*Reproduced from* Peterson LR, Soto PF, Herrero P, et al. Sex differences in myocardial oxygen and glucose metabolism. J Nucl Cardiol 2007;14(4):573–81; with permission).

following exercise-induced ischemia in the absence of either perfusion deficits or ECG abnormalities.[66] Similar observations have been made with SPECT using BMIPP. Results of numerous studies have demonstrated in patients who had acute chest pain that abnormalities in myocardial BMIPP uptake may persist 24 to 36 hours following the resolution of symptoms (**Fig. 7**).[67,68] Moreover, this "metabolic fingerprint" is superior to perfusion imaging for either identifying coronary artery disease as the cause of the chest pain or assigning prognosis.[67] The persistence of the metabolic defect increases the flexibility of radiotracer administration because it allows for delivery of a unit dose after the patient has already been evaluated; this is in contrast to the use of perfusion radiotracers, which frequently must be available on-site because of the narrow time window from the resolution of symptoms and normalization of the flow deficit. Based on these observations, BMIPP is currently undergoing Phase 3 evaluation for acute chest pain imaging. Metabolic imaging with either FDG or BMIPP has also been used for direct ischemia detection during stress testing. The belief is that abnormalities in vasodilator reserve with perfusion tracers will underestimate ischemia if oxygen supply remains balanced. Results of initial studies in which FDG was injected during exercise seems to support this contention with a greater detection rate for moderately severe

coronary artery stenoses compared with perfusion imaging.[15] Despite the promising results with these radiotracers, numerous questions remain as to the optimal imaging protocols, the impact of alterations in the plasma substrate environment on diagnostic accuracy, whether added diagnostic and prognostic information is provided over perfusion imaging, and whether this information alters clinical management.

HYPERTENSION/LEFT VENTRICULAR HYPERTROPHY

There is well-established linkage between abnormalities in myocardial substrate metabolism and left ventricular hypertrophy. In animal models of pressure-overload left ventricular hypertrophy there is a reduction in the expression of beta-oxidation enzymes, leading to a decrease in myocardial fatty acid oxidation and an increase in glucose use.[69,70] Moreover, interventions in animals that involve inhibition of mitochondrial fatty acid beta oxidation result in cardiac hypertrophy.[70] In humans, variants in genes regulating key aspects of myocardial fatty acid metabolism ranging from PPARα to various key beta-oxidative enzymes are associated with left ventricular hypertrophy.[71,72]

This metabolic shift has been confirmed in vivo in an animal model of hypertrophy.[73] PET with

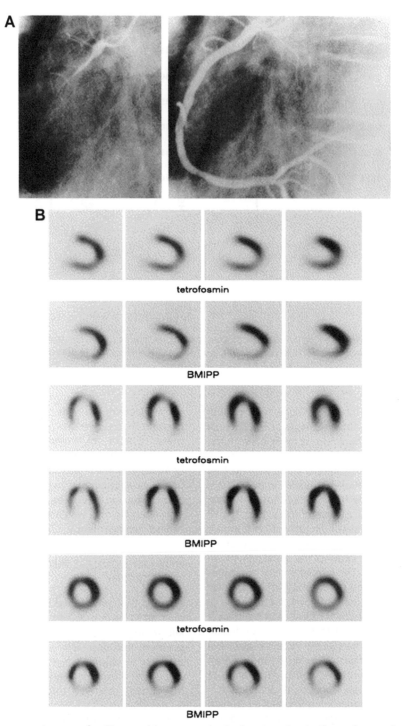

Fig. 7. (*A*) Coronary angiogram of a 48-year-old woman who had rest angina in the early morning. Seven days later, coronary angiography shows no significant stenosis in either coronary artery. After injection of ergonovine maleate into the right coronary artery, total spasm was provoked (*left*), with severe chest pain and electrocardiographic changes. After isosorbide dinitrate was injected, the spasm was completely resolved (*right*). (*B*) Series of rest tetrofosmin perfusion and BMIPP SPECT images. No significant abnormal perfusion is observed on the rest tetrofosmin images at the time of hospital admission. The BMIPP images show reduced uptake in the inferior region on the next day (*Reproduced from* Kawai Y, Tsukamoto E, Nozaki Y, et al. Significance of reduced uptake of iodinated fatty acid analog for the evaluation of patients with acute chest pain. J Am Coll Cardiol 2001;38(7):1888–94; with permission).

FDG demonstrated myocardial glucose uptake tracked directly with increasing hypertrophy. Similar results have been found in humans. PET with ^{11}C-palmitate in humans has shown that reduction in myocardial fatty acid oxidation is an independent predictor of left ventricular mass in hypertension.[74] Combining measurements of left ventricular myocardial external work (either by echocardiography or MRI) with measurements of MVO_2 performed by PET with ^{11}C-acetate or ^{15}O-oxygen, it is possible to estimate cardiac efficiency.[23,75] Using this approach in patients who have hypertension-induced left ventricular hypertrophy has shown that the decline in myocardial fatty acid metabolism is associated with a decline in efficiency, a condition that may increase the potential for the development of heart failure. PET has also been used to phenotype patients who have hypertrophic cardiomyopathy attributable to a known specific variant in the α-tropomyosin gene.[76] It was observed that increased myocardial perfusion, fatty acid metabolism, and efficiency characterize patients who have mild hypertrophy, whereas these metabolic alterations decrease as hypertrophy becomes more advanced. The results may represent differential penetrance of the gene variant or the effect of modifier genes, potentially helping in their identification. Although requiring further study in larger patient populations, this study suggests that metabolic imaging may identify relevant gene variants without waiting for more end-stage manifestations, such as left ventricular remodeling and dysfunction, to occur.

NONISCHEMIC DILATED CARDIOMYOPATHY

In addition to left ventricular hypertrophy, alterations in myocardial substrate metabolism have been implicated in the pathogenesis of contractile dysfunction and heart failure. Animal models of heart failure have shown that in the progression from cardiac hypertrophy to ventricular dysfunction, the expression of genes encoding for enzymes regulating beta oxidation is coordinately decreased, resulting in a shift in myocardial substrate metabolism to primarily glucose use, similar to that seen in the fetal heart.[69,77,78] These metabolic changes are paralleled by re-expression of fetal isoforms of various contractile and calcium regulatory proteins. The reactivation of the metabolic fetal gene program may have numerous detrimental consequences on myocardial contractile function ranging from energy deprivation to the inability to process fatty acids leading to accumulation of nonoxidized toxic fatty acid derivatives, resulting in lipotoxicity. Alterations in myocardial

substrate use are now becoming attractive targets for novel treatments for heart failure with prime examples being the partial fatty acid oxidation antagonists and the insulin sensitizer glucagon-like peptide-1.[79]

The down-regulation in myocardial fatty acid metabolism leading to an overdependence on glucose use in heart failure has been well documented using PET and SPECT techniques. For example, PET using ^{11}C-palmitate and ^{11}C-glucose demonstrated that myocardial fatty acid uptake and oxidation are lower in patients who have nonischemic dilated cardiomyopathy when compared with age-matched controls. In contrast myocardial glucose use was higher in the cardiomyopathic patients.[42] The metabolic findings cannot be explained by differences in plasma substrates or insulin, blood flow, or MVO_2. Similarly, SPECT with BMIPP demonstrated reduced myocardial uptake and increased clearance radiotracer in patients who had dilated cardiomyopathy compared with controls.[80] Moreover, the magnitude of the perturbations correlated with other measurements of heart failure severity, such as left ventricular size and plasma b-natriuretic peptide levels. PET has also been used to provide mechanistic insights into the myocardial metabolic perturbations associated with heart failure. For example, abrupt lowering of fatty acid delivery with acipimox results in reduced fatty acid uptake, MVO_2, and cardiac work and no change cardiac efficiency in normal volunteers.[81] In contrast, patients who had nonischemic dilated cardiomyopathy exhibited a decrease in myocardial fatty acid uptake and cardiac work, no change in MVO_2, and a decline in efficiency. Although limited by a small sample size, these results seem to reinforce to the central role of loss of flexibility in myocardial substrate metabolism in the pathogenesis of heart failure with even minor changes in substrate delivery having detrimental consequences on cardiac energy transduction.

Metabolic imaging has also been used to study the mechanisms responsible for the effectiveness of treatment in cardiomyopathy. For example, the efficacy of β-blocker therapy in treatment of patients who have heart failure is well established. Treatment with the selective β-blocker metoprolol results in a reduction in oxidative metabolism and an improvement in cardiac efficiency as measured by PET in patients who have left ventricular dysfunction.[82] With similar PET techniques, myocardial efficiency has been shown to be improved in patients who have heart failure who undergo either exercise training or cardiac resynchronization therapy, implicating improved myocardial energetics as a potential mechanism.[83,84] Moreover, treatment with cardiac resynchronization therapy resulted in homogenization of initially heterogeneously distributed glucose metabolism.[85] There is significant interest in the partial fatty acid oxidation inhibitors for the treatment of heart failure. Theoretically, decreasing myocardial fatty acid oxidation should increase the oxidation of glucose leading to a more favorable energetic state and improved left ventricular function. In a recent study, the administration of trimetazidine to patients who had dilated cardiomyopathy resulted in a significant improvement in left ventricular ejection fraction.[86] The improvement in left ventricular function seemed to reflect the complex interplay between a mild decrease in myocardial fatty acid oxidation, improved whole-body insulin resistance, and synergistic effects with β-blockade. Metabolic imaging can also be used to predict the response to specific therapies in patients who have heart failure. For example, in patients who have dilated cardiomyopathy, the percent of glucose uptake, as measured by PET with FDG, can be used as a predictor for the effectiveness of β-blocker therapy.[87] Moreover, in patients who have ischemic cardiomyopathy the extent of viable myocardium as measured with PET and FDG correlated with the hemodynamic response after cardiac resynchronization therapy suggesting a role for PET in discriminating responders from nonresponders.[88]

DIABETES MELLITUS

Cardiovascular disease is the leading cause of morbidity and mortality in patients who have diabetes mellitus.[89] The mechanisms by which diabetes mellitus confers this increased cardiovascular risk are multifactorial and complex with possibilities including an increased prevalence of hyperlipidemia and hypertension, impaired fibrinolysis, abnormal myocardial endothelial function, and reduced sympathetic neuronal function. There is a burgeoning body of evidence to suggest that abnormalities in myocardial substrate metabolism contribute to the cardiovascular abnormalities observed in patients who have diabetes.[90,91] The metabolic phenotype in diabetes is an overdependence on fatty acid metabolism and a decrease in glucose use. Multiple mechanisms contribute to this phenotype. These include increased plasma delivery of fatty acids because of peripheral insulin resistance, decreased insulin signaling, and activation of key transcriptional pathways, such as the PPARα/PGC-1 signaling network.[90,92,93] Both insulin-mediated glucose transport and glucose

transporter expression decline in diabetes mellitus. Rates of myocardial glucose uptake are frequently normal, however, because of the presence of hyperglycemia. Further metabolism of extracted glucose declines. The increase in myocardial fatty acid use results in increased citrate levels, which inhibit phosphofructokinase. Glucose oxidation is inhibited at the level of pyruvate dehydrogenase complex because of increased mitochondrial acetyl-CoA levels and the phosphorylation of pyruvate dehydrogenase kinase 4 by PPARα activation. Consequently, the maintenance of myocardial glucose uptake but decrease in downstream metabolism results in an accumulation of glucose metabolites. Potential detrimental effects associated with this shift in metabolism include: impaired mechanical function due to the inability to increase glucose metabolism in response to increase myocardial work, depletion of tricarboxylic acid cycle intermediates due to reduced anaplerosis, electrical instability and apoptosis, a greater sensitivity to myocardial ischemia, and myocardial lipid accumulation or lipotoxicity leading to increased apoptosis.

Small animal imaging has helped clarify the mechanisms responsible for the metabolic alterations that occur in diabetes mellitus. Potential mechanisms underlying diabetic cardiomyopathy have been studied in transgenic mice. For example, mice with cardiac-restricted overexpression of PPARα demonstrate a metabolic phenotype that is similar to diabetic hearts.[94] Small animal PET studies with ^{11}C-palmitate and FDG in these mice demonstrate an increase in fatty acid uptake and oxidation and an abnormal suppression of glucose uptake. In contrast, in mice with cardiac-restricted overexpression of PPARβ/δ small animal PET measurements demonstrated an increase glucose uptake and reduced fatty acid uptake and oxidation.[95] Taken in sum these observations demonstrate that PPARα and PPARβ/δ drive different metabolic regulatory programs in the heart and that imaging can help characterize genetic manipulations in mouse heart. From an imaging perspective, however, these studies also demonstrate the challenges in imaging the mouse heart because of its small size as only semiquantitative measurements of tracer uptake were performed. Quantitative measures of myocardial substrate metabolism are now possible with small animal PET in rat heart, however. For example, rates of myocardial glucose uptake correlate directly and closely with GLUT 4 gene expression in the Zucker-Diabetic-Fat (ZDF) rat, a model of type 2 diabetes mellitus.[96] Moreover, rates of myocardial glucose uptake and fatty acid uptake and oxidation measured with

PET in the same disease model demonstrated the importance of increased fatty acid delivery to defining the metabolic phenotype in diabetes (**Fig. 8**).[97]

Numerous imaging studies have been performed in humans to assess the impact of diabetes mellitus on myocardial glucose metabolism. These studies have been primarily limited to PET using FDG.[98–100] In general, rates of myocardial glucose uptake are reduced in patients who have either type 1 or type 2 diabetes mellitus compared with those who do not have diabetes except under conditions of marked hyperglycemia or supraphysiologic levels in plasma insulin, such as occurs with a hyperinsulinemic-euglycemic clamp. Increased myocardial fatty acid uptake measured by arterial-coronary sinus balance studies has been reported in humans who have type 1 diabetes mellitus without coronary artery disease.[101] Although the impact of plasma levels of free fatty acids on the level of myocardial fatty acid uptake was not determined, a negative correlation between myocardial glucose uptake and plasma fatty acid levels was observed. Recently, studies using PET and ^{11}C-plamitate and ^{11}C-glucose in patients who have type 1 diabetes mellitus have helped clarify the myocardial metabolic phenotype in this disease. For example, patients who had diabetes exhibited higher levels of fatty acid uptake and oxidation compared with those who did not have diabetes primarily because of increased plasma fatty acid levels. In contrast, glucose uptake was reduced in these patients primarily because of decreased glucose transport mechanisms.[43] Moreover, the metabolic fate of extracted glucose is impaired in diabetes with reduced rates of glycolysis and glucose oxidation, which become more pronounced with increases in cardiac work induced by dobutamine (**Fig. 9**).[102] The diabetic myocardium is responsive to changes in plasma insulin and fatty acid levels, but at a cost. Higher insulin levels are needed to achieve the same level of glucose uptake and glucose oxidation compared with those who do not have diabetes consistent with myocardial insulin resistance.

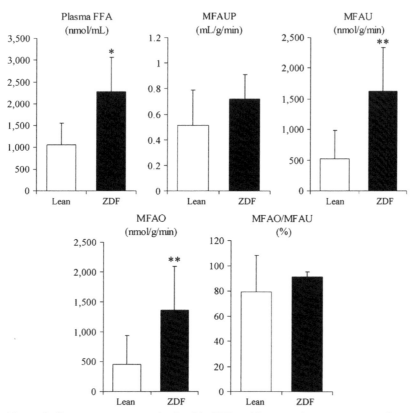

Fig. 8. Fatty acid metabolism measurements obtained in ZDF and lean rats by compartmental modeling of ^{11}C-palmitate PET data. MFAO, myocardial fatty acid oxidation; MFAO/MFAU, myocardial FFA that was oxidized; MFAU, myocardial fatty acid use; MFAUP, myocardial fatty acid uptake. *$P<.001$; **$P<.01$ (*Reproduced from Welch MJ, Lewis JS, Kim J, et al. Assessment of myocardial metabolism in diabetic rats using small-animal PET: a feasibility study. J Nucl Med 2006;47(4):689–97; reprinted by permission of the Society for Nuclear Medicine.*)

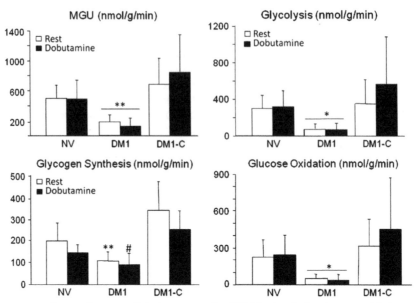

Fig. 9. Measurements of overall myocardial glucose uptake (MGU), glycolysis, glucose oxidation, and glycogen synthesis for normal volunteers (NV), patients who had type 1 diabetes studied under baseline metabolic conditions (DM1), and patients who had diabetes studied during hyperinsulinemic-euglycemic clamp (DM1-C), at rest (*open bars*) and during dobutamine (*solid bars*) (*Reproduced from* Herrero P, McGill JB, Lesniak D, et al. PET detection of the impact of dobutamine on myocardial glucose metabolism in women with type 1 diabetes mellitus. J Nucl Cardiol 2008;15(6):598–604; with permission).

Similarly, in response to higher fatty acid plasma levels, myocardial fatty acid uptake is increased, but at a cost of a greater esterification rate.[102,103]

The increase in plasma fatty acids is an attractive target to reduce the overdependence of the myocardium on fatty acid metabolism and perhaps improve energetics and function of the left ventricle. For example, the use of the insulin sensitizing agent troglitazone in ZDF rats results in reduced plasma fatty acid levels, decreased myocardial lipid accumulation, reduced apoptosis, and improved left ventricular function.[104] PET with FDG studies in patients who had type 2 diabetes mellitus, before and 26 weeks after treatment with rosiglitazone, demonstrated nearly a 40% increase in insulin-stimulated myocardial glucose uptake, implying reduced fatty acid uptake, which was attributed in large part to suppression in plasma fatty acid levels.[105] Of note, similar metabolic changes were not seen with the biguanide metformin, whose mechanism of action is designed to reduce hepatic glucose production. The metabolic response could not be predicted by changes in the plasma glucose or HgbA1C levels. Metabolic imaging can thus be used to follow the effects of therapies designed to alter myocardial substrate metabolism in patients who have diseases, such as diabetes mellitus, in which more readily available clinical parameters are not predictive of a therapeutic response.

OBESITY AND INSULIN RESISTANCE

It is now apparent that a significant increase in body mass index (BMI) induces marked increases in myocardial fatty acid metabolism. For example, in either dietary-induced or transgenic models of obesity, myocardial fatty acid uptake and oxidation are significantly increased.[104,106] This increase, at least initially, reflects the increase in fatty acid delivery to the heart due to increased lipolysis from visceral/abdominal and subcutaneous fat stores secondary to insulin resistance. Similar to diabetes mellitus, the increased delivery of fatty acids likely initiates a cascade of events that lead to increased fatty acid metabolism. Ultimately, fatty acid uptake may exceed oxidation leading to extracted fatty acids entering non-oxidative pathways most likely initially forming triglycerides. The accumulation of the neutral fats or triglycerides may ultimately become detrimental.[104]

Imaging of obese young women with PET and ^{11}C-acetate and ^{11}C-palmitate has demonstrated that an increase in BMI is associated with a shift in myocardial substrate metabolism toward greater fatty acid use. Moreover, this dependence on myocardial fatty acid metabolism increased with worsening insulin resistance.[44] Of note, little change in myocardial glucose metabolism was observed. Paralleling the preferential use of fatty acids was an increase in MVO$_2$ and a decrease in energy transduction. These findings suggest that metabolic changes in obesity may play a role in the pathogenesis of cardiac dysfunction. Of note, the myocardial metabolic response to

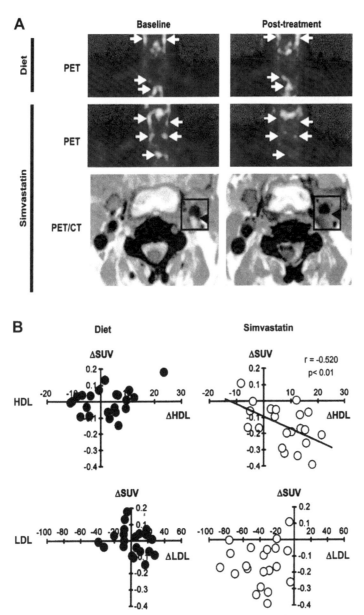

Fig.10. (A) Effects of simvastatin on 18FDG uptake in atherosclerotic plaque inflammation. Representative 18FDG-PET images at baseline and after 3 months of treatment (post-treatment) with dietary management alone (diet) or simvastatin. (Top) Dietary management alone had no effect on 18FDG uptake (arrows) in the aortic arch and the carotid arteries. (Middle) 18F-FDG uptakes were attenuated by simvastatin treatment. (Bottom) The co-registered images of 18FDG-PET and CT clearly show that the plaque 18FDG uptakes (arrowheads) disappeared after 3-month treatment with simvastatin. (B) Correlations of changes in plaque 18F-FDG uptakes (ΔSUV) with alterations in HDL cholesterol (ΔHDL, mg/dL) and LDL cholesterol (ΔLDL, mg/dL) after 3-month treatment with dietary management alone (diet) or simvastatin. ΔSUV had a significant correlation only with ΔHDL in the statin group (LDL) cholesterol (A) and high-density lipoprotein (HDL) cholesterol (Reproduced from Tahara N, Kai H, Ishibashi M, et al. Simvastatin attenuates plaque inflammation: evaluation by fluorodeoxyglucose positron emission tomography. J Am Coll Cardiol 2006;48(9):1825–31; with permission).

obesity seems gender dependent.[55] For example, using similar PET techniques it has been recently demonstrated that in contrast to obese women, obese men had a greater impairment in myocardial glucose metabolism per level of plasma insulin, suggesting greater myocardial insulin resistance. In addition, obesity had less effect on myocardial fatty acid metabolism in men. In contrast, MVO_2 was higher in the obese women compared with obese men. This seems to be a complex interplay between gender and obesity in influencing myocardial substrate metabolism.

BEYOND THE MYOCARDIUM—VASCULAR IMAGING

Atherosclerosis is a dynamic immune inflammatory process. It is characterized by cycles of intense activity and progression followed by intervals of stabilization. A common result of this process is coronary artery luminal stenosis that compromises myocardial blood flow and induces ischemia during stress. The most devastating event is acute plaque rupture with thrombosis leading to myocardial infarction and frequently sudden cardiac death. Moreover, for many patients acute plaque rupture is the initial clinical event. Despite the plethora of currently available imaging tools to detect and characterize the extent and severity coronary atherosclerosis, none of them identify patients who have active disease and who are at risk for plaque rupture. To this end, FDG is being evaluated for the detection of "biologically active" atherosclerosis based on the premise that the tracer accumulates in activated macrophages, which are a key component of atherosclerotic plaque. Several groups have established that inflamed arterial vessels have increased uptake of FDG as measured by PET. The increased uptake has been noted in animal models of atherosclerosis, and demonstrated and verified in humans who have atherosclerosis of the carotid artery and aorta.[107–110] Moreover, a significant correlation between FDG uptake and macrophage staining and CD68 staining has recently been established. A decrease in carotid artery FDG uptake is correlative with an increase in plasma high-density lipoprotein levels following statin therapy (**Fig. 10**).[109] Many questions remain, such as the site of localization of radiotracer (eg, plaque or smooth muscle), the suitability of the method for evaluating the coronary arteries, and whether the information provides more refined risk stratification compared with other more widely applicable methods or if it alters therapy.

FUTURE NEEDS

The continued growth of metabolic imaging will require advances in several areas. First is the continued improvement in instrumentation design, at the human level and at the level of imaging of small animals. For example, accurate tracer quantification may be possible with new SPECT/CT systems where accurate attenuation correction can be performed. Advances in PET detector design and post-detector electronics will result in improved counting statistics, which should improve the ability to perform more complex compartmental modeling permitting more complete characterization of the metabolism of a given substrate. Second, there is a key need for the development of new radiopharmaceuticals that permit characterization of key metabolic pathways, such as uptake, storage, or oxidation, that are linked to disease manifestations. Moreover, new radiopharmaceuticals are needed to provide insights into the pleiotropic aspects of metabolism, such as the relationships between substrate metabolism and cell growth, cell survival, and energy transduction. Third, the availability of radiopharmaceuticals radiolabeled with either F-18 or I-123 will be needed for the performance of appropriately powered clinical trials designed to answer key questions about metabolic imaging regarding diagnostic accuracy, risk stratification, and monitoring of therapy in specific patient populations. Taken together, these advances will facilitate the translation of metabolic imaging to the clinic.

REFERENCES

1. Bing RJ. The metabolism of the heart. Harvey Lect 1955;50:27–70.
2. Neely JR, Morgan HE. Relationship between carbohydrate and lipid metabolism and the energy balance of heart muscle. Annu Rev Physiol 1974; 36:413–59.
3. Goodwin GW, Taegtmeyer H. Regulation of fatty acid oxidation of the heart by MCD and ACC during contractile stimulation. Am J Phys 1999;277(4 Pt 1): E772–7.
4. McGarry JD, Brown NF. The mitochondrial carnitine palmitoyltransferase system. From concept to molecular analysis. Eur J Biochem 1997;244(1): 1–14.
5. McGarry JD, Mannaerts GP, Foster DW. A possible role for malonyl-CoA in the regulation of hepatic fatty acid oxidation and ketogenesis. J Clin Invest 1977;60(1):265–70.
6. Sugden MC, Holness MJ. Recent advances in mechanisms regulating glucose oxidation at the

level of the pyruvate dehydrogenase complex by PDKs. Am J Physiol Endocrinol Metab 2003; 284(5):E855–62.

7. Young ME, Goodwin GW, Ying J, et al. Regulation of cardiac and skeletal muscle malonyl-CoA decarboxylase by fatty acids. Am J Physiol Endocrinol Metab 2001;280(3):E471–9.

8. Kelly DP. PPARs of the heart: three is a crowd. Circ Res 2003;92(5):482–4.

9. Finck BN, Han X, Courtois M, et al. A critical role for PPARalpha-mediated lipotoxicity in the pathogenesis of diabetic cardiomyopathy: modulation by dietary fat content. Proc Natl Acad Sci U S A 2003;100(3):1226–31.

10. Depre C, Shipley GL, Chen W, et al. Unloaded heart in vivo replicates fetal gene expression of cardiac hypertrophy. Nat Med 1998;4(11):1269–75.

11. Szczepaniak LS, Babcock EE, Schick F, et al. Measurement of intracellular triglyceride stores by H spectroscopy: validation in vivo. Am J Phys 1999;276(5 Pt 1):E977–89.

12. Yoshida T. The rate of phosphocreatine hydrolysis and resynthesis in exercising muscle in humans using 31P-MRS. J Physiol Anthropol Appl Human Sci 2002;21(5):247–55.

13. Lewandowski ED. Cardiac carbon 13 magnetic resonance spectroscopy: on the horizon or over the rainbow? J Nucl Cardiol 2002;9(4):419–28.

14. Bottomley PA, Weiss RG. Non-invasive magnetic-resonance detection of creatine depletion in nonviable infarcted myocardium. Lancet 1998; 351(9104):714–8.

15. He ZX, Shi RF, Wu YJ, et al. Direct imaging of exercise-induced myocardial ischemia with fluorine-18-labeled deoxyglucose and Tc-99m-sestamibi in coronary artery disease. Circulation 2003;108(10):1208–13.

16. DeGrado TR, Holden JE, Ng CK, et al. Quantitative analysis of myocardial kinetics of 15-p-[iodine-125] iodophenylpentadecanoic acid. J Nucl Med 1989; 30(7):1211–8.

17. Dormehl IC, Hugo N, Rossouw D, et al. Planar myocardial imaging in the baboon model with iodine-123-15-(iodophenyl)pentadecanoic acid (IPPA) and iodine-123-15-(P-iodophenyl)-3-R,S-methylpentadecanoic acid (BMIPP), using time-activity curves for evaluation of metabolism. Nucl Med Biol 1995;22(7):837–47.

18. Eckelman WC, Babich JW. Synthesis and validation of fatty acid analogs radiolabeled by nonisotopic substitution. J Nucl Cardiol 2007;14(Suppl 3): S100–9.

19. Reske SN, Sauer W, Machulla HJ, et al. Metabolism of 15 (p 123I iodophenyl-)pentadecanoic acid in heart muscle and noncardiac tissues. Eur J Nucl Med 1985;10(5–6):228–34.

20. Ambrose KR, Owen BA, Goodman MM, et al. Evaluation of the metabolism in rat hearts of two new radioiodinated 3-methyl-branched fatty acid myocardial imaging agents. Eur J Nucl Med 1987;12(10):486–91.

21. Goodman MM, Kirsch G, Knapp FF Jr. Synthesis and evaluation of radioiodinated terminal p-iodophenyl-substituted alpha- and beta-methyl-branched fatty acids. J Med Chem 1984;27(3): 390–7.

22. Iida H, Rhodes CG, Araujo LI, et al. Noninvasive quantification of regional myocardial metabolic rate for oxygen by use of 15O2 inhalation and positron emission tomography. Theory, error analysis, and application in humans. Circulation 1996; 94(4):792–807.

23. Laine H, Katoh C, Luotolahti M, et al. Myocardial oxygen consumption is unchanged but efficiency is reduced in patients with essential hypertension and left ventricular hypertrophy. Circulation 1999; 100(24):2425–30.

24. Yamamoto Y, de Silva R, Rhodes CG, et al. Noninvasive quantification of regional myocardial metabolic rate of oxygen by 15O2 inhalation and positron emission tomography. Experimental validation. Circulation 1996;94(4):808–16.

25. Armbrecht JJ, Buxton DB, Schelbert HR. Validation of [1-11C]acetate as a tracer for noninvasive assessment of oxidative metabolism with positron emission tomography in normal, ischemic, postischemic, and hyperemic canine myocardium. Circulation 1990;81(5):1594–605.

26. Brown M, Marshall DR, Sobel BE, et al. Delineation of myocardial oxygen utilization with carbon-11-labeled acetate. Circulation 1987;76(3):687–96.

27. Brown MA, Myears DW, Bergmann SR. Noninvasive assessment of canine myocardial oxidative metabolism with carbon-11 acetate and positron emission tomography. J Am Coll Cardiol 1988; 12(4):1054–63.

28. Buck A, Wolpers HG, Hutchins GD, et al. Effect of carbon-11-acetate recirculation on estimates of myocardial oxygen consumption by PET. J Nucl Med 1991;32(10):1950–7.

29. Sun KT, Yeatman LA, Buxton DB, et al. Simultaneous measurement of myocardial oxygen consumption and blood flow using [1-carbon-11]acetate. J Nucl Med 1998;39(2):272–80.

30. Choi Y, Hawkins RA, Huang SC, et al. Parametric images of myocardial metabolic rate of glucose generated from dynamic cardiac PET and 2-[18F]fluoro-2-deoxy-d-glucose studies. J Nucl Med 1991;32(4):733–8.

31. Gambert S, Vergely C, Filomenko R, et al. Adverse effects of free fatty acid associated with increased oxidative stress in postischemic isolated rat hearts. Mol Cell Biochem 2006;283(1–2):147–52.

32. Iozzo P, Chareonthaitawee P, Di Terlizzi M, et al. Regional myocardial blood flow and glucose

utilization during fasting and physiological hyperin-sulinemia in humans. Am J Physiol Endocrinol Metab 2002;282(5):E1163–71.

33. Krivokapich J, Huang SC, Selin CE, et al. Fluoro-deoxyglucose rate constants, lumped constant, and glucose metabolic rate in rabbit heart. Am J Phys 1987;252(4 Pt 2):H777–87.

34. Botker HE, Bottcher M, Schmitz O, et al. Glucose uptake and lumped constant variability in normal human hearts determined with [18F]fluorodeoxy-glucose. J Nucl Cardiol 1997;4(2 Pt 1):125–32.

35. Hariharan R, Bray M, Ganim R, et al. Fundamental limitations of [18F]2-deoxy-2-fluoro-D-glucose for assessing myocardial glucose uptake. Circulation 1995;91(9):2435–44.

36. Hashimoto K, Nishimura T, Imahashi KI, et al. Lumped constant for deoxyglucose is decreased when myocardial glucose uptake is enhanced. Am J Phys 1999;276(1 Pt 2):H129–33.

37. Herrero P, Sharp TL, Dence C, et al. Comparison of 1-(11)C-glucose and (18)F-FDG for quantifying myocardial glucose use with PET. J Nucl Med 2002;43(11):1530–41.

38. Herrero P, Weinheimer CJ, Dence C, et al. Quantifica-tion of myocardial glucose utilization by PET and 1-carbon-11-glucose. J Nucl Cardiol 2002;9(1):5–14.

39. Herrero P, Kisrieva-Ware Z, Dence CS, et al. PET measurements of myocardial glucose metabolism with 1-11C-glucose and kinetic modeling. J Nucl Med 2007;48(6):955–64.

40. Herrero P, Dence CS, Coggan AR, et al. L-3-11C-lactate as a PET tracer of myocardial lactate metabolism: a feasibility study. J Nucl Med 2007; 48(12):2046–55.

41. Bergmann SR, Weinheimer CJ, Markham J, et al. Quantitation of myocardial fatty acid metabolism using PET. J Nucl Med 1996;37(10):1723–30.

42. Davila-Roman VG, Vedala G, Herrero P, et al. Altered myocardial fatty acid and glucose metabo-lism in idiopathic dilated cardiomyopathy. J Am Coll Cardiol 2002;40(2):271–7.

43. Herrero P, Peterson LR, McGill JB, et al. Increased myocardial fatty acid metabolism in patients with type 1 diabetes mellitus. J Am Coll Cardiol 2006; 47(3):598–604.

44. Peterson LR, Herrero P, Schechtman KB, et al. Effect of obesity and insulin resistance on myocar-dial substrate metabolism and efficiency in young women. Circulation 2004;109(18):2191–6.

45. DeGrado TR. Synthesis of 14(R,S)-[18F]fluoro-6-thia-heptadecanoic acid (FTHA). J Labelled Comp Radiopharm 1991;29:989–95.

46. DeGrado TR, Coenen HH, Stocklin G. 14(R,S)-[18F]fluoro-6-thia-heptadecanoic acid (FTHA): evaluation in mouse of a new probe of myocardial utilization of long chain fatty acids. J Nucl Med 1991;32(10):1888–96.

47. Schulz G, von Dahl J, Kaiser HJ, et al. Imaging of beta-oxidation by static PET with 14(R,S)-[18F]-flu-oro-6-thiaheptadecanoic acid (FTHA) in patients with advanced coronary heart disease: a compar-ison with 18FDG-PET and 99Tcm-MIBI SPET. Nucl Med Commun 1996;17(12):1057–64.

48. Taylor M, Wallhaus TR, Degrado TR, et al. An eval-uation of myocardial fatty acid and glucose uptake using PET with [18F]fluoro-6-thia-heptadecanoic acid and [18F]FDG in patients with congestive heart failure. J Nucl Med 2001;42(1):55–62.

49. DeGrado TR, Wang S, Holden JE, et al. Synthesis and preliminary evaluation of (18)F-labeled 4-thia palmitate as a PET tracer of myocardial fatty acid oxidation. Nucl Med Biol 2000;27(3):221–31.

50. DeGrado TR, Kitapci MT, Wang S, et al. Validation of 18F-fluoro-4-thia-palmitate as a PET probe for myocardial fatty acid oxidation: effects of hypoxia and composition of exogenous fatty acids. J Nucl Med 2006;47(1):173–81.

51. Shoup TM, Elmaleh DR, Bonab AA, et al. Evaluation of trans-9-18F-fluoro-3,4-Methyleneheptadecanoic acid as a PET tracer for myocardial fatty acid imaging. J Nucl Med 2005;46(2):297–304.

52. Desrois M, Sidell RJ, Gauguier D, et al. Gender differences in hypertrophy, insulin resistance and ischemic injury in the aging type 2 diabetic rat heart. J Mol Cell Cardiol 2004;37(2):547–55.

53. Dyck JR, Lopaschuk GD. Glucose metabolism, H+ production and Na+/H+-exchanger mRNA levels in ischemic hearts from diabetic rats. Mol Cell Bio-chem 1998;180(1–2):85–93.

54. Peterson LR, Soto PF, Herrero P, et al. Sex differ-ences in myocardial oxygen and glucose metabo-lism. J Nucl Cardiol 2007;14(4):573–81.

55. Peterson LR, Soto PM, Herrero P, et al. Impact of gender on the myocardial metabolic response to obesity. JACC CU Imag 2008;1:424–33.

56. Abu-Erreish GM, Neely JR, Whitmer JT, et al. Fatty acid oxidation by isolated perfused working hearts of aged rats. Am J Phys 1977;232(3):E258–62.

57. McMillin JB, Taffet GE, Taegtmeyer H, et al. Mito-chondrial metabolism and substrate competition in the aging Fischer rat heart. Cardiovasc Res 1993;27(12):2222–8.

58. Iemitsu M, Miyauchi T, Maeda S, et al. Aging-induced decrease in the PPAR-alpha level in hearts is improved by exercise training. Am J Physiol Heart Circ Physiol 2002;283(5):H1750–60.

59. Odiet JA, Boerrigter ME, Wei JY. Carnitine palmityl transferase-I activity in the aging mouse heart. Mech Ageing Dev 1995;79(2–3):127–36.

60. Paradies G, Ruggiero FM, Gadaleta MN, et al. The effect of aging and acetyl-L-carnitine on the activity of the phosphate carrier and on the phospholipid composition in rat heart mitochondria. Biochim Bio-phys Acta 1992;1103(2):324–6.

61. Kates AM, Herrero P, Dence C, et al. Impact of aging on substrate metabolism by the human heart. J Am Coll Cardiol 2003;41:293–9.

62. Soto PF, Herrero P, Kates AM, et al. Impact of aging on myocardial metabolic response to dobutamine. Am J Physiol Heart Circ Physiol 2003;285:2158–64.

63. Soto PF, Herrero P, Schechtman KB, et al. Exercise training impacts the myocardial metabolism of older individuals in a gender-specific manner. Am J Physiol Heart Circ Physiol 2008;295(2):H842–50.

64. Lopaschuk G. Regulation of carbohydrate metabolism in ischemia and reperfusion. Am Heart J 2000; 139(2 Pt 3):S115–9.

65. Araujo LI, Camici P, Spinks TJ, et al. Abnormalities in myocardial metabolism in patients with unstable angina as assessed by positron emission tomography. Cardiovasc Drugs Ther 1988;2(1):41–6.

66. Camici P, Araujo LI, Spinks T, et al. Increased uptake of 18F-fluorodeoxyglucose in postischemic myocardium of patients with exercise-induced angina. Circulation 1986;74(1):81–8.

67. Kawai Y, Tsukamoto E, Nozaki Y, et al. Significance of reduced uptake of iodinated fatty acid analogue for the evaluation of patients with acute chest pain. J Am Coll Cardiol 2001;38(7):1888–94.

68. Tamaki N. Role of BMIPP imaging for risk stratification in patients with coronary artery disease. J Nucl Cardiol 2005;12(2):148–50.

69. Barger PM, Kelly DP. Fatty acid utilization in the hypertrophied and failing heart: molecular regulatory mechanisms. Am J Med Sci 1999;318(1): 36–42.

70. Rupp H, Jacob R. Metabolically-modulated growth and phenotype of the rat heart. Eur Heart J 1992; 13(Suppl D):56–61.

71. Blair E, Redwood C, Ashrafian H, et al. Mutations in the gamma(2) subunit of AMP-activated protein kinase cause familial hypertrophic cardiomyopathy: evidence for the central role of energy compromise in disease pathogenesis. Hum Mol Genet 2001;10(11):1215–20.

72. Jamshidi Y, Montgomery HE, Hense HW, et al. Peroxisome proliferator–activated receptor alpha gene regulates left ventricular growth in response to exercise and hypertension. Circulation 2002; 105(8):950–5.

73. Handa N, Magata Y, Mukai T, et al. Quantitative FDG-uptake by positron emission tomography in progressive hypertrophy of rat hearts in vivo. Ann Nucl Med 2007;21(10):569–76.

74. de las Fuentes L, Herrero P, Peterson LR, et al. Myocardial fatty acid metabolism: independent predictor of left ventricular mass in hypertensive heart disease. Hypertension 2003;41(1):83–7.

75. de las Fuentes L, Soto PF, Cupps BP, et al. Hypertensive left ventricular hypertrophy is associated with abnormal myocardial fatty acid metabolism

76. Tuunanen H, Kuusisto J, Toikka J, et al. Myocardial perfusion, oxidative metabolism, and free fatty acid uptake in patients with hypertrophic cardiomyopathy attributable to the Asp175Asn mutation in the alpha-tropomyosin gene: a positron emission tomography study. J Nucl Cardiol 2007;14(3):354–65.

77. Buttrick PM, Kaplan M, Leinwand LA, et al. Alterations in gene expression in the rat heart after chronic pathological and physiological loads. J Mol Cell Cardiol 1994;26(1):61–7.

78. Sack MN, Kelly DP. The energy substrate switch during development of heart failure: gene regulatory mechanisms [Review]. Int J Mol Med 1998; 1(1):17–24.

79. Taegtmeyer H. Cardiac metabolism as a target for the treatment of heart failure. Circulation 2004; 110(8):894–6.

80. Nakae I, Matsuo S, Koh T, et al. Iodine-123 BMIPP scintigraphy in the evaluation of patients with heart failure. Acta Radiol 2006;47(8):810–6.

81. Tuunanen H, Engblom E, Naum A, et al. Decreased myocardial free fatty acid uptake in patients with idiopathic dilated cardiomyopathy: evidence of relationship with insulin resistance and left ventricular dysfunction. J Card Fail 2006;12(8):644–52.

82. Beanlands RSB, Nahmias C, Gordon E, et al. The effects of b$_1$-blockade on oxidative metabolism and the metabolic cost of ventricular work in patients with left ventricular dysfunction: a double-blind, placebo-controlled, positron-emission tomography study. Circulation 2000;102:2070–5.

83. Stolen KQ, Kemppainen J, Ukkonen H, et al. Exercise training improves biventricular oxidative metabolism and left ventricular efficiency in patients with dilated cardiomyopathy. J Am Coll Cardiol 2003;41(3):460–7.

84. Sundell J, Engblom E, Koistinen J, et al. The effects of cardiac resynchronization therapy on left ventricular function, myocardial energetics, and metabolic reserve in patients with dilated cardiomyopathy and heart failure. J Am Coll Cardiol 2004;43(6): 1027–33.

85. Nowak B, Sinha AM, Schaefer WM, et al. Cardiac resynchronization therapy homogenizes myocardial glucose metabolism and perfusion in dilated cardiomyopathy and left bundle branch block. J Am Coll Cardiol 2003;41(9):1523–8.

86. Tuunanen H, Engblom E, Naum A, et al. Trimetazidine, a metabolic modulator, has cardiac and extracardiac benefits in idiopathic dilated cardiomyopathy. Circulation 2008;118(12):1250–8.

87. Hasegawa S, Kusuoka H, Maruyama K, et al. Myocardial positron emission computed tomographic images obtained with fluorine-18 fluoro-2-deoxyglucose predict the response of idiopathic

dilated cardiomyopathy patients to beta-blockers. J Am Coll Cardiol 2004;43(2):224–33.

88. van Campen CM, Visser FC, van der Weerdt AP, et al. FDG PET as a predictor of response to re-synchronisation therapy in patients with ischaemic cardiomyopathy. Eur J Nucl Med Mol Imaging 2007;34(3):309–15.

89. Kannel WB, Hjortland M, Castelli WP. Role of diabetes in congestive heart failure: the Framingham study. Am J Cardiol 1974;34:29–34.

90. Stanley WC, Lopaschuk GD, McCormack JG. Regulation of energy substrate metabolism in the diabetic heart. Cardiovasc Res 1997;34(1):25–33.

91. Rodrigues B, Cam MC, McNeill JH. Myocardial substrate metabolism: implications for diabetic cardiomyopathy. J Mol Cell Cardiol 1995;27: 169–79.

92. Taegtmeyer H, McNulty P, Young ME. Adaptation and maladaptation of the heart in diabetes: part I: general concepts. Circulation 2002;105(14):1727–33.

93. Young ME, McNulty P, Taegtmeyer H. Adaptation and maladaptation of the heart in diabetes: part II: potential mechanisms. Circulation 2002; 105(15):1861–70.

94. Finck BN, Lehman JJ, Leone TC, et al. The cardiac phenotype induced by PPARalpha overexpression mimics that caused by diabetes mellitus. J Clin Invest 2002;109(1):121–30.

95. Burkart EM, Sambandam N, Han X, et al. Nuclear receptors PPARbeta/delta and PPARalpha direct distinct metabolic regulatory programs in the mouse heart. J Clin Invest 2007;117(12):3930–9.

96. Shoghi KI, Gropler RJ, Sharp T, et al. Time course of alterations in myocardial glucose utilization in the Zucker diabetic fatty rat with correlation to gene expression of glucose transporters: a small-animal PET investigation. J Nucl Med 2008;49(8):1320–7.

97. Welch MJ, Lewis JS, Kim J, et al. Assessment of myocardial metabolism in diabetic rats using small-animal PET: a feasibility study. J Nucl Med 2006;47(4):689–97.

98. Monti LD, Landoni C, Setola E, et al. Myocardial insulin resistance associated with chronic hypertri-glyceridemia and increased FFA levels in Type 2 diabetic patients. Am J Physiol Heart Circ Physiol 2004;287(3):H1225–31.

99. Monti LD, Lucignani G, Landoni C, et al. Myocardial glucose uptake evaluated by positron emission tomography and fluorodeoxyglucose during hyperglycemic clamp in IDDM patients. Role of free fatty acid and insulin levels. Diabetes 1995; 44(5):537–42.

100. vom Dahl J, Herman WH, Hicks RJ, et al. Myocardial glucose uptake in patients with insulin-dependent diabetes mellitus assessed quantitatively by dynamic positron emission tomography. Circulation 1993;88(2):395–404.

101. Avogaro A, Nosadini R, Doria A, et al. Myocardial metabolism in insulin-deficient diabetic humans without coronary artery disease. Am J Phys 1990; 258(4 Pt 1):E606–18.

102. Herrero P, McGill JB, Lesniak D, et al. PET detection of the impact of dobutamine on myocardial glucose metabolism in women with type 1 diabetes mellitus. J Nucl Cardiol 2008;15(6):598–604.

103. Peterson LR, Herrero P, McGill J, et al. Fatty acids and insulin modulate myocardial substrate metabolism in humans with type 1 diabetes. Diabetes 2008;57(1):32–40.

104. Zhou YT, Grayburn P, Karim A, et al. Lipotoxic heart disease in obese rats: implications for human obesity. Proc Natl Acad Sci U S A 2000;97(4):1784–9.

105. Hallsten K, Virtanen KA, Lonnqvist F, et al. Enhancement of insulin-stimulated myocardial glucose uptake in patients with Type 2 diabetes treated with rosiglitazone. Diabet Med 2004; 21(12):1280–7.

106. Commerford SR, Pagliassotti MJ, Melby CL, et al. Fat oxidation, lipolysis, and free fatty acid cycling in obesity-prone and obesity-resistant rats. Am J Physiol Endocrinol Metab 2000;279(4):E875–85.

107. Ogawa M, Ishino S, Mukai T, et al. (18)F-FDG accumulation in atherosclerotic plaques: immunohistochemical and PET imaging study. J Nucl Med 2004;45(7):1245–50.

108. Rudd JH, Warburton EA, Fryer TD, et al. Imaging atherosclerotic plaque inflammation with [18F]-fluorodeoxyglucose positron emission tomography. Circulation 2002;105(23):2708–11.

109. Tahara N, Kai H, Ishibashi M, et al. Simvastatin attenuates plaque inflammation: evaluation by fluorodeoxyglucose positron emission tomography. J Am Coll Cardiol 2006;48(9):1825–31.

110. Tawakol A, Migrino RQ, Bashian GG, et al. In vivo 18F-fluorodeoxyglucose positron emission tomography imaging provides a noninvasive measure of carotid plaque inflammation in patients. J Am Coll Cardiol 2006;48(9):1818–24.

Cardiac Neuronal Imaging at the Edge of Clinical Application

Mark I. Travin, MD

KEYWORDS

• Autonomic • Imaging • Nuclear • Cardiac • MIBG • HED

Neuronal innervation plays a crucial role in cardiac function. The heart is richly innervated with sympathetic and parasympathetic fibers that work in conjunction with circulating catecholamine mediators, such as norepinephrine (NE), to tightly regulate cardiac output at rest and during periods of increased cardiac demand. An impairment of cardiac autonomic function, most often the result of cardiac disease (although sometimes secondary to primary neurologic abnormalities), can reflect the severity of the condition, and in many cases is associated with and likely contributing to worsening of the clinical condition, increasing the potential for life-threatening cardiac arrhythmias and death. Because cardiac autonomic function involves numerous molecular processes, use of radiotracers for imaging is an ideal method of assessment.

CARDIAC NEURONAL ANATOMY

Cardiac neural autonomic function is controlled by regulatory centers in the midbrain, hypothalamus, pons, and medulla that integrate input signals from other parts of the brain and receptors throughout the body. From the brain, efferent signals follow descending pathways in the spinal cord, and synapse with preganglionic fibers that leave the spinal cord at levels T1–L3, subsequently synapsing with paravertebral stellate ganglia. Left stellate postganglionic fibers innervate the right ventricle, whereas right postganglionic fibers innervate anterior and lateral left ventricle. In the heart sympathetic nerves follow the coronary arteries in the subepicardium and then penetrate the myocardium. The major chemical mediator of sympathetic function is NE.[1,2]

Parasympathetic fibers are scarce in comparison with sympathetic fibers. They originate in the medulla and follow the vagus nerves. In the heart they start epicardially, cross the atrioventricular (AV) groove, and penetrate the myocardium, located thereafter in the subendocardium. Parasympathetic output controls sinoatrial and AV nodal function. Parasympathetic fibers predominantly innervate the atria and are scare in the ventricle (densest in the inferior wall). The chemical mediator of parasympathetic function is acetylcholine.

Most published literature and current clinical applicability of autonomic radionuclide imaging is of the sympathetic system, with parasympathetic imaging studies limited mostly to animals. The following discussion therefore deals predominantly with cardiac sympathetic imaging.

RADIONUCLIDE TRACERS FOR IMAGING CARDIAC SYMPATHETIC INNERVATION

Imaging of cardiac sympathetic innervation focuses on the synaptic junction, shown in **Fig. 1**. Most of the radiotracers developed and investigated to this point image presynaptic anatomy and function, although newer tracers that bind to postsynaptic α and β receptors are also being designed and investigated. All cardiac neuronal radiotracers are considered investigational for cardiac imaging at the time of this writing.

The sympathetic mediator NE is synthesized by a series of steps originating with tyrosine, and is stored at high concentrations in presynaptic

Department of Nuclear Medicine, Montefiore Medical Center, 111 East 210th Street, Bronx, NY 10467 2490, USA

E-mail address: mtravin@montefiore.org

Cardiol Clin 27 (2009) 311–327

doi:10.1016/j.ccl.2008.12.007

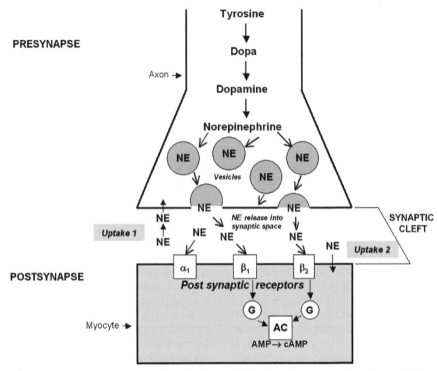

Fig. 1. Sympathetic neuronal synapse. AC, adenyl cyclase; AMP, adenosine monophosphate; cAMP, cyclic adenosine monophosphate; G, G proteins; NE, norepinephrine.

vesicles. In response to a stimulus, the NE-containing vesicles are released into the synaptic space and bind to postsynaptic β_1, β_2, and α receptors, enhancing adenyl cyclase activity through intermediary G proteins, resulting in the desired cardiac stimulatory effects.[3,4] As part of tight control of sympathetic physiology, NE is then taken back up into the presynaptic terminal by way of a transporter protein–mediated, sodium-, energy-, and temperature-dependent process (ie, "uptake-1") for storage or catabolic disposal, in effect terminating the sympathetic response. Some synaptic NE is also taken up by the nonneuronal postsynaptic cells, probably by sodium-independent passive diffusion (ie, the "uptake-2" system).[5,6]

Synthesis and administration of radiolabeled modifications or radiolabeled analogs of the various molecules along the NE production pathway allows imaging along with qualitative and quantitative assessment of neuron function. For example, a radiolabeled modification of the intermediary compound dopamine (ie, ^{18}F-dopamine) has shown promise as a potential PET agent for neuronal imaging.[7] Most of the experimental and clinical work on neuronal imaging has been with radiolabeled analogs, both single photon emission computed tomography (SPECT) and

positron emission tomography (PET), of the end product, NE. Guanethidine is a false neurotransmitter analog of NE that when administered is taken up by the uptake-1 pathway. Chemical modification of guanethidine produces a molecule that can be labeled with radioactive iodine—meta-iodobenzylguanidine (mIBG)—and therefore imaged. When first developed in the late 1970s, mIBG was labeled with ^{131}I and was used for detection of neural crest tumors, neuroblastomas, and pheochromocytomas. ^{131}I-mIBG imaging of such tumors is at the time of this writing the only US Food and Drug Administration (FDA)–approved use of radiolabeled mIBG in the United States. Because ^{131}I gives off relatively high-energy (365 keV) γ emissions, emits β^- particles, and has a relatively long half-life of about 8.02 days, ^{123}I labeling has been developed and is preferred. ^{123}I emits predominantly γ photons with energies of 159 keV and has a half-life of 13.2 hours, therefore being easily imaged and well tolerated. ^{123}I-mIBG has been used extensively in Europe and Japan for cardiac imaging, but is currently not FDA approved in the United States for cardiac imaging and is therefore considered to be investigational.

As an analog of NE and guanethidine, intravenously administered ^{123}I-mIBG diffuses into the synaptic space and is taken up and accumulates in the presynaptic nerve terminal by way of the uptake-1 pathway. Although [123]I-*m*IBG seems to share the same uptake, storage, and release mechanisms as NE, unlike NE [123]I-*m*IBG is not catabolized by monoamine oxidase (MAO) or catechol-*o*-methyltransferase, allowing it to localize in myocardial sympathetic nerve endings to a higher cytoplasmic concentration than NE.[6,8–10] There is also the potential for the non-neuronal uptake-2 process to occur, but this seems minimal at the relatively low concentrations used for human cardiac imaging.

There are also various PET analogs of NE that are under investigation.[5] Compared with [123]I-*m*IBG, these tracers are more similar to NE in composition thereby having distinct biologic advantages, and as PET tracers they have better physical properties for imaging. The most commonly used neuronal PET tracer has been ^{11}C-meta-hydroxyephedrine (HED). Among the advantages of ^{11}C-HED compared with [123]I-*m*IBG is higher uptake-1 selectivity (ie, lower nonspecific nonneuronal uptake), resulting in better differentiation between innervated and denervated myocardium, recently found to be of particular advantage in evaluating neuronal heterogeneity in hibernating myocardium.[11] ^{11}C-HED also seems to have more homogeneous uptake than [123]I-*m*IBG (less heterogeneity in the inferior wall). Other less well-studied ^{11}C neuronal tracers include ^{11}C-epinephrine and ^{11}C-phenyl-ephrine. The latter is rapidly metabolized by MAO and as a result could potentially play a role in assessment of vesicular storage function. **Table 1** lists these and other presynaptic tracers under use or investigation for presynaptic neuronal imaging.[5,12,13]

CARDIAC IMAGING WITH [123]I-*m*IBG

[123]I-*m*IBG is the most studied radiotracer for cardiac neuronal imaging. Tracer injection is performed at rest and needs only minimal preparation. Medications that might interfere with catecholamine uptake, such as various antidepressants, antipsychotics, and some calcium channel blockers, should be held for 24 hours before tracer injection and imaging.

There is disagreement regarding the need for administration of thyroid-blocking agents before [123]I-*m*IBG administration. Historically such blockade has been undertaken to shield the thyroid from exposure to unbound radionuclide impurities, such as [124]I and [125]I. With modern production methods the amount of such unbound impurities, and unbound ^{123}I, is minimal, and thus

many investigators believe that such pretreatment is unnecessary. This issue will be clarified further when and if [123]I-*m*IBG obtains FDA approval for cardiac and oncologic imaging.

The amount of tracer activity to administer has not been formally established. In several published investigations a dose of 3 to 5 mCi (111–185 MBq) of [123]I-*m*IBG over 1-minute period has been used, and this is generally satisfactory for planar image analysis. Because it is often difficult to obtain satisfactory SPECT images using these tracer doses in patients who have severe cardiac dysfunction and heart failure, a dose of up to 10 mCi (370 MBq) may be appropriate and is under investigation.[3]

Parameters for planar and SPECT acquisition of [123]I-*m*IBG are not formally established, but current methods are described in various published reviews.[1,14] Planar images are obtained in the anterior view for 10 minutes using an energy window of 159 keV ± 20%. SPECT images are obtained using the 159 keV ± 20% energy window by way of a 180° circular acquisition from 45° right anterior oblique to 45° left posterior oblique, using a total of 60 stops (30 stops per head if done with a dual-headed camera) at 30 seconds per stop.

Although low-energy collimators have been customarily used for [123]I-*m*IBG acquisition, multiple, low-abundance higher-energy photon emissions (including one of 529 keV) that are emitted by ^{123}I more freely penetrate the septa and degrade image quality. Work is under way using a measured point spread function to perform three-dimensional deconvolution of the septal penetration to compensate for this effect and improve image accuracy, particularly for quantitative parameters.[15]

Planar and SPECT images are routinely obtained at approximately 15 minutes following [123]I-*m*IBG administration (early), and again 3 to 5 hours later (delayed). Although some believe that only the delayed image should be used for interpretation and analysis because it represents actual neuronal uptake (as opposed to interstitial uptake for the early images), studies mostly from Japan have shown that tracer washout between early and delayed images provides important additional information.

[123]I-*m*IBG IMAGE INTERPRETATION

Although most published data describe the prognostic usefulness of global myocardial tracer uptake and washout parameters on planar images, one can also perform SPECT imaging to assess regional tracer uptake. When coupled with rest imaging using a standard SPECT

Table 1
Radiotracers for imaging of presynaptic sympathetic innervation

Tracer	SPECT/ PET	Metabolized by MAO	Development Stage	Comments
I-123 metaiodobenzylguanidine (MIBG)	SPECT	No	Clinical	Most extensively studied, wide potential clinical applications. Limitations from normal variants and attenuation as a SPECT agent
C-11 metahydroxyephedrine (HED)	PET	No	Clinical	Most widely used PET tracer. More homogenous uptake than MIBG, with fewer inferior defects in normal patients
C-11 epinephrine	PET	Yes	Clinical	A more physiologic tracer for evaluation of presynaptic function with respect to uptake, vesicular storage, and metabolism
C-11 phenylephrine	PET	Yes	Clinical	Vesicular storage necessary to protect from rapid metabolism by neuronal MAO. Potential use to assess function/impairment of vesicular storage function
F-18 6-fluorodopamine	PET	Yes	Clinical	Had been used mainly to identify cardiac involvement from neurologic diseases. Allows assessment of uptake and washout of NE. Difficult to produce
F-18 6-flurometaraminol	PET	Yes	Experimental	Low specific activity. Potent vasoactive properties
F-18 (−)-6-fluoronorepinephrine	PET	Yes	Experimental	High cardiac uptake and retention shown in baboons
F-18 para-fluorobenzylguanidine (PFBG)	PET	No	Experimental	PET analog of ^{123}I-MIBG, with potential for quantitation. Considerable nonneuronal retention by uptake-2 mechanism. May depend less on flow for uptake
F-18 fluoroidobenzylguanidine	PET	No	Experimental	Greater lipophilicity than PFBG—more similar to MIBG
Br-76 metabromobenzylguanidine	PET	No	Experimental	Low uptake-1 selectivity

Abbreviations: MAO, Monoamine oxidase; NE, Norepinephrine; PET, Positron emission tomography; SPECT, Single photon emission computer tomography.
  Data from Bengel FM, Schwaiger M. Assessment of cardiac sympathetic neuronal function using PET imaging. J Nucl Cardiol 2004;11:605.

perfusion tracer, regional analysis can identify areas of neuronal/perfusion mismatch that may have denervation supersensitivity and increase the risk for cardiac arrhythmias.[16]

The standard measure of global ^{123}I-mIBG uptake is the heart mediastinal ratio (HMR), derived through regions of interest over the heart and upper mediastinum, created in various ways [17–19] but all seeming to give similar results in any given patient study. Normal values for HMR range from 1.9 to 2.8, with a mean of about 2.2.[10]

Another frequently measured quantity from planar images is ^{123}I-mIBG washout.[18,20] The washout ratio may reflect turnover of catecholamines attributable to sympathetic drive. A normal washout value in control subjects is reported to be 9.6% ± 8.5%.

Although ideally cardiac [123]I-*m*IBG uptake would be homogeneous in normal individuals, there are variations that seem unrelated to cardiac disease. Gill and colleagues[21] and Morozumi and colleagues[22] have shown that in normal subjects there is relatively less uptake (12%–18%) of [123]I-*m*IBG in the septum and especially the inferior wall compared with the anterior and lateral walls, attributed to differences in regional myocardial autonomic innervation. Furthermore, these heterogeneities are reported to be more pronounced in older subjects and in men.[23] It has been proposed that such regional variation may be the result of increased vagal tone in the inferior wall, supported in a study by Estorch and colleagues[24] finding that in athletes who have sinus bradycardia, [123]I-*m*IBG uptake is lower in the inferior wall. Such relative decreased inferior uptake seems not to be present when using the PET tracer ^{11}C-HED, but is present to a mild degree when ^{11}C-epinephrine is used.[25] The reported normal variant decrease in inferior wall uptake of [123]I-*m*IBG may thus in part be the result of attenuation of a SPECT tracer or differences in the characteristics of the various autonomic tracers, but likely also true physiologic changes. Such variations need to be investigated further, particularly if autonomic radiotracer imaging is to be used to follow patient response to therapies.

ASSESSMENT OF PATIENTS WHO HAVE CONGESTIVE HEART FAILURE

Although congestive heart failure (CHF) had in the past been largely considered a condition of abnormal cardiac output resulting in hemodynamic pressure abnormalities during ventricular filling and emptying, with therapies directed accordingly, the current approach focuses on understanding and directing treatment at the neurohormonal changes that accompany and worsen heart failure. In response to decreased cardiac function, there is activation of the sympathetic adrenergic system (SAS) and the renin-angiotensin system (RAS), causing the release of various vasoactive mediators (endothelin, vasopressin, cytokines), leading to down-regulation of receptors, myocardial remodeling and fibrosis, and apoptosis and necrosis, all of which then further worsen cardiac function and stimulate more neurohormonal activation, a cycle that if not broken results in a downward spiraling clinical course.

The initial SAS response to CHF is designed to compensate for decreased cardiac function by increasing heart rate, contractility, and venous return to the heart. Nevertheless, this increased sympathetic activity can eventually lead to harmful effects, including precipitation of arrhythmias, decreased myocardial catecholamine levels, down-regulation of β-receptors, increased plasma NE, and further activation of the RAS. High levels of circulating catecholamines can lead to myocardial structural changes, such as remodeling, hypertrophy, and changes in extracellular matrix, accompanied by myocyte death.[26]

At the cellular level, there is initially an increase in NE release into the synaptic cleft, promoting an increase in the NE transporter 1 (uptake-1, NET-1) process. Eventually the NET-1 system is overwhelmed, with a reduction in NET-1 carrier density, leading to increased spillover of NE into plasma, likely accounting for the increased washout seen with [123]I-*m*IBG imaging in patients who have heart failure. With progression of cardiac dysfunction there is diminished presynaptic function from loss of neurons and down-regulation of NET-1, likely accounting for decreased global radiotracer uptake in advanced stages of heart failure.[27]

A key role for assessing cardiac [123]I-*m*IBG washout in patients who had CHF was reported by Ogita and colleagues.[18] In 79 patients who had CHF and a left ventricular ejection fraction (LVEF) less than 40%, those who had washout 27% or greater (2 standard deviations higher than 9.6% ± 8.5% determined from a group of 20 controls) had a 35% cardiac death rate over 52 months, compared with 0 deaths for patients who had lower tracer washout. There was also a greater than threefold increase in hospital admissions for CHF in the high washout group. A later study from the same group reported that increased washout predicts sudden death.[28]

A consistent finding associated with a poor prognosis in patients who have advanced heart failure is a decreased HMR.[29–31] The finding was initially reported by Merlet and colleagues[32] in a prospective study of 90 patients who had moderate to severe CHF and LVEF less than 45% (mean 22%). Patients who had an HMR less than 1.2 had 6- and 12-month survivals of 60% and 40%, respectively, compared with a 100% 12-month survival for patients who had a higher ratio. By multivariate analysis, HMR was a better predictor of mortality than LVEF. A subsequent report from this group studying 112 patients who had idiopathic dilated cardiomyopathy also showed cardiac [123]I-*m*IBG uptake to be independent of and better than LVEF in predicting cardiac death.[31] A study by Nakata and colleagues[33] of about 400 patients showed a progressive worsening of survival as the HMR decreased, and that HMR was a more powerful predictor of cardiac death than New York Heart Association (NYHA) class, age, prior myocardial infarction (MI), and LVEF. Most recently Agostini and colleagues[34] reviewed the records of 290 patients who had heart failure in six centers in Europe and quantitatively reanalyzed [123]I-*m*IBG studies the patients had. Logistic regression showed that the only significant predictors of major cardiac events (cardiac death, transplant, and potentially fatal arrhythmias) over 24 months were LVEF and HMR. Particularly striking was the ability of HMR to risk stratify patients who had LVEF 35% or less, with event rates ranging from less than 5% for those who had HMR 2.18 or greater, to more than 50% for those who had HMR 1.45 or less, illustrated in **Fig. 2**. A large, prospective international multicenter study of more than 1000 patients that looks comprehensively into the prognostic value of [123]I-*m*IBG parameters in patients who have class II-III CHF (ADMIRE-HF: Adreview Myocardial Imaging for Risk Evaluation in Heart Failure) is currently in progress.[35]

There have been concerns that the cause of congestive heart failure, especially whether it is ischemic versus nonischemic, may affect the usefulness of [123]I-*m*IBG imaging. As discussed subsequently, ischemic heart disease can by itself, without CHF, result in [123]I-*m*IBG abnormalities, and thus contribute to different findings and implications of image results in these two settings. It seems, however, that regardless of the initial cause of heart failure, as the condition progresses there is a common state in which the characteristic cardiac autonomic abnormalities are seen on [123]I-*m*IBG imaging and remain strong correlates of prognosis. In a study of 76 patients who had ischemic cardiomyopathies and 56 patients who had idiopathic cardiomyopathies, Wakabayashi and colleagues[36] showed that for both groups late HMR was the most powerful independent predictor of lethal clinical outcome (although there were different HMR threshold values: 1.50 for ischemic compared with 2.02 for idiopathic cardiomyopathies).

[123]I-*m*IBG IMAGING TO FOLLOW AND GUIDE THERAPY IN PATIENTS WHO HAVE HEART FAILURE

To become of widespread clinical use, [123]I-*m*IBG imaging will need to help guide therapy in a way that other perhaps less expensive and more readily available testing techniques do not. Given the high costs of health care in the modern era, using an expensive test simply to show that sick patients are at high risk is not likely to be widely accepted.

One promising use of [123]I-*m*IBG imaging in patients who have heart failure is the monitoring of the response to various pharmacologic treatments. Studies have consistently shown that cardiac [123]I-*m*IBG images improve after therapy with β-blockers.[17,37–40] In a small study of 18 patients who had idiopathic dilated cardiomyopathy, Merlet and colleagues[37] showed that increased cardiac [123]I-*m*IBG uptake after 6 months of metoprolol therapy was associated with concomitant improvements in NYHA class and increased LVEF. In a subsequent double-blind, multicenter, placebo-controlled study from this same group, for 64 patients who had CHF before and after 6 months of carvedilol therapy or placebo, there was an increase in both planar and tomographic myocardial [123]I-*m*IBG uptake associated with decreased ventricular volumes and increased LVEF in the carvedilol-treated patients but not in those receiving placebo.[39] In this particular study there was no change in cardiopulmonary exercise capacity nor were there any changes in circulating catecholamine levels, suggesting that improvements in [123]I-*m*IBG imaging parameters may identify patients responding to therapy who would not otherwise be identified by alternative means. Slightly different results were obtained by Gerson and colleagues[40] who, although finding increased cardiac [123]I-*m*IBG uptake in 22 patients treated with carvedilol (more so if the baseline HMR was lower), did not find a clear association with improvement in LVEF.

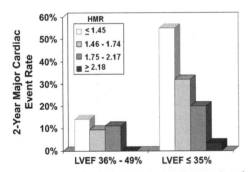

Fig. 2. Major cardiac event rates over 2 years in relation to left ventricular ejection fraction (LVEF) and [123]I-*m*IBG heart mediastinal ratio HMR in patients who had New York Heart Association class II-IV heart failure. Major cardiac events included cardiac death, cardiac transplant, and potentially fatal arrhythmias (implantable cardioverter defibrillator discharge). (*Adapted from* Agostini D, Verberne HJ, Burchert W, et al. I-123-*m*IBG myocardial imaging for assessment of risk for a major cardiac event in heart failure patients: insights from a retrospective European multicenter study. Eur J Nucl Med Mol Imaging 2008;35:542; with permission.)

Although changes in autonomic function response to β-blockers is not entirely surprising, various other medications that do not directly influence cardiac sympathetic function also lead to improvements in [123]I-*m*IBG image findings. For example medications that affect the RAS system also improve cardiac [123]I-*m*IBG uptake. Takeishi and colleagues[41] showed an increase in HMR and a decrease in tracer washout in 19 NYHA class II-III patients treated with enalapril. Toyama and colleagues[42] reported an improvement in HMR and a decrease in planar image defect scores in 24 patients who had dilated cardiomyopathy treated with angiotensin-converting enzyme inhibitors (ACE-I), although there was less of an effect compared with patients who instead received metoprolol. Kasama and colleagues[43,44] showed that adding the ARB valsartan to an ACE-I improved [123]I-*m*IBG parameters accompanied by an increase in LVEF and an improvement in NYHA functional class. They subsequently showed similar improvements with spironolactone.

Because function of the RAS is related to function of the SAS, it follows that ACE-I and ARBs would affect [123]I-*m*IBG imaging. Amiodarone, however, an antiarrhythmic medication that would not be expected to directly influence cardiac sympathetic function, has also been shown to improve [123]I-*m*IBG parameters in patients who have advanced CHF.[45] Whether these image findings are the result of other effects of amiodarone that may directly affect cardiac sympathetic function (eg, noncompetitive inhibition of α-adrenergic receptors, influence on thyroid hormone metabolism, or protection against oxidative stress), or instead an indirect effect from overall cardiac improvement, is unclear.

It is important to consider how the aforementioned could provide a way for cardiac [123]I-*m*IBG imaging to direct therapy. Although some have investigated the use of autonomic imaging to identify patients who have CHF who would most benefit from β-blockers,[46,47] given the overlap of predictive values in such studies and the high benefit-to-risk ratio of therapies, such as carvedilol and ACE inhibitors, it is unlikely that an [123]I-*m*IBG study result would preclude use of these therapies.[26] Alternatively, [123]I-*m*IBG imaging might become useful by indicating whether or not medical therapy is working satisfactorily, thereby helping to guide the use of higher risk and usually more expensive invasive interventions. A study by Matsui and colleagues[48] of 85 patients who had dilated cardiomyopathy and LVEF less than 45% showed that among 19 clinical, serum, and image variables, a worsening HMR after 6 months of optimized medical therapy had, with brain natriuretic peptide (BNP), the highest predictive value for cardiac death, with a sensitivity of 92% and a specificity of 73%. It is possible that institution of additional or alternate therapies in the patients who had worsening HMR could have improved outcome.

An increasingly used therapeutic approach to patients who have severe symptomatic CHF is cardiac resynchronization therapy (CRT). Although CRT has been shown to reduce cardiac morbidity and mortality in patients who have chronic CHF,[49] not all patients who meet currently recommended criteria improve with CRT,[50,51] and thus better ways are needed to decide who is likely to benefit. In a study of 30 patients on comprehensive medical therapy for chronic NYHA III-IV CHF and classic indications for CRT, D'Orio Nishioka and colleagues[52] showed that an HMR greater than 1.36 was an effective and the only independent predictor of response to CRT (sensitivity 75%, specificity 71%).

Many patients who have CHF deteriorate to the point at which cardiac transplantation is the only option, but of course this therapy is limited by various factors, particularly donor heart availability. Although peak exercise oxygen consumption is often a key factor prioritizing who should receive a transplant, in a study of 112 patients who had idiopathic dilated cardiomyopathy, Merlet and colleagues[31] found that HMR was a better predictor of patient outcome than peak V_{O_2}, suggesting that [123]I-*m*IBG could be better method of prioritizing patients for transplant. More work is needed on this issue, and needs also to include investigation of the potential use of [123]I-*m*IBG to guide left ventricular assist device (LVAD) therapy.

[123]I-*m*IBG IMAGING TO ASSESS THE NEED FOR AN IMPLANTABLE DEFIBRILLATOR

Although for many patients who have advanced CHF pump failure is the cause of death, up to 50% of deaths are instead sudden and unexpected, the most common mechanism likely being ventricular tachycardia (VT) or ventricular fibrillation.[53] To reduce sudden cardiac death (SCD) and thereby enhance patient survival in patients who have CHF, it is currently accepted that patients who meet defined criteria are best treated with an implantable cardioverter defibrillator (ICD), shown to significantly reduce SCD and enhance overall patient survival.[54] In SCD-HeFT (Sudden Cardiac Death in Heart Failure Trial), an ICD led to a 23% 5-year death reduction in patients who had NYHA class II-III CHF and LVEF less than 35%.[55]

Currently LVEF is used for selecting who should receive an ICD, but based on this criterion in SCD-HeFT, 14 patients need to be treated to save 1 life.[56] It is clear that LVEF alone has limited ability to predict SCD.[57] Given the potentially adverse clinical consequences of ICD implantation, including operative complications, device malfunction, pain, psychiatric problems associated with shocks, lifestyle restrictions, and a cost of about $28,000 for the device,[58] a better approach for deciding who should get an ICD is needed.

Although mechanisms of cardiac arrhythmias are complex and multifactorial, the cardiac autonomic nervous system plays a crucial role,[4,59] suggesting that ^{123}I-mIBG imaging could help identify patients at risk for arrhythmic SCD and thereby be a potential guide for selecting patients who would benefit from an ICD. Early dog work showed that artificial creation of focal areas of cardiac denervation resulted in regional ^{123}I-mIBG defects associated with production of supersensitive action potential refractory periods.[16] Subsequent work from this group showed an association between focal ^{123}I-mIBG defects and ventricular arrhythmias on Holter monitoring following MI.[60,61]

Because performing clinical research studies on the occurrence of sudden cardiac death is difficult, particularly given that ascertaining a definitive arrhythmic cause of death is often not possible, a suitable group to investigate the association of cardiac ^{123}I-mIBG findings with life-threatening ventricular arrhythmias would be patients who already have an ICD. Although occurrence of an ICD shock in these patients does not necessarily mean that they would have experienced SCD if not for the device, it is probably the best method available at this time. Using this approach, Arora

and colleagues[62] performed a pilot study on 17 patients with advanced CHF who already had an ICD, deliberately selecting a balanced group of patients with and without prior ICD discharges, and correlated cardiac image finding with the occurrence of the discharges. As expected, a reduced late HMR (threshold 1.54) was associated with increased likelihood of an ICD discharge, with a positive predictive value of 71% and a negative predictive value of 17%. Combining autonomic imaging with another measure of cardiac autonomic function (ie, the low frequency [lf] component of heart rate variability [HRV] ECG analysis) none of 3 patients who had both a high HMR and high lf component had an ICD discharge, whereas all 4 patients who had a low HMR and a low lf component did. In addition, patients who had ICD discharges had more extensive ^{123}I-mIBG/perfusion (Tc-99m sestamibi) mismatches on SPECT imaging, shown in **Fig. 3**. Representative images from this study are seen in **Fig. 4**.

A subsequent study by Nagahara and colleagues[63] of 54 prospectively followed ICD patients showed that SCD or an ICD discharge triggered by a potentially lethal arrhythmia strongly correlated with late HMR (hazard ratio = 0.141, $P = .008$) independent of numerous other variables, including LVEF. Combining HMR with LVEF or BNP gave additional predictive power. Finally, Kioka and colleagues[28] reported an association of high ^{123}I-mIBG washout and SCD.

In summary, reported studies consistently show that cardiac neuronal imaging provides better predictive potential for SCD in patients who have CHF than the currently accepted LVEF standard. The published studies are small

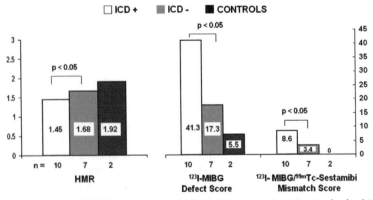

Fig. 3. ^{123}I-mIBG results in relation to the occurrence of ICD discharges in 17 patients who had ICDs and 2 control patients who did not have heart disease. Compared with patients who did not have ICD discharge (ICD −), patients with a discharge (ICD +) had a lower mean HMR, a higher mean neuronal tracer defect score, and a higher mean neuronal tracer uptake/perfusion tracer mismatch score. (*Data from* Arora R, Ferrick KJ, Nakata T, et al. I-123 MIBG imaging and heart rate variability analysis to predict the need for an implantable cardioverter defibrillator. J Nucl Cardiol 2003;10:121–31.)

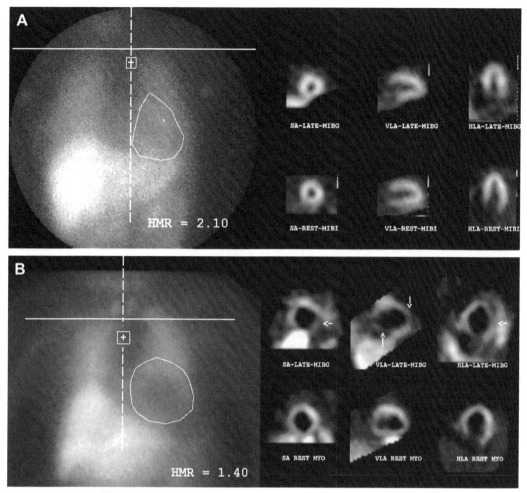

Fig. 4. Representative ^{123}I-*m*IBG images. (*A*) Images from a normal patient showing normal HMR (left-sided planar images) and absence of neuronal or perfusion tracer defects (right-sided SPECT images). (*B*) Abnormal images showing a reduced HMR (left-sided planar images) and neuronal/perfusion mismatches (right-sided SPECT images) in the lateral wall (←), distal anterior and apical walls (↓), and the mid-basal inferior wall (↑). HLA, horizontal long axis; MIBG, ^{123}I-metaiodobenzylguanidine; MIBI, ^{99m}Tc-sestamibi; MYO, ^{99m}Tc-tetrofosmin (myoview); SA, short axis; VLA, vertical long axis.[62]

and need further validation, however, before meriting wider acceptance. A high negative predictive value is crucial. At the same time, it remains to be seen whether an algorithm of neuronal imaging can be developed to efficiently and effectively identify seemingly lower risk patients, such as patients who have CHF who have high LVEFs and patients who have subclinical cardiac conditions who make up the vast majority of patients who experience SCD.[64] Furthermore, it will be important to determine how radionuclide imaging compares with other noninvasive modalities, such as HRV or electrocardiographic microvolt T-wave alternans.[65] A combination of several variables may turn out to be most useful.

NEURONAL IMAGING IN PATIENTS FOLLOWING HEART TRANSPLANT

For patients who have advanced CHF, when medical, CRT, ICD, and LVAD therapy reach the end of their benefit, cardiac transplantation may offer the only chance for long-term survival. During cardiac transplantation, postganglionic sympathetic fibers of the donor heart are interrupted, resulting in complete sympathetic denervation of the transplanted heart. The new heart thus has an impaired response to the demands of exercise. Over time, though, at least some sympathetic reinnervation occurs,[66,67] and can be assessed with cardiac neuronal imaging.[68] In a study of 20 posttransplant patients, Bengel and colleagues[69] used

[11]C-HED imaging to demonstrate progressive cardiac reinnervation, low within the first 12 to 18 months posttransplant, but progressively increasing thereafter up to at least 15 years later, and to as much as 66% of the left ventricle. A follow-up study showed a correlation between ^{11}C-HED measured reinnervation and an enhanced contractile response to exercise with improved exercise times.[70]

[123]I-mIBG IMAGING IN PATIENTS WHO HAVE ISCHEMIC HEART DISEASE

Ischemia or infarction from coronary artery disease (CAD) affects cardiac autonomic function in several ways.[71] One involves the triggering of cardiac reflex responses by stimulation of mechanosensitive and chemosensitive sensory nerve endings in ischemic myocardium, illustrated for example by inferoposterior ischemia/infarction leading to bradycardia and hypotension, and anterior ischemia/infarction causing tachycardia and hypertension. More relevant to the discussion here, though, is the effect of ischemia/infarction on impulse transmission through the sympathetic nerve trunks that course along the coronary arterial pathways before penetrating the myocardium. Myocardial ischemia/infarction disrupts sympathetic transmission, in which case myocardium distal to and beyond the site of injury but not otherwise involved in the ischemic process may be affected, resulting in perfused and viable, but denervated, myocardium. Such areas exhibit denervation supersensitivity and are prone to arrhythmias. The ^{123}I-mIBG defect pattern may depend on the type of infarction in that, using a dog model, Dae and colleagues[72] showed that although transmural injury results in distal ^{123}I-mIBG defects, nontransmural infarction instead often results in ^{123}I-mIBG defects localized to the region of infarct, probably from damage to penetrating sympathetic fibers in the subendocardial region but sparing the subepicardial nerve trunks. The situation becomes more complex in the setting of mixtures of ischemic and infarcted tissue that can occur in various directions and distributions. With regard to effects on cardiac pathophysiology and predisposition to arrhythmias, one must also consider the varying effects of ischemia/injury on parasympathetic function because vagal fibers, after the AV node, for the most part traverse the subendocardial layers.

In patient studies following acute MI, areas of sympathetic denervation are larger than areas of myocardial necrosis, with these regions of viable but sympathetically denervated myocardium seeming to predispose patients to ventricular arrhythmias.[60,61,73,74] The pathophysiology of the post-MI state was more recently assessed by Simões and colleagues[75] who performed ^{123}I-mIBG and ^{201}Tl imaging in 67 consecutive patients 14 days after the infarct. A total of 90% of the patients had MIBG/Tl mismatches whose presence correlated with prolonged QTc intervals and delayed depolarization on signal-averaged ECG, both predisposing to lethal arrhythmias. Nevertheless, over a 4.3-year follow-up, event rates were too low (2 deaths) to show any prognostic significance. The post-MI pathophysiologic cardiac neuronal state was further investigated in a study by Sasano and colleagues[76] of six pigs that had artificially produced LAD infarcts, demonstrating reduced myocardial voltage and increased inducibility of sustained VT in those that had larger areas of perfusion/innervation mismatch. Cardiac neuronal imaging may thus help identify post-MI patients who are most at risk for lethal ventricular arrhythmias, and who therefore may benefit from ICD therapy. The physiologic and histologic changes occurring post-MI are extremely complex, however, and need more investigation.

Another potential use of neuronal imaging in patients who have CAD is the identification of abnormalities after the acute ischemic insult has resolved. For example, after an episode of acute ischemia, myocardial perfusion may be restored and a perfusion defect no longer present, but the myocytes may not have totally returned to their baseline normal metabolic and functioning state. Recent work has shown that fatty acid radiotracers, such as ^{123}I-BMIPP (β-methyl-p-[^{123}I]-iodophenyl-pentadecanoic acid), often show abnormalities of metabolism in areas that were previously ischemic, so-called "ischemic memory."[77,78] For ^{123}I-BMIPP ischemic memory is possible because metabolic cellular abnormalities persist after resolution of acute ischemia. A similar situation may occur in the setting of neuronal imaging, because sympathetic nerves do not return to normal function for some time after the ischemic insult has resolved. Experimental animal studies have shown that temporal sympathetic denervation from myocardial ischemia may last from 8 to 17 weeks after myocardial ischemia.[71] In a study by Tomoda and colleagues,[79] 24 ± 12 days after an ischemic attack, only 4 of 8 patients who had non–Q-wave MI had a Tl perfusion defect, whereas all 8 had an ^{123}I-mIBG defect; although none of 12 patients who had unstable angina had a Tl-201 defect, 7 of 12 had an ^{123}I-mIBG defect. Watanabe and colleagues[80] performed rest ^{123}I-BMIPP and rest ^{123}I-mIBG studies on 50 patients within 2 weeks of documented vasospastic angina on cardiac catheterization, and found that tracer defects were seen in 86% of ^{123}I-BMIPP images and in 100% of the ^{123}I-mIBG images despite no TI-201 perfusion abnormalities appreciated.

Another potential use of ^{123}I-mIBG imaging is the detection of subclinical CAD. In an interesting study by Simula and colleagues,[81] 30 asymptomatic volunteers with a strong family history of disease underwent quantitative coronary angiography, stress ^{99m}Tc-sestamibi, and rest ^{123}I-mIBG studies. Although all subjects had normal sestamibi studies, 3 had stenoses less than 30% and 6 had stenoses 50% or greater. LAD stenosis severity (range 0%–54%) correlated directly with delayed MIBG uptake and inversely with MIBG washout, particularly in the anteroseptal region, consistent with an enhanced sympathetic response in the early stages of coronary disease. The authors postulated that subclinical endothelial dysfunction in these patients caused episodes of vasoconstriction, resulting in activation of local neurohormonal sequences of events that affected local sympathetic output and produced the image findings.

In summary, ischemic heart disease produces various effects on sympathetic innervation that can be imaged with radiotracers, with the potential to provide better understanding of the clinical situation and thereby allow more rapid and effective therapies. Much work is still needed in this area.

NEURONAL IMAGING IN PATIENTS WHO HAVE DIABETES MELLITUS

Autonomic neuropathy is a common complication of diabetes mellitus (DM), occurring in 20% to 35% of patients at presentation, and is associated with a worsened prognosis.[82,83] Although diabetic autonomic neuropathy has been customarily diagnosed with bedside maneuvers and ECG techniques (eg, Valsalva, heart rate and blood pressure response to postural changes, HRV), radiotracer imaging shows promise in more easily detecting autonomic dysfunction, often before clinical manifestations appear.[14] Langer and colleagues[84] performed ^{123}I-mIBG/^{99m}Tc-sestamibi dual isotope tomographic imaging in 65 asymptomatic patients who had type II DM and found greatly diminished tracer in all segments and in areas of MIBG/sestamibi mismatch, including in some patients who did not have clinical evidence of autonomic problems. Similarly, Hattori and colleagues[85] found ^{123}I-mIBG SPECT defects in most (60%) of 31 patients who had type II DM, but also reported abnormalities in patients who did not have clinical evidence of neuropathy, appearing initially in the inferior wall

and then gradually spreading to adjacent segments in patients who had mild and severe neuropathies, with the latter also showing a lower HMR on delayed images.

Stevens and colleagues[86] found abnormalities of ^{11}C-HED retention in 40% of autonomic neuropathy–free patients who had diabetes, again first appearing in the inferior wall and then spreading to other parts of the heart in patients who had mild or severe clinical neuropathies. In patients who had severe neuropathies, increased absolute tracer retention (hyperinnervation) was seen in proximal myocardial segments in combination with more decreased retention (denervation) in distal segments, an innervation pattern that could result in electrical stability and predispose to life-threatening arrhythmias.

The promise of using autonomic imaging to identify higher risk patients who had DM was supported in a study by Nagamachi[87] of 144 type II patients who did not have evidence of organic heart disease, followed for a mean of 7.2 years. By multivariate analysis, a combination of decreased delayed-image HMR and an abnormality on HRV predicted cardiac events (hospitalization for cardiac events, such as arrhythmia, CHF, MI), whereas abnormal delayed HMR alone was an independent predictor of all-cause mortality.

Further work is needed to determine how valuable and practical neuronal imaging could be in people who have diabetes, especially those who do not have manifestations of end-organ damage. In some cases neuronal imaging may identify patients who have subclinical ischemic coronary disease and need aggressive management, and may find patients who have autonomic heterogeneities predisposing to lethal arrhythmias.

NEURONAL IMAGING IN PATIENTS WHO HAVE PRIMARY ARRHYTHMIC DISEASES

Although lethal or potentially lethal ventricular arrhythmias are most often the result of organic heart disease, in about 5% of cases the arrhythmias are from primary electrical abnormalities, sometimes apparent from the ECG and sometimes not.[88] Mitrani and colleagues[89] saw that in 9 patients who presented with VT but had structurally normal hearts, 5 (55%) had regional sympathetic denervation compared with none of 9 control patients. Gill and colleagues[90] found asymmetrical uptake of ^{123}I-mIBG (less uptake in septum) in 7 (47%) of 15 patients who had VT and "clinically normal" hearts, particularly obvious in patients who had exercise-induced VT.

Particular neuronal tracer uptake abnormalities are seen in some of the more specifically characterized primary arrhythmic disorders. Schäfers and colleagues[91] found an abnormal volume of distribution of [11]C[HED] uptake in patients who had idiopathic right ventricular outflow tract tachycardia, and decreased uptake of the postsynaptic tracer [11][C]CGP12177 indicating reduced density of postsynaptic β-adrenoceptor density. Neuronal tracer uptake in Brugada syndrome is especially interesting in that ^{123}I-mIBG defects seem localized to the inferior and inferoseptal walls, suggesting that a local dominance of parasympathetic tone in these affected regions may be related to these patients' propensity to arrhythmogenesis.[92]

POST-CHEMOTHERAPY

Given the enhanced sensitivity of sympathetic nerves to myocardial insults, ^{123}I-mIBG imaging has been investigated as a potential method of assessing cardiac damage from chemotherapeutic agents. In studies with rats, Wakasugi and colleagues[93] showed that doxorubicin administration resulted in a decrease in cardiac uptake of ^{125}I-mIBG, preceding a decrease in LVEF. In humans, Olmos and colleagues[94] reported decreased cardiac uptake of ^{123}I-mIBG as the cumulative dose of doxorubicin increased, followed by subsequent deterioration in LVEF. Carrió and colleagues[95] showed that at a cumulative doxorubicin dose of 240 to 300 mg/m^2 there was a correlation of cardiac ^{123}I-mIBG abnormalities with cardiac uptake of ^{111}In-antimyosin antibody, but in this study there was no clear association between decreased ^{123}I-mIBG uptake and severe LV functional impairment. The potential role of ^{123}I-mIBG imaging in following patients with chemotherapy therefore shows promise, but still needs to be investigated further, particularly determining how it would add in a significant way to currently used monitoring techniques.

IMAGING OF POSTSYNAPTIC RECEPTORS

Although to this point the vast majority of cardiac neuronal investigative and clinical work has been on presynaptic imaging, postsynaptic processes also play an important role in cardiac function. Postsynaptic receptors, consisting of β and α receptors, transmit sympathetic signals to the target tissues, with the β receptors regulating chronotropic, dromotropic, and inotropic cardiac effects, and the α receptors controlling vascular tone and myocardial contractility.[5] Studying these receptors with radiotracer imaging has been difficult because of the challenge of synthesizing

tracers with sufficient target specificity and low nonspecific binding.[12]

Some clinical work has been done with ^{11}C-CGP12177, a nonselective, hydrophilic β-receptor antagonist that produces good-quality cardiac PET images. Recent work by Caldwell and colleagues[96] studied 13 patients who had ischemic CHF and 25 age-matched healthy controls using ^{11}C-HED for presynaptic imaging and ^{11}C-CGP12177 to assess postsynaptic β-adrenergic receptor (BAR) density. Although patients who had CHF had a decrease in ^{11}C-HED and in BAR density compared with controls, the decrease in HED uptake was significantly greater, resulting in marked presynaptic/postsynaptic mismatch, especially in the inferior and lateral walls. Of 4 patients who had an adverse event over 18 months, 3 had a mean mismatch score greater than 6 standard deviations above the mean of healthy subjects.

Cardiac neuronal pathophysiology is more complex than just imaging presynaptic function, and using neuronal imaging to predict outcomes such as arrhythmic death will likely require more comprehensive assessment. Because synthesis of ^{11}C-CGP12177 is laborious and demanding, other potential postsynaptic imaging tracers, both β and α, are under investigation, and are shown in **Table 2**.[5,12]

IMAGING OF CARDIAC PARASYMPATHETIC FUNCTION

Abnormalities of parasympathetic activity also contribute to cardiac pathophysiology. For example, parasympathetic innervation and activation can induce and maintain atrial fibrillation, whereas ablation can induce parasympathetic denervation and improve clinical outcome.[97,98] Unfortunately, radiotracer imaging of the cardiac parasympathetic innervation is difficult for various reasons, including low density of cholinergic neurons in the heart and rapid degradation of acetylcholine making tracer design difficult. Among tracers under investigation are ^{18}F-FEOBV (a vesamicol derivative), ^{11}C-MQNB (a postsynaptic muscarine receptor antagonist), and 2-deoxy-2-[^{18}F]fluoro-d-glucose-A85380 (visualizes nicotinic acetylcholine receptors).[12]

SUMMARY

Imaging of the cardiac neuronal system with radiotracers shows promise as a potentially powerful tool to evaluate patients who have various cardiac conditions and to direct patient management in guiding pharmacologic therapy, implanting

Table 2
Radiotracers for imaging of postsynaptic sympathetic innervation

Tracer	Receptor Type	Subtype	Comments
C-11 CGP12177	β	Nonselective	Clinical studies available and promising, with good quality images. Difficult synthesis.
C-11 CGP12388	β	Nonselective	Easier synthesis than C-11 CGP12177. Some studies in humans
F-18 fluorocarazolol	β	Nonselective	Lipophilic, poor heart–lung contrast
C-11 CGP26505	β	1	Low specific binding
C-11 bisoprolol	β	1	Low specific binding
C-11 formoterol	β	2	Low specific binding
C-11 procaterol	β	2	Low specific binding
C-11 prazosin	α	1	Low specific binding
C-11 GB67	α	1	Analog of prazosin. Good tracer uptake found in small human studies, with high selectivity

Data from Bengel FM, Schwaiger M. Assessment of cardiac sympathetic neuronal function using PET imaging. J Nucl Cardiol 2004;11:607.

mechanical devices, and determining the need for cardiac transplant. Given that radiotracer imaging allows visualization and quantitative measurements of the underlying molecular aspects of cardiac disease, it should provide a perspective that other cardiac tests cannot.

REFERENCES

1. Carrió I. Cardiac neurotransmission imaging. J Nucl Med 2001;42(7):1062–76.
2. Zipes DP. Autonomic Modulation of Cardiac Arrhythmias. In: Zipes DP, Jalife J, editors. Cardiac electrophysiology: from cell to bedside. 2nd edition. Philadelphia: W.B. Saunders Company; 1995. p. 441–2.
3. Flotats A, Carrio I. Cardiac neurotransmission SPECT imaging. J Nucl Cardiol 2004;11:587–602.
4. Verrier RL, Antzelevich C. Autonomic aspects of arrhythmogenesis: the enduring and the new. Curr Opin Cardiol 2004;19:2–11.
5. Bengel FM, Schwaiger M. Assessment of cardiac sympathetic neuronal function using PET imaging. J Nucl Cardiol 2004;11:603–16.
6. Sisson JC, Wieland DM. Radiolabelled meta-iodobenzylguanidine pharmacology: pharmacology and clinical studies. Am J Physiol Imaging 1986;1:96–103.
7. Goldstein DS, Holmes CS, Dendi R, et al. Orthostatic hypotension from sympathetic denervation in Parkinson's disease. Neurology 2002;58:1247–55.
8. Kline RC, Swanson DP, Wieland DM, et al. Myocardial imaging in man with I-123 metaiodobenzylguanidine. J Nucl Med 1981;22:129–32.
9. Wieland DM, Brown LE, Rogers WL, et al. Myocardial imaging with a radioiodinated norepinephrine storage analog. J Nucl Med 1981;22:22–31.
10. Hattori N, Schwaiger M. Metaiodobenzylguanidine scintigraphy of the heart. What have we learned clinically? Eur J Nucl Med 2000;27:1–6.
11. Luisi AJ, Suzuki G, deKemp R, et al. Regional ^{11}C-hydroxyephedrine retention in hibernating myocardium: chronic inhomogeneity of sympathetic innervation in the absence of infarction. J Nucl Med 2005;46:1368–74.
12. Lautamäki R, Tipre D, Bengel FM. Cardiac sympathetic neuronal imaging using PET. Eur J Nucl Med Mol Imaging 2007;34:S74–85.
13. Langer O, Halldin C. PET and SPECT tracers for mapping the cardiac nervous system. Eur J Nucl Med Mol Imaging 2002;29:416–34.
14. Patel AD, Iskandrian AE. MIBG imaging. J Nucl Cardiol 2002;9:75–94.
15. Chen JI, Garcia EV, Galt JR, et al. Optimized acquisition and processing protocols for I-123 cardiac SPECT imaging. J Nucl Cardiol 2006;13:251–60.
16. Minardo JD, Tuli MM, Mock BH, et al. Scintigraphic and electrophysiologic evidence of canine myocardial sympathetic denervation and reinnervation produced by myocardial infarction or phenol application. Circulation 1988;78:1008–19.
17. Agostini D, Belin A, Amar MH, et al. Improvement of cardiac neuronal function after carvedilol treatment in dilated cardiomyopathy: a ^{123}I-MIBG scintigraphic study. J Nucl Med 2000;41:845–51.
18. Ogita H, Shimonagata T, Fukunami M, et al. Prognostic significance of cardiac ^{123}I metaiodobenzylguanidine imaging for mortality and morbidity in

patients with chronic heart failure: a prospective study. Heart 2001;86:656–60.

19. Yamada T, Shimonagata T, Fukunami M, et al. Comparison of the prognostic value of cardiac iodine-123 metaiodobenzylguanidine imaging and heart rate variability in patients with chronic heart failure. J Am Coll Cardiol 2003;41:231–8.

20. Somsen GA, Verberne HJ, Fleury E, et al. Normal values and within-subject variability of cardiac I-123 MIBG scintigraphy in healthy individuals: implications for clinical studies. J Nucl Cardiol 2004;11:126–33.

21. Gill JS, Hunter GJ, Gane G, et al. Heterogeneity of the human myocardial sympathetic innervation: in vivo demonstration by iodine 123-labeled metaiodobenzylguanidine scintigraphy. Am Heart J 1993;126:390–8.

22. Morozumi T, Kusuoka H, Fukuchi K, et al. Myocardial iodine-123-metaiodobenzylguanidine images and autonomic nerve activity in normal subjects. J Nucl Med 1997;38:49–52.

23. Tsuchimochi S, Tamaki N, Tadamura E, et al. Age and gender differences in normal myocardial adrenergic neuronal function evaluated by iodine-123-MIBG imaging. J Nucl Med 1995;36:969–74.

24. Estorch M, Serra-Grima R, Flotats A, et al. Myocardial sympathetic innervation in the athlete's sinus bradycardia: is there selective inferior myocardial wall denervation? J Nucl Cardiol 2000;7:354–8.

25. Bülow HH, Nekolla SG, Schwaiger M, et al. Comparison of the normal distribution of three tracers used for evaluation of the presynaptic sympathetic neuron. J Nucl Cardiol 2003;10:S44.

26. Udelson JE, Shafer CD, Carrió I. Radionuclide imaging in heart failure: assessing etiology and outcomes and implications for management. J Nucl Cardiol 2002;9:S40–52.

27. Chen GP, Tabibiazar R, Branch KR, et al. Cardiac receptor physiology and imaging: an update. J Nucl Cardiol 2005;12:714–30.

28. Kioka H, Yamada T, Mine T, et al. Prediction of sudden death in patients with mild-to-moderate chronic heart failure by using cardiac iodine-123 metaiodobenzylguanidine imaging. Heart 2007;93:1213–8.

29. Anastasiou-Nana MI, Terrovitis JV, Athanasoulis T, et al. Prognostic value of iodine-123-metaiodobenzylguanidine myocardial uptake and heart rate variability in chronic congestive heart failure secondary to ischemic or idiopathic dilated cardiomyopathy. Am J Cardiol 2005;96:427–31.

30. Arimoto T, Takeishi Y, Niizeki T, et al. Cardiac sympathetic denervation and ongoing myocardial damage for prognosis in early stages of heart failure. J Card Fail 2007;13:34–41.

31. Merlet P, Benvenuti C, Moyse D, et al. Prognostic value of MIBG imaging in idiopathic dilated cardiomyopathy. J Nucl Med 1999;40:917–23.

32. Merlet P, Valette H, Dubois-Randé J, et al. Prognostic value of cardiac metaiodobenzylguanidine in patients with heart failure. J Nucl Med 1992;33:471–7.

33. Nakata T, Miyamoto K, Doi A, et al. Cardiac death prediction and impaired cardiac sympathetic innervation assessed by MIBG in patients with failing and nonfailing hearts. J Nucl Cardiol 1998;5:579–90.

34. Agostini D, Verberne HJ, Burchert W, et al. I-123-mIBG myocardial imaging for assessment of risk for a major cardiac event in heart failure patients: insights from a retrospective European multicenter study. Eur J Nucl Med Mol Imaging 2008;35:535–46.

35. Jacobson AF, Lombard J, Banerjee G, et al. 123-I-mIBG scintigraphy to predict risk for adverse cardiac outcomes in heart failure patients: design of two prospective multicenter international trials. J Nucl Cardiol 2009;16:113–21.

36. Wakabayashi T, Nakata T, Hashimoto A, et al. Assessment of underlying etiology and cardiac sympathetic innervation to identify patients at high risk of cardiac death. J Nucl Med 2001;42:1757–67.

37. Merlet P, Pouillart F, Dubois-Randé J, et al. Sympathetic nerve alterations assessed with ^{123}I-MIBG in the failing human heart. J Nucl Med 1999;40:224–31.

38. Lotze U, Kaepplinger S, Kober A, et al. Recovery of the cardiac adrenergic nervous system after long-term β-blocker therapy in idiopathic dilated cardiomyopathy: assessment by increase in myocardial ^{123}I-metaiodobenzylguanidine uptake. J Nucl Med 2001;42:49–54.

39. Cohen-Solal A, Rouzet F, Berdeaux A, et al. Effects of carvedilol on myocardial sympathetic innervation in patients with chronic heart failure. J Nucl Med 2005;46:1796–803.

40. Gerson MC, Craft LL, McGuire N, et al. Carvedilol improves left ventricular function in heart failure patients with idiopathic dilated cardiomyopathy and a wide range of sympathetic nervous system function as measured by iodine 123 metaiodobenzylguanidine. J Nucl Cardiol 2002;9:608–15.

41. Takeishi Y, Atsumi H, Fujiwara S, et al. ACE inhibition reduces cardiac iodine-123-MIBG release in heart failure. J Nucl Med 1997;38:1085–9.

42. Toyama T, Aihara Y, Iwasaki T, et al. Cardiac sympathetic activity estimated by ^{123}I-MIBG myocardial imaging in patients with dilated cardiomyopathy after β-blocker or angiotensin-converting enzyme inhibitor therapy. J Nucl Med 1999;40:217–23.

43. Kasama S, Toyama T, Kumakura H, et al. Addition of valsartan to an angiotensin-converting enzyme inhibitor improves cardiac sympathetic nerve activity and left ventricular function in patients with congestive heart failure. J Nucl Med 2003;44:884–90.

44. Kasama S, Toyama T, Kumakura H, et al. Spironolactone improves cardiac sympathetic nerve activity and symptoms in patients with congestive heart failure. J Nucl Med 2002;43:1279–85.

45. Toyama T, Hoshizaki H, Seki R, et al. Efficacy of amiodarone treatment on cardiac symptom, function, and sympathetic nerve activity in patients with dilated cardiomyopathy: comparison with β-blocker therapy. J Nucl Cardiol 2004;11:134–41.

46. Suwa M, Otake Y, Moriguchi A, et al. Iodine-123 metaiodobenzylguanidine myocardial scintigraphy for prediction of response to β-blocker therapy in patients with dilated cardiomyopathy. Am Heart J 1997;133:353–8.

47. Choi JY, Lee KH, Hong KP, et al. Iodine-123 MIBG imaging before treatment of heart failure with carvedilol to predict improvement of left ventricular function and exercise capacity. J Nucl Cardiol 2001;8:4–9.

48. Matsui T, Tsutamoto T, Maeda K, et al. Prognostic value of repeated ^{123}I-metaiodobenzylguanidine imaging in patients with dilated cardiomyopathy with congestive heart failure before and after optimized treatments—comparison with neurohumoral factors. Circ J 2002;66:537–43.

49. Cleland JG, Daubert JC, Erdmann E, et al. The effect of cardiac resynchronization on morbidity and mortality in heart failure. N Engl J Med 2005;352:1539–49.

50. Swedberg K, Cleland J, Dargie H, et al. Guidelines for the diagnosis and treatment of chronic failure: executive summary (update 2005): The Task Force for the Diagnosis and Treatment of Chronic Heart Failure of the European Society of Cardiology. Eur Heart J 2005;26:1115–40.

51. Yu CM, Zhang Q, Fung JW, et al. A novel tool to assess systolic asynchrony and identify responders of cardiac resynchronization therapy by tissue synchronization imaging. J Am Coll Cardiol 2005; 45:677–84.

52. D'Orio Nishioka SA, Filho MM, Soares Brandão SC, et al. Cardiac sympathetic activity pre and post resynchronization therapy evaluated by ^{123}I-MIBG myocardial scintigraphy. J Nucl Cardiol 2007;14:852–9.

53. Tomaselli GF, Zipes DP. What causes sudden death in heart failure? Circ Res 2004;95:754–63.

54. Zipes DP, Camm AJ, Borggrefe M, et al. ACC/AHA/ESC 2006 guidelines for management of patients with ventricular arrhythmias and the prevention of sudden cardiac death—executive summary: a report of the American College of Cardiology/American Heart Association Task Force and the European Society of Cardiology Committee for Practice Guidelines Writing Committee to Develop Guidelines for Management of Patients with Ventricular Arrhythmias and the Prevention of Sudden Cardiac Death. J Am Coll Cardiol 2006;48:1064–108.

55. Bardy GH, Lee KL, Mark DB, et al. Amiodarone or an implantable defibrillator for congestive heart failure. N Engl J Med 2005;352:225–37.

56. Fisher JD, Hector HE. Relative and absolute benefits: main results should be reported in absolute terms. Pacing Clin Electrophysiol 2007;30:935–7.

57. Buxton AE, Lee KL, Hafley GE, et al. For the MUSTT Investigators. Limitations of ejection fraction for prediction of sudden death risk in patients with coronary artery disease. J Am Coll Cardiol 2007;50:1150–7.

58. Sanders GD, Hlatky MA, Owens DK. Cost-effectiveness of implantable cardioverter-defibrillators. N Engl J Med 2005;353:1471–80.

59. Barron HV, Lesh MD. Autonomic nervous system and sudden cardiac death. J Am Coll Cardiol 1996;27:1053–60.

60. Stanton MS, Tuli MM, Radtke NL, et al. Regional sympathetic denervation after MI in humans detected noninvasively using I-123-MIBG. J Am Coll Cardiol 1989;14:1519–26.

61. McGhie AI, Corbett JR, Akers MS, et al. Regional cardiac adrenergic function using I-123 MIBG SPECT imaging after acute myocardial infarction. Am J Cardiol 1991;67:236–42.

62. Arora R, Ferrick KJ, Nakata T, et al. I-123 MIBG imaging and heart rate variability analysis to predict the need for an implantable cardioverter defibrillator. J Nucl Cardiol 2003;10:121–31.

63. Nagahara D, Nakata T, Hashimoto A, et al. Predicting the need for an implantable cardioverter defibrillator using cardiac metaiodobenzylguanidine activity together with plasma natriuretic peptide concentration or left ventricular function. J Nucl Med 2008;49:225–33.

64. Exner DV, Klein GJ, Prystowsky EN. Primary prevention of sudden death with implantable defibrillator therapy in patients with cardiac disease: can we afford to do it? (Can we afford not to?). Circulation 2001;104:1564–70.

65. Chow T, Kereiakes DJ, Bartone C, et al. Microvolt T-wave alternans identified patients with ischemic cardiomyopathy who benefit from implantable cardioverter-defibrillator therapy. J Am Coll Cardiol 2007; 49:50–8.

66. Wilson RF, Christensen BV, Olivari MT, et al. Evidence for structural sympathetic reinnervation after orthotopic cardiac transplantation in humans. Circulation 1991;38:1210–20.

67. Hunt S. Reinnervation of the transplanted heart—why is it important? N Engl J Med 2001;345:762–4.

68. Schwaiger M, Hutchins GD, Kalff V, et al. Evidence for regional catecholamine uptake and storage sites in the transplanted human heart by positron emission tomography. J Clin Invest 1991;87:1681–90.

69. Bengel FM, Ueberfuhr P, Ziegler SI, et al. Serial assessment of sympathetic reinnervation after

orthotopic heart transplantation. A longitudinal study using PET and C-11 hydroxyephedrine. Circulation 1999;99:1866–71.

70. Bengel FM, Ueberfuhr P, Schiepel N, et al. Effect of sympathetic reinnervation on cardiac performance after heart transplantation. N Engl J Med 2001;345:731–8.

71. Zipes DP. Influence of myocardial ischemia and infarction on autonomic innervation of heart. Circulation 1990;82:1095–105.

72. Dae MW, Herre JM, O'Connell JW, et al. Scintigraphic assessment of sympathetic innervation after transmural versus nontransmural myocardial infarction. J Am Coll Cardiol 1991;17:1416–23.

73. Matsunari I, Schricke U, Bengel FM, et al. Extent of cardiac sympathetic neuronal damage is determined by the area of ischemia in patients with acute coronary syndrome. Circulation 2000;101:2579–85.

74. Bengel FM, Barthel P, Matsunari I, et al. Kinetics of ^{123}I-MIBG after acute myocardial infarction and reperfusion therapy. J Nucl Med 1999;40:904–10.

75. Simões MV, Barthel P, Matsunari I, et al. Presence of sympathetically denervated but viable myocardium and its electrophysiologic correlates after early revascularised, acute myocardial infarction. Eur Heart J 2004;25:551–7.

76. Sasano T, Abraham R, Chang KC, et al. Abnormal sympathetic innervation of viable myocardium and the substrate of ventricular tachycardia after myocardial infarction. J Am Coll Cardiol 2008;51:2266–75.

77. Kawai Y, Tsukamoto E, Nozaki Y, et al. Significance of reduced uptake of iodinated fatty acid analogue for the evaluation of patients with acute chest pain. J Am Coll Cardiol 2001;38:1888–94.

78. Dilsizian V, Bateman TM, Bergmann SR, et al. Metabolic imaging with β-methyl-p-^{123}I]-iodophenyl-pentadecanoic acid identifies ischemic memory after demand ischemia. Circulation 2005;112:2169–74.

79. Tomoda H, Yoshioka K, Shiina Y, et al. Regional sympathetic denervation detected by iodine 123 metaiodobenzylguanidine in non-Q-wave myocardial infarction and unstable angina. Am Heart J 1994;128:452–8.

80. Watanabe K, Takahashi T, Miyajima S, et al. Myocardial sympathetic denervation, fatty acid metabolism, and left ventricular wall motion in vasospastic angina. J Nucl Med 2002;43:1476–81.

81. Simula S, Vanninen E, Viitanen L, et al. Cardiac adrenergic innervation is affected in asymptomatic subjects with very early stage of coronary disease. J Nucl Med 2002;43:1–7.

82. Ewing DJ, Campbell IW, Clarke BF. The natural history of diabetic autonomic neuropathy. QJM 1980;49:95–108.

83. Dyrberg T, Benn J, Christianses JS, et al. Prevalence of autonomic neuropathy measured by simple bedside tests. Diabetologia 1981;20:190–4.

84. Langer A, Freeman MR, Josse RG, et al. Metaiodobenzylguanidine imaging in diabetes mellitus: assessment of cardiac sympathetic denervation and its relation to autonomic dysfunction and silent myocardial ischemia. J Am Coll Cardiol 1995;25:610–8.

85. Hattori N, Tamaki N, Hayashi T, et al. Regional abnormality of iodine-123-MIBG in diabetic hearts. J Nucl Med 1996;27:1985–90.

86. Stevens MJ, Raffel DM, Allman KC, et al. Cardiac sympathetic dysinnervation in diabetes. Implications for enhanced cardiovascular risk. Circulation 1998;98:961–8.

87. Nagamachi S, Fujita S, Nishii R, et al. Prognostic value of cardiac I-123 metaiodobenzylguanidine imaging in patients with non-insulin-dependent diabetes mellitus. J Nucl Cardiol 2006;13:34–42.

88. Huikuri HV, Castellanos A, Myerburg RJ. Sudden death due to cardiac arrhythmias. N Engl J Med 2001;345:1473–82.

89. Mitrani RD, Klein LS, Miles WM, et al. Regional cardiac sympathetic denervation in patients with ventricular tachycardia in the absence of coronary artery disease. J Am Coll Cardiol 1993;22:1344–53.

90. Gill JS, Hunter GJ, Gane J, et al. Asymmetry of cardiac ^{123}I] meta-iodobenzylguanidine scans in patients with ventricular tachycardia and a "clinically normal" heart. Br Heart J 1993;69:6–13.

91. Schäfers M, Lerch H, Wichter T, et al. Cardiac sympathetic innervation in patients with idiopathic right ventricular outflow tract tachycardia. J Am Coll Cardiol 1998;32:181–6.

92. Wichter T, Matheja P, Eckardt L, et al. Cardiac autonomic dysfunction in Brugada syndrome. Circulation 2002;105:702–6.

93. Wakasugi S, Fischman AJ, Babich JW, et al. Metaiodobenzylguanidine: evaluation of its potential as a tracer for monitoring doxorubicin cardiomyopathy. J Nucl Med 1993;34:1282–6.

94. Valdés Olmos RA, ten Bokkel Huinink WW, ten Hoeve RFA, et al. Assessment of anthracycline-related myocardial adrenergic derangement by ^{123}I]Metaiodobenzylguanidine scintigraphy. Eur J Cancer 1995;31:26–31.

95. Carrió I, Estorch M, Berná L, et al. Assessment of anthracycline-related myocardial adrenergic Indium-111-antimyosin and iodine-123-MIBG studies in early assessment of doxorubicin cardiotoxicity. J Nucl Med 1995;36:2024–49.

96. Caldwell JH, Link JM, Levy WC, et al. Evidence for pre- to postsynaptic mismatch of the cardiac

sympathetic nervous system in ischemic congestive heart failure. J Nucl Med 2008;49:234–41.

97. Arora R, Ng J, Ulphani J, et al. Unique autonomic profile of the pulmonary veins and posterior left atrium. J Am Coll Cardiol 2007;49:1340–8.

98. Lellouche N, Buch E, Celigoj A, et al. Functional characterization of atrial electrograms in sinus rhythm delineates sites of parasympathetic innervation in patients with paroxysmal atrial fibrillation. J Am Coll Cardiol 2007;50:1324–31.

New Molecular Imaging Targets to Characterize Myocardial Biology

Alan R. Morrison, MD, PhD, Albert J. Sinusas, MD*

KEYWORDS

- Molecular imaging • Angiogenesis • Inflammation
- Ventricular remodeling • Apoptosis
- Radionuclide imaging • SPECT/CT • PET/CT

ROLE OF MOLECULAR IMAGING

As a greater understanding of the complex molecular interactions that take place within an organism in the physiologic and pathologic states develops, there is an opportunity to design more precise and effective medical therapies that carry less of a burden of side effects and invasive injuries. This evolution of truly individualized health care will require enough knowledge of an individual's genome and proteome to model molecular interactions from levels of gene expression to the complex milieu and kinetics of protein expression and post-translational modification that occur in physiologic and pathologic processes. New therapies that target specific molecular pathways can then be developed to affect outcomes before disease burden affects the health and productivity of an individual in question. To track disease and intervention, a parallel engineering of tools to image specific molecular events must take place that allows assessment of the in vivo state before and after any intervention is performed. This article reviews the molecular-based nuclear imaging approaches for evaluation of critical processes within the myocardium, such as angiogenesis, apoptosis, inflammation, and ventricular remodeling.

APPROACHES TO MOLECULAR IMAGING

The application of imaging using biologically targeted markers (ie, molecular imaging) has several requirements.[1] Selection of a molecular target that adequately represents the process being studied is critical to the specificity of any imaging approach. The next requirement is a readily synthesizable probe that binds to the target molecule with a high degree of specificity. Last, an imaging technology that provides the best combination of sensitivity and resolution (spatial and temporal) to identify and localize the probe within the target organ system must be available. Molecular imaging approaches are currently being developed for most of the imaging modalities, including nuclear, magnetic resonance, CT, optical fluorescence, bioluminescence, and ultrasound.[2] Although each modality carries strengths and weaknesses, the practical limitations of cost and widespread availability will likely be what allow any modality to be adapted for clinical use. The focus of this article is the specific applications of the nuclear imaging approaches.

NUCLEAR IMAGING

Single photon emission computed tomography (SPECT) and positron emission tomography (PET) are imaging techniques that make use of radiolabeled probes and have been used for more than 3 decades. Radiolabeling has the unique advantage of augmenting low signal intensity objects. For example, PET can detect picomolar and nanomolar concentrations of a molecule of interest.[2] Although SPECT offers the advantage of decreased cost and widespread availability, PET offers the advantages of increased sensitivity with the ability to quantitate and repetitively image through tracers with ultrashort half-lives.

Yale University School of Medicine, Section of Cardiovascular Medicine, 3FMP, P.O. Box 208017, New Haven, CT 06520-8017, USA
* Corresponding author.
E-mail address: albert.sinusas@yale.edu (A.J. Sinusas).

Cardiol Clin 27 (2009) 329–344
doi:10.1016/j.ccl.2008.12.008

Traditionally, nuclear imaging modalities have been limited by attenuation artifacts from soft tissue and partial volume effects. More recent systems combining CT imaging with either SPECT or PET have allowed for attenuation correction, leading to improved imaging quantification.

The article reviews several important areas of active cardiovascular research in which nuclear-based molecular imaging have been used, including the processes of angiogenesis, apoptosis, inflammation, and ventricular remodeling. Key molecular events or signaling proteins involved in each process that were identified through basic research have served as targets for imaging. Some molecular signals overlap between biologic processes, which emphasizes the importance of understanding the setting in which a molecular event takes place.

PROCESSES WITHIN THE MYOCARDIUM
Angiogenesis

Atherosclerotic disease can lead to chronic ischemia in areas of myocardium, which may stimulate an angiogenic response to restore perfusion. Angiogenesis is defined as the process of sprouting new capillaries from preexisting microvessels.[3] There is a great interest in understanding the processes of angiogenesis to design therapeutic treatments that allow revascularization through a stimulated angiogenic response. This angiogenic process often occurs in association with arteriogenesis, which represents the remodeling of larger preexisting vascular channels or collateral vessels feeding the microvascular network. The goal for any revascularization strategy would be to initiate angiogenesis and arteriogenesis to create an effective blood delivery system. There is a large body of literature devoted to understanding these phenomena.[4] Angiogenesis seems to be stimulated by external processes, such as ischemia, hypoxia, inflammation, and shear stress. Several cell types are involved in the process, including endothelial cells, smooth muscle cells, blood-derived macrophages, circulating stem cells, and the interaction of these cells within the tissue of extracellular matrix proteins. Potential targets for molecular imaging of angiogenesis can be divided into three major categories.[5] Non-endothelial targets, such as molecules associated with monocytes, macrophages, and stem cells, fall into one category. The second category includes endothelial cell targets, such as vascular endothelial growth factor (VEGF), integrins, CD13, and syndecan-4. Extracellular matrix proteins compose the final group of molecules that might serve as targets.

Biology of angiogenesis

Hypoxia, the imbalance between oxygen delivery and demand in a given tissue, can be a potent stimulator of angiogenesis. Hypoxic conditions, such as myocardial ischemia or infarction, result in up-regulation of the transcriptional activator hypoxia-inducible factor 1 (HIF-1).[6] Up-regulation of HIF-1 leads to transcription of vascular endothelial growth factor (VEGF) and the VEGF receptors (VEGFRs) Flt-1 (VEGFR-1) and FLK-1 (VEGFR-2).[7–10] When VEGF binds to these receptors on the surface of endothelial cells, a signal is transduced through their tyrosine kinase activity. This signal initiates a series of processes that results in endothelial cell proliferation, migration, survival, and angiogenesis.[11] The process also involves the activation molecules, such as integrins and matrix metalloproteinases (MMPs), and the recruitment of inflammatory cells, such as macrophages.

Integrins are a family of heterodimeric ($\alpha\beta$) cell-surface receptors that mediate divalent cation-dependent cell–cell and cell–matrix adhesion and signaling through tightly regulated interactions with their respective ligands.[12] During angiogenesis, endothelial cells make use of integrins to adhere to one another and the extracellular matrix to construct and extend new vessels. Integrins are capable of mediating an array of cellular processes, including cell adhesion, migration, proliferation, differentiation, and survival by way of several signal transduction pathways.[13,14] Activation of c-Jun NH2-terminal kinase (JNK) and extracellular signal-regulated kinase (ERK) may lead to endothelial cell-induced remodeling of the extracellular matrix in response to mechanical stimuli. Specifically, the endothelial cell integrin, $\alpha_v\beta_3$, allows cells to interact with the extracellular matrix in a way that aids in endothelial cell migration.[15] Through outside-in signaling, integrin $\alpha_v\beta_3$ also plays a critical role in the survival of cells undergoing angiogenesis.[16]

Other molecules have been identified in this schema of endothelial cell activation. Syndecan-4 is a transmembrane heparin sulfate carrying core protein that promotes VEGF to VEGFR binding and signaling by activation of protein kinase C.[17] CD13, a cell surface antigen that is expressed in endothelial cells, is an aminopeptidase that serves as a membrane-bound metalloproteinase that seems to be essential for capillary tube formation.[18]

Molecular targets used for radiotracer-based imaging of angiogenesis

Vascular endothelial growth factor receptors VEGFRs have been targeted for imaging in models of ischemia-induced angiogenesis. Radiolabeled-VEGF$_{121}$ has been used to effectively identify angiogenesis in a rabbit model of hindlimb ischemia.[19] In this study, KDR and Flt-1 receptor expression was increased in the immunohistochemistry analysis of the skeletal muscle, supporting the theoretic hypoxic-driven angiogenic response. One concern of the study is the biodistribution of the radiotracer, which revealed 20-fold higher levels in critical organs (liver, kidneys) compared with ischemic limb, which is presumably related to relative VEGFR density in these organ systems.

A PET tracer, ^{64}Cu-6DOTA-VEGF$_{121}$, was recently developed for imaging angiogenesis in a rat model of myocardial infarction (**Fig. 1**).[20] Rats underwent ligation of the left coronary artery and subsequent PET imaging at various time points post myocardial infarction. The investigators hypothesized that this tracer would detect early angiogenic signals because ischemia drives VEGFR expression. Coregistration of images was performed using CT, and the zone of infarct was demonstrated using ^{18}F-labeled deoxyglucose (FDG) uptake. The study demonstrated that ^{64}Cu-6DOTA-VEGF$_{121}$–specific signal was present in the infarct region and peaked on day 3 consistent with the changing levels of VEGFR

expression in the tissue as analyzed by immunofluorescence microscopy.

Another type of cardiac-specific reporter has been developed as a gene expression system for use in rats with microPET imaging.[21] Briefly, the system involves adenovirus delivery of mutated thymidine kinase under the control of a cytomegalovirus promoter that drives expression in myocardial cells. The reporter probe is ^{18}F-FHBG, which crosses the myocardial membrane and gets phosphorylated by the thymidine kinase. Phosphorylation essentially traps the ^{18}F-FHGB in the myocardium for subsequent microPET imaging. Early studies revealed that the localized site of the mutated thymidine kinase, HSV1-sr39tk, corresponded closely with that defined by postmortem autoradiography, histology, and immunohistochemistry.[22] Other studies have demonstrated the feasibility of using a similar reporter system in pigs using a clinical PET scanner.[23] The reporter system was then linked to VEGF to assess feasibility of developing an approach that links therapy and imaging.[24] Early experiments with rat embryonic cardiomyocytes revealed a strong correlation that both the mutated

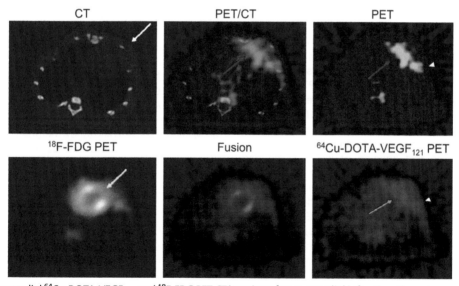

Fig. 1. Myocardial ^{64}Cu-DOTA-VEGF$_{121}$ and ^{18}F-FDG PET-CT imaging after myocardial infarction. Upper images demonstrate co-registered images of microCT (*left*), PET (*right*), and fused PET/CT image (*center*) in a representative animal after myocardial infarction. The ^{64}Cu-DOTA-VEGF$_{121}$ signal is detected by PET in the anterolateral myocardium (PET and fused images, *red arrow*). Intercostal muscle layer is designated on microCT image with a white arrow. There is some increased uptake in area of surgical wound (PET image, *arrowhead*). Lower images demonstrate ^{64}Cu-DOTA-VEGF$_{121}$ (*left*), ^{18}F-FDG (*right*), and ^{64}Cu-DOTAVEGF$_{121}$/^{18}F-FDG fused image (*middle*). ^{18}F-FDG scan shows that coronary artery ligation resulted in development of a scar by lack of ^{18}F-FDG uptake (*yellow arrow*) and that uptake of ^{64}Cu-DOTA-VEGF$_{121}$ occurs in the region of that scar (*turquoise arrow*). Fusion of both scans results in complementation of ^{18}F-FDG and ^{64}Cu-DOTA-VEGF$_{121}$ signals. Again, increased uptake in area of surgical wound is designated with an arrowhead. (*Reprinted from* Rodriguez-Porcel M, Cai W, Gheysens O, et al. Imaging of VEGF receptor in a rat myocardial infarction model using PET. J Nucl Med. 2008;49:667–73; reprinted by permission of the Society for Nuclear Medicine.)

thymidine kinase and VEGF were expressed in the same cells. Further studies involved injection of the VEGF/thymidine kinase reporter system in models of ischemia. Using microPET, cardiac transgene expression was assessed and the in vivo imaging correlated well with ex vivo tissue studies for gamma counting, thymidine kinase activity, and VEGF levels. There appeared to be increased capillaries and small blood vessels in the VEGF-treated myocardium; however, there was no improvement in perfusion assessed by nitrogen-13 ammonia imaging or metabolism assessed with ^{18}F-FDG imaging. These studies suggest that a reporter system can be developed to help visualize the effectiveness of delivering VEGF gene therapies for stimulation of angiogenesis.

Integrin $\alpha_v\beta_3$ Imaging angiogenic vessels through targeting of $\alpha_v\beta_3$ integrin was first proposed through a series of magnetic resonance imaging studies using a monoclonal antibody to $\alpha_v\beta_3$ tagged with a paramagnetic contrast agent.[25] Such studies were complicated by poor clearance of the tracer from the blood pool. Later studies made use of several $\alpha_v\beta_3$ antagonists that were radiolabeled.[26,27] These studies made use of the arginine-glycine-aspartate (RGD)–binding sequence on integrins by synthesizing RGD analogs.

An ^{111}In-labeled quinolone (^{111}In-RP748) revealed high affinity and selectivity for $\alpha_v\beta_3$ integrin in adhesion assays.[28] Subsequent studies using a cy3-labeled homolog of ^{111}In-RP748 demonstrated preferential binding to activated $\alpha_v\beta_3$ integrins on endothelial cells in culture, with localization to cell–cell contact points.[29] Initial studies with this agent focused on imaging tumor angiogenesis, although the first imaging of ischemia-induced myocardial angiogenesis using ^{111}In-RP748 was performed in rat and canine models of infarction.[30] In these studies, ^{111}In-RP748 demonstrated favorable kinetics for in vivo SPECT imaging ischemia-induced angiogenesis of the heart. Relative ^{111}In-RP748 activity was markedly increased in the infarcted region acutely and persisted for at least 3 weeks post reperfusion.[30,31] Targeted imaging with ^{111}In-RP748 has demonstrated integrin $\alpha_v\beta_3$ activation early postinfarction, suggesting a role for this technique in early detection of angiogenesis and for detection of chronic ischemia (**Fig. 2**).[31]

Other experiments, using a ^{99m}Tc-labeled peptide, NC100692, in the rodent model of hindlimb ischemia for targeting of $\alpha_v\beta_3$ integrin, have also been performed and support the value of integrin imaging in models of peripheral arterial disease.[32] The recent imaging of $\alpha_v\beta_3$ integrin by the PET imaging tracer ^{18}F-Galakto-RGD in a patient who had a transmural myocardial infarction 2 weeks prior demonstrates the feasibility of detecting angiogenesis in the myocardium in humans.[33]

Apoptosis Versus Necrosis

Apoptosis is the physiologic process of programmed cell death, whereby organisms selectively target cells to be eliminated when they are no longer needed. The cardiovascular pathologies of cardiomyopathy, heart failure, myocarditis, and myocardial infarction are associated with increased levels of apoptosis, particularly in the myocyte. On the other hand, a subset of cell death that occurs as an outcome of these pathologic processes outside of programmed cellular mechanisms is termed necrosis. A recent study evaluating a role of apoptosis and necrosis in the setting of acute myocardial infarction revealed a potential therapeutic role for cyclosporine.[34] The intervention is hypothesized to minimize peri-infarct, reperfusion-related cell death that takes place in the setting of revascularization. It is estimated that 30% of cardiomyocytes in the injured myocardium become apoptotic as a result of ischemia reperfusion injury, and animal models of acute infarction demonstrate that up to 50% of the final size of the infarct can be related to lethal reperfusion injury.[35,36] In other animal studies, inhibition of apoptosis with caspase inhibitors is cardioprotective.[37–39] There are also some data to suggest early apoptosis may be the pathologic substrate that leads from ischemia to necrosis.[40] An ability to assess cell death anywhere along the spectrum of apoptosis to necrosis would allow investigators to fine tune a therapeutic regimen and optimize the outcome. In targeting these pathologies for new interventions, it has become apparent that better in vivo imaging techniques for detection of apoptosis will be required.

Biology of apoptosis and necrosis
The earliest studies of apoptosis evolved around histologic assessment of the cells undergoing cell death. The earliest descriptions included the microscopic visualization of chromatin condensation, dissolution of nuclear membrane, nuclear shrinkage, and formation of apoptotic bodies that were cleared by phagocytic cells.[41–43] Over time it became clear that programmed cell death is central to the development and maintenance of homeostasis of a wide array of organisms.[44] In addition, cell death plays a role in the pathology of various disease states.[45] Depending on the initiating signals, there are two major pathways for cell death: intrinsic and extrinsic.[46] The intrinsic pathway is generated from within the cell through DNA damage, mitochondrial signals,

and oncogene activation, leading to activation of caspase enzymes, cysteine proteases that cleave after aspartate residues. The extrinsic pathway is initiated through extracellular signals that target cell membrane receptors, such as Fas, a death receptor. The culmination of this event through either pathway is the activation of a key effector, caspase-3.[47]

Soon after the activation of caspase-3, the energy-dependent asymmetric distribution of phospholipids that enables the definition of various subregions within the lipid bilayer of cell membranes is lost. This loss leads to increased phosphatidyl serine (PS) on the outer cell membrane from its typical location on the inner cell membrane.[48] In part, this is the result of increased calcium levels and decreased amounts of ATP that block the translocase enzyme responsible for maintenance of PS. The exposure of PS on the surface of the cell makes it a target for binding the protein, annexin V.[49] Annexin V binds to PS in a calcium-dependent manner, which has led to an in vitro assay of fasligand–initiated cell death through binding of annexin V.[48,50]

The first application of annexin binding to identify phosphatidyl serine on the surface of cells in a cardiovascular model came from a mouse model of acute myocardial infarction.[51] In this study, the left anterior descending coronary artery of a series of mice was ligated shortly after the injection of biotinylated annexin V. Immunohistochemical analysis of the tissue distal to the site of ligation revealed annexin A5 binding in an area of cell death. DNA laddering confirmed programmed cell death to be occurring in the same region as the annexin A5 binding.

As myocardial ischemia or infarction persists, cells move from early apoptotic signals to complete necrosis. Breakdown of mitochondrial respiration and loss of membrane potential lead to the accumulation of calcium in the mitochondria of infarcted or severely injured myocardium.[52,53] With loss of membrane potential cellular structures also begin to dissipate. Positively charged histones and other organelle proteins are exposed from the protection of their membrane barriers. These changes in early necrotic tissue have been used for imaging techniques that seek to identify early necrosis in acute myocardial infarctions and are discussed in more detail later.

Molecular targets used for radiotracer-based imaging in apoptosis and necrosis
Annexin V Initial studies using annexin A5 for imaging purposes involved ^{99m}Tc labeling. The goal was to image the distribution of cells expressing PS noninvasively with a standard gamma camera. Radiolabeling involved derivatization of annexin A5 with hydrazinonicotinamine (HYNIC),

which binds to reduced ^{99m}Tc.[54] The initial studies were performed in mice with fulminant hepatic apoptosis through the injection of an anti-Fas antibody, which initiates an apoptotic cascade, particularly in hepatocytes.[55] Concomitant TUNEL studies confirmed localization of annexin A5 with apoptotic cells.

^{99m}Tc-labeled annexin V was used in humans to detect in vivo cell death in patients presenting with myocardial infarction (**Fig. 3**).[56] Patients presenting with their first myocardial infarction within 6 hours of symptom onset underwent standard revascularization with percutaneous intervention. Within 2 hours of revascularization, SPECT imaging was performed using ^{99m}Tc-labeled annexin V. This procedure was followed by perfusion imaging 6 to 8 weeks after discharge using ^{99m}Tc-sestamibi. Regional retention of ^{99m}Tc-labeled annexin V correlated with the perfusion defect identified 6 to 8 weeks after discharge, providing a proof of concept that annexin-V imaging can be used for noninvasive detection of myocardial cell death.

Annexin V imaging has also been used to differentiate between benign and malignant cardiac tumors given the high proliferation and cell death rates associated with malignancy.[57]

Heart transplant rejection is characterized by perivascular and interstitial mononuclear inflammatory infiltrates associated with myocyte apoptosis and necrosis.[58] In a study of 18 patients undergoing apoptotic imaging within 1 year of cardiac transplantation, annexin-V retention correlated with the severity of rejection.[59] Patients who had a negative scan had a concomitant negative biopsy. Of the 5 patients who had a positive scan, 3 patients demonstrated regional uptake and 2 patients demonstrated diffuse uptake. The annexin-V scans correlated to the degree of severity of rejection by biopsy specimens. The authors suggested that serial annexin-V imaging for apoptotic cells could be used as a surrogate for detection of allograft rejection in place of serial biopsies in patients following heart transplantation.

Myocarditis is another area of pathologic condition in which apoptosis is known to occur.[60] In a rat model of autoimmune myocarditis, ^{99m}Tc-labeled annexin V retention corresponded to histologic TUNEL staining for areas of myocardial apoptosis. These areas could be differentiated from areas of inflammation by ^{14}C-labeled deoxyglucose that corresponded to foci of inflammation. This finding suggests that one could differentiate between inflammation and active apoptosis with molecular imaging. To date, no studies have attempted to use this technique in conjunction with FDG-PET in human cases of myocarditis.

Caspase inhibitors Because phosphatidyl serine can be exposed on the surface of cells in physiologic conditions other than apoptosis, there is interest in developing more specific apoptosis tracers. Recently, caspase-3 inhibitors have been synthesized and labeled with ^{18}F as potential PET tracers for in vivo imaging of apoptosis (see Fig. 3).[61,62] These caspase-3–targeted tracers have shown favorable biodistribution and clearance. MicroPET imaging in a murine model of hepatic apoptosis has shown specificity of the tracer to the liver; however, more studies are needed to assess binding relative to activated caspase density. In addition, further analysis in

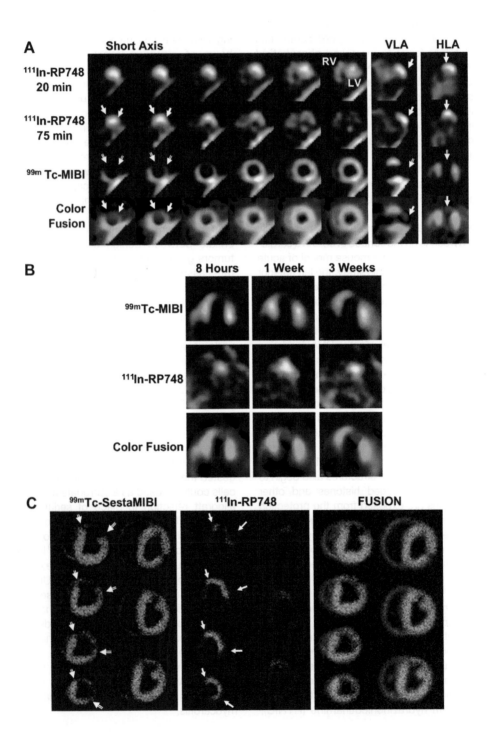

cardiovascular models is necessary to determine feasibility of using this new class of tracers for cardiac applications in humans.

Pyrophosphate and glucarate The in vivo noninvasive detection of myocardial infarction allows for early diagnosis and treatment in patients when electrocardiographic changes may not be evident or when biomarkers may not distinguish between ischemic injury associated with acute plaque rupture that may be treatable with mechanical revascularization versus unstable angina and demand-related ischemia. In addition to visualizing apoptosis, several studies have demonstrated that certain agents allow for the visualization of ongoing myocardial necrosis as a mechanism of identifying acute infarction potentially even in the presence of prior myocardial infarction. ^{99m}Tc-labeled pyrophosphate has been shown to bind to areas of necrosis and is believed to bind exposed mitochondrial calcium.[52,53] ^{99m}Tc-pyrophosphate has a moderate degree of sensitivity for acute infarction depending on the presence of Q-wave infarction or a non-ST elevation infarction.[63] The specificity for acute myocardial infarction is considered to be between 60% to 80%. The primary reason that ^{99m}Tc-pyrophosphate has not gained widespread clinical use is the limitation in the detection of early infarction. In fact, depending on the residual degree of perfusion to the infarct zone, the test may not be positive for the first 24 hours.

[99m]Tc-glucarate imaging provides an alternative to ^{99m}Tc-pyrophosphate imaging for the detection of acute infarction.[53] ^{99m}Tc-glucarate enters the necrotic cells by passive diffusion following breakdown of the sarcolemma, and binds to exposed histones in the nucleus of the myocytes. Canine models for ischemia and infarction reveal a high affinity of ^{99m}Tc-glucarate for necrotic tissue over ischemic but viable myocardium.[64] In a rabbit model of infarction, ^{99m}Tc-glucarate did not accumulate in areas of ischemia and could be imaged in areas of infarction as early as 10 minutes post reperfusion and within 30 to 60 minutes in nonreperfused zones.[65] Initial data in patients revealed that ^{99m}Tc-glucarate is able to noninvasively diagnose myocardial infarction in patients presenting with chest pain with a sensitivity that depends on the onset of symptoms, specifically within the first 9 hours of symptom onset.[66] ^{99m}Tc-glucarate does have a rapid blood clearance and good target-to-background signal. ^{99m}Tc-glucarate imaging is currently under investigation as a tool to detect early infarction in several clinical trials.

Inflammation

Inflammation plays an important role in many cardiovascular processes, including myocardial infarction, reperfusion injury, angiogenesis, apoptosis, cardiac allograft rejection, and myocarditis. Radiolabeling leukocytes with ^{99m}Tc or ^{111}In has been performed in the past and requires removal of blood and in vitro labeling techniques before reinjection for imaging.[67,68] These techniques carry concern for nonspecific activation of the cells that may interfere with the localization in vivo.[67] Ga-citrate has also been used but has been shown to be relatively nonspecific.[69] FDG PET imaging takes advantage of increased metabolic activity of inflammatory cells but can also be relatively nonspecific because a change in glucose uptake can be associated with other tissues and disease processes, including tumors.[70,71] There is tremendous interest in

---

Fig. 2. In vivo and ex vivo ^{111}In-RP748 and ^{99m}Tc-sestamibi (^{99m}Tc-MIBI) images from dogs with chronic infarction. (*A*) Serial in vivo ^{111}In-RP748 SPECT short axis, vertical long axis (VLA), and horizontal long axis (HLA) images in a dog 3 weeks post LAD infarction at 20 minutes and 75 minutes postinjection in standard format. ^{111}In-RP748 SPECT images were registered with ^{99m}Tc-MIBI perfusion images (*third row*). The 75-minute ^{111}In-RP748 SPECT images were colored red and fused with MIBI images (*green*) to better demonstrate localization of ^{111}In-RP748 activity within the heart (color fusion, *bottom row*). Right ventricular (RV) and left ventricular (LV) blood pool activity are seen at 20 minutes. Filled arrows indicate region of increased ^{111}In-RP748 uptake in anterior wall, which corresponds to the anteroapical ^{99m}Tc-sestamibi perfusion defect (*open arrow*). (*B*) Sequential ^{99m}Tc-sestamibi (*top row*) and ^{111}In-RP748 in vivo SPECT HLA images at 90 minutes postinjection (*middle row*) from a dog at 8 hours (Acute), and 1 and 3 weeks post LAD infarction. Increased myocardial ^{111}In-RP748 uptake is seen in anteroapical wall at all three time points, although it appears to be maximal at 1 week postinfarction. Color fusion ^{99m}Tc-MIBI (*green*) and ^{111}In-RP748 (*red*) images (*bottom row*) demonstrate ^{111}In-RP748 uptake within ^{99m}Tc-MIBI perfusion defect. (*C*) Ex vivo ^{99m}Tc-sestamibi (*left*) and ^{111}In-RP748 (*center*) images of myocardial slices from a dog 3 weeks post LAD occlusion, with color fusion image on right. Short axis slices are oriented with anterior wall on top, RV on left. Open arrows indicate anterior location of nontransmural perfusion defect region, and filled arrows indicate corresponds area of increased ^{111}In-RP748 uptake. (*Reprinted from* Meoli DF, Sadeghi MM, Krasilnikova S, et al. Noninvasive imaging of myocardial angiogenesis following experimental myocardial infarction. J Clin Invest 2004;113:1684–91; with permission.)

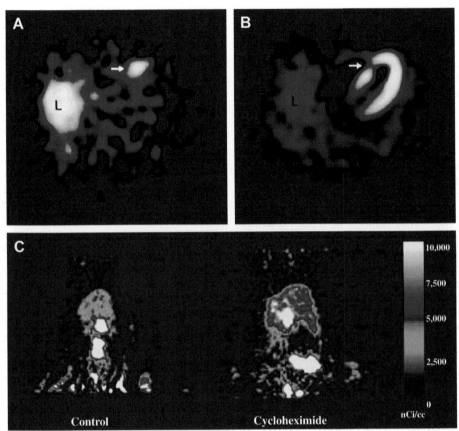

Fig. 3. In vivo imaging of apoptosis. (*A, B*) Transverse tomographic images of acute anteroseptal infarction in a patient. (*A*) Arrow shows increased ^{99m}Tc-labelled annexin-V uptake in the anteroseptal region 22 hours after reperfusion. (*B*) Perfusion scintigraphy with sestamibi 6 to 8 weeks after discharge shows an irreversible perfusion defect that coincides with the area of increased ^{99m}Tc-labeled annexin-V uptake (*arrow*). (*Reprinted from* Hofstra L, Liem IH, Dumont EA, et al. Visualisation of cell death in vivo in patients with acute myocardial infarction. Lancet 2000;359:209–12; with permission.) (*C*) Whole-body microPET images of caspase-3–specific inhibitor, ^{18}F-WC-II-89, distribution in a control rat (*left*) and cycloheximide-treated rat (*right*). Images were summed from 10 to 60 minutes after intravenous injection of approximately 150 μCi of ^{18}F-WC-II-89. (*Reprinted from* Zhou D, Chu W, Rothfuss J, et al. Synthesis, radiolabeling, and in vivo evaluation of an 18F-labeled isatin analog for imaging caspase-3 activation in apoptosis. Bioorg Med Chem Lett 2006;16:5041–6; with permission.)

developing more specific noninvasive imaging techniques to detect inflammation in myocardium.

Molecular targets used for radiotracer-based imaging of inflammatory-mediated processes
Antimyosin antibody Injury to myocytes in the setting of inflammation leads to the disruption of cellular membranes and the release of myosin heavy chain. To take advantage of this extracellular exposure of myosin in the setting of inflammation and necrosis, monoclonal antibody to myosin was generated in hopes of applying this for imaging. Early attempts to visualize myosin used ^{111}In-labeled antimyosin antibodies to visualize myocyte damage in myocardial infarction.[72] Other studies used ^{99m}Tc-labeled monoclonal antibody fragments to quantitate the degree of myosin exposure

in patients in the setting of acute myocardial infarction and correlate it with necrosis.[73] Inflammation associated with myocarditis, an inflammatory process not associated with ischemia, were also performed using ^{111}In-antimyosin antibodies.[74,75] Using antimyosin antibody imaging, patients who had dilated cardiomyopathy and lower ejection fractions revealed positive studies, suggesting a role for this in stratifying appropriate patients for cardiac transplantation. Although these initial studies showed promise, the background antibody binding to necrotic debris in the cell was high, and therefore the specificity of ^{111}In-labeled antimyosin antibody turned out to be low (25%–50%).[76]

Antitenascin-C antibody Another monoclonal antibody against an extracellular matrix protein tenascin-C, which seems to be involved in wound healing and inflammation, has been identified as a potential imaging agent. In rodent models of myocarditis, ^{111}In-labeled antitenascin-C localizes to the sites of myocardial inflammation.[77] Using a dual isotope SPECT approach with ^{111}In-antitenascin-C and ^{99m}Tc-sestamibi, the antibody localized to the injured septal wall by in vivo imaging.

LTB$_4$ receptor LTB$_4$ is a lipid mediator synthesized from arachidonic acid and secreted by neutrophils, macrophages, and endothelial cells as a potent chemotactic agent.[78,79] The LTB$_4$ receptor can be found on neutrophils, and signaling through this receptor stimulates endothelial adhesion and superoxide production. Recently, a radiolabeled LTB$_4$ receptor antagonist, ^{99m}Tc-RP517, was developed for in vivo imaging of inflammation.[80,81] ^{99m}Tc-RP517 localized to sites of inflammation induced by *Staphylococcus aureus* and *Escherichia coli* infection, and chemical (phorbol-ester)–induced bowel inflammation.

When prepared with human peripheral whole blood in vitro, fluorinated RP517 localized to neutrophils by fluorescence-activated cell sorter (FACs) analysis.[82] This analysis confirmed the potential to label human blood neutrophils with ^{99m}Tc-labeled RP517. In an attempt to characterize the in vivo imaging ability of ^{99m}Tc-RP517, a canine model of postischemic myocardial inflammation was used. ^{99m}Tc-RP517 was injected into open-chest dogs before occlusion and reperfusion. There was an inverse relationship between radiotracer uptake and occlusion flow, suggesting localization of the imaging agent to the site of ischemic inflammation (**Fig. 4**). Ex vivo segment analysis revealed that ^{99m}Tc-RP517 correlated with the neutrophil enzyme myeloperoxidase. Intramyocardial injection of TNFα also correlated with ^{99m}Tc-RP517 uptake and concomitant myeloperoxidase activity, again supporting localization to the site of inflammation. One concern regarding the application of ^{99m}Tc-RP517 is the lipophilic nature of the molecule, resulting in high hepatobiliary clearance and thus large amounts of gastrointestinal uptake. To overcome this, alternative constructs of the LTB$_4$ antagonist are currently being evaluated.[83]

Ventricular Remodeling

Ventricular remodeling is a complex biologic process that involves inflammation, repair, and healing with specific biochemical and structural alterations in the myocardial infarct and peri-infarct regions and the remote regions.[84,85] The process is one of adaptation to form a scar that allows a degree of mechanical stability. The remodeling process involves several key cell types and structural elements, including myocardial cells, endothelial cells, inflammatory cells, and the extracellular matrix.

Biology of myocardial remodeling
Early in the first weeks after a myocardial infarction, an innate immune response initiates a complex process of wound healing in the necrotic tissue. This process evolves into a more chronic remodeling process that can involve hypertrophy, chamber dilation, and, depending on the success of healing, heart failure.[85]

MMPs are a family of zinc-containing enzymes that play a key role in ventricular remodeling by degradation of the extracellular matrix.[86,87] MMPs play an integral role in infarct expansion and left ventricular dilation. Gene deletion of MMPs has been demonstrated to have some cardioprotective effects from ventricular dilation and rupture postinfarct.[88] Pharmacologic inhibition of MMPs has also been shown to decrease left ventricular dilation in infarct models.[89–91]

Factor XIII has been shown to be crucial in organizing the new matrix of the scar by involvement with extracellular matrix turnover and regulation of inflammatory cascades.[92,93] Mice with decreased levels of factor XIII demonstrate increased ventricular dilation and postinfarct rupture. Patients who had infarct rupture were demonstrated to have lower levels of factor XIII in their myocardium. Factor XIII is activated by thrombin and often decreased in the setting of acute myocardial infarction in part because of therapeutic inhibition of thrombin. It is hypothesized that supplementing factor XIII activity may have a beneficial role in postinfarct remodeling.

A critical system that is locally activated during remodeling and contributes to the progression to heart failure is the renin-angiotensin system.[94] As healing and remodeling are unsuccessful in the failing heart, there is increased expression of pro-renin, renin, and angiotensin-converting enzyme (ACE). Activation of this system through signaling pathways mediated by the angiotensin II type I receptor (AT1) leads to myocyte hypertrophy, interstitial and perivascular collagen deposition, and myocyte apoptosis.[95] Inhibition of this pathway has been demonstrated to reverse the functional abnormalities associated with this negative remodeling.

Molecular targets used for radiotracer-based imaging of left ventricular remodeling
Matrix metalloproteinases By radiolabeling molecules that target MMPs, such as pharmacologic inhibitors that specifically bind to the catalytic

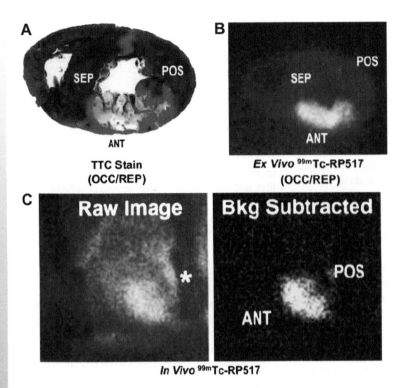

Fig. 4. Imaging ischemic inflammation with the LTB$_4$ receptor antagonist, RP517. TTC-stained heart slice (*A*) and ex vivo ^{99m}Tc-RP517 image (*B*) of the same heart slice. (*C*) Raw (*left*) and background subtracted (*right*) in vivo ^{99m}Tc-RP517 images acquired from a dog 60 minutes after reperfusion. Background subtraction was performed to eliminate the surgically related tracer uptake in the field of view. The shadow on the raw image denoted by an asterisk is the metal rib spreader. Note that focal ^{99m}Tc-RP517 uptake was readily observed in the inflamed anteroseptal region of the heart on ex vivo and in vivo images. Tracer uptake was negligible in the normal, posterior wall. (*Reprinted from* Riou LM, Ruiz M, Sullivan GW, et al. Assessment of myocardial inflammation produced by experimental coronary occlusion and reperfusion with 99mTc-RP517, a new leukotriene B4 receptor antagonist that preferentially labels neutrophils in vivo. Circulation 2002;106:592–8; with permission.)

domain, MMP activation postinfarct can be visualized in vivo (**Fig. 5**).[96] Initial studies involved nonimaging techniques with ^{111}In-labeled broad-spectrum MMP inhibitor (RP782), a molecule that selectively targets activated MMPs. This MMP-targeted agent demonstrated a favorable biodistribution in a murine model of myocardial infarction. One week after myocardial infarction, ^{111}In-RP782 localized primarily within the infarct region, although a lesser increase in retention was seen in the remote noninfarcted regions of the heart, consistent with global MMP activation and remodeling.

Further imaging studies were performed using ^{99m}Tc-labeled analog of RP782 (^{99m}Tc-RP805) and hybrid SPECT/CT imaging with a dual isotope protocol involving ^{99m}Tc-RP805 imaging and adjunctive ^{201}Tl- perfusion imaging. The dual isotope imaging studies revealed MMP activation within the perfusion defect region. This finding suggests that MMP activation is taking place primarily within the sites of injury and is proof of concept that molecules that target MMP activation might be used to evaluate ventricular remodeling and therapeutic interventions directed at inhibition of MMP activation.

Factor XIII ^{111}In-DOTA-FXIII is a radiolabeled glutaminase factor XIII substrate analog that factor XIII recognizes and cross-links to extracellular matrix proteins (**Fig. 6**).[93] ^{111}In-DOTA-FXIII accumulates in areas of increased factor XIII activity. In a murine model of myocardial infarction, this ^{111}In-labeled peptide substrate was demonstrated to be decreased in infarcts of animals treated with the direct thrombin inhibitor, dalteparin. Moreover, dalteparin treatment increased the risk for infarct rupture. Conversely, mice treated with factor XIII intravenously exhibited increased factor XIII activity in the infarct zone and demonstrated more rapid inflammatory turnover of neutrophils and increased recruitment of macrophages to the site of infarction. There was also increased collagen synthesis and capillary density in the factor XIII-treated animals, suggesting improved healing postinfarction.

Angiotensin-converting enzyme inhibitors and angiotensin II type I antagonists Several ACE inhibitors and AT1 antagonists have been radiolabeled for molecular imaging techniques.[94] In a study of explanted hearts from patients who had ischemic cardiomyopathy, ^{18}F-fluorobenzoyl-lisinopril was used to assess ACE levels in infarcted myocardium and fibrosed tissue.[97] The study demonstrated that the radiolabeled ACE inhibitor bound with some degree of specificity to areas adjacent to the infarct.

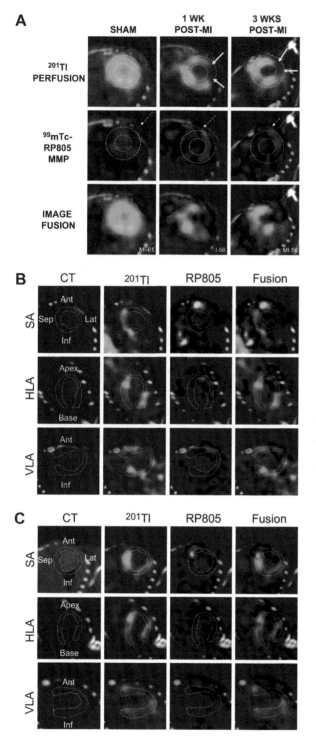

Fig. 5. Imaging of MMP activity postinfarction. Hybrid microSPECT/CT reconstructed short-axis images were acquired without contrast (*A*) in control sham-operated mouse (*left*) and selected mice at 1 week (*middle*) and 3 weeks (*right*) after myocardial infarction, after injection of [201]Tl (*top row, green*) and ^{99m}Tc-RP805 (*middle row, red*). A black-and-white (B&W) and multicolor fusion image is shown on bottom. Control heart demonstrates normal myocardial perfusion and no focal ^{99m}Tc-RP805 uptake within the heart, although some uptake is seen in chest wall at the thoracotomy site (*dashed arrows*). All post–myocardial infarction mice have a large anterolateral ^{201}Tl perfusion defect (*yellow arrows*) and focal uptake of ^{99m}Tc-RP805 in defect area. A dashed circle is drawn around the heart to demonstrate localization of ^{99m}Tc-RP805, the MMP radiotracer, within the infarcted area of the heart. Some activity is also seen in the peri-infarct border zone. Additional microSPECT/CT images were acquired by use of a higher-resolution SPECT detector after the administration of contrast, at 1 week (*B*) and 3 weeks (*C*) after MI. The contrast agent permitted better definition of the LV myocardium, which is highlighted by white dotted line. Representative short-axis (SA), horizontal long-axis (HLA), and vertical long-axis (VLA) images are shown. Focal uptake of ^{99m}Tc-RP805 is seen within the central infarct and peri-infarct regions, which again correspond to ^{201}Tl perfusion defect. (*Reprinted from* Su H, Spinale FG, Dobrucki LW et al. Noninvasive targeted imaging of MMP activation in a murine model of postinfarction remodeling. *Circulation* 2005;112:3157–67; with permission.)

Other studies using AT1 antagonists have demonstrated a differential between ACE activity and AT1 levels.[98] In an ovine model of heart failure, ACE activity was primarily in the vascular endothelium, whereas AT1 was up-regulated in the myofibroblasts of the infarct region. In a murine model of acute myocardial infarction, a ^{99m}Tc-labeled AT1 receptor peptide analog was developed and demonstrated specificity to the myofibroblasts that localized to the infarct region in the

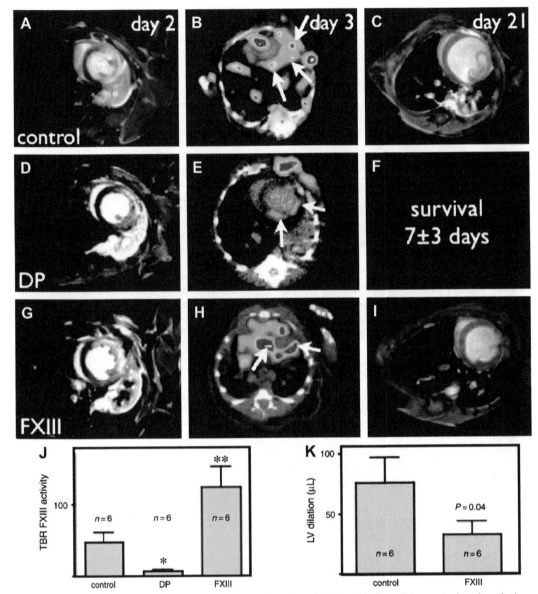

Fig. 6. In vivo molecular imaging of transglutaminase factor XIII (FXIII) activity predicts survival and evolution of heart failure. (*A–I*) Longitudinal imaging study (MRI day 2, SPECT-CT day 3, second MRI day 21); on day 2 (*A, D, G*), late enhancement MRI showed similar infarct size in all groups. FXIII-treatment led to higher SPECT signal (*H, J*). In dalteparin-treated mice, the SPECT signal was lower (*E, J*). Serial MRI showed attenuated left ventricular (LV) dilation in FXIII-treated mice (*K*). Due to reduced survival in dalteparin (DP)-treated mice, the second MRI on day 21 was not acquired (*F*). *P<.05, **P<.001. (*Reprinted from* Nahrendorf M, Aikawa E, Figueiredo JL, et al. Transglutaminase activity in acute infarcts predicts healing outcome and left ventricular remodelling: implications for FXIII therapy and antithrombin use in myocardial infarction. Eur Heart J 2008;29:445–54; with permission.)

weeks following the infarction. These early studies suggest that the neurohormonal changes that take place within an infarction may be used to identify those at risk for developing significant heart failure after myocardial infarction. Much more work is needed to assess the feasibility of these agents for imaging of postinfarction remodeling in clinical trials.

SUMMARY

In summary, molecular imaging represents a targeted approach to noninvasively assess biologic processes in vivo. The goal of molecular imaging is to develop an approach to studying not only the disease process but also more importantly the efficacy of an individually tailored therapeutic regimen. The relatively high sensitivity of radiotracer-based imaging approaches, such as SPECT and PET, have been of great use in the practical application of molecular imaging techniques. Research has demonstrated the feasibility of specific targeted imaging approaches in the evaluation of angiogenesis, apoptosis, inflammation, and ventricular remodeling. Combining nuclear (SPECT or PET) and CT imaging modalities should help overcome issues of attenuation or partial volume effects and improve quantitative accuracy. The evolution of hybrid imaging systems and imaging protocols that include application of dual isotopes for monitoring physiologic parameters (metabolism or perfusion) with targeted molecular probes shows promise in the areas of myocardial infarction and angiogenesis. Tailoring gene therapy with PET reporter constructs should allow for optimization of therapeutic efficacy in the areas of angiogenesis. The role for apoptotic imaging in understanding reperfusion injury and the effects of therapeutic interventions, or in identifying the presence and severity of graft rejection following cardiac transplantation without the need for biopsy, shows some promise. Imaging the activation of MMPs, active factor XIII, or the levels of neurohormonal activation during ventricular remodeling may guide therapeutic regimens that could help positively influence outcomes postinfarction. In conclusion, targeted radiotracer-based molecular imaging is clearly feasible and may play an important role in the evaluation and management of cardiovascular disease, including the future investigation of novel genetic or cell-based therapeutic interventions.

REFERENCES

1. Pichler A, Piwnica-Worms D, et al. Overview of cardiovascular molecular imaging. In: Gropler RJ, Glover DK, Sinusas AJ, et al, editors. Cardiovascular molecular imaging. New York: Informa Healthcare U.S.A., Inc; 2007. p. 1–8.

2. Sinusas AJ, Bengel F, Nahrendorf M, et al. Multimodality cardiovascular molecular imaging, part I. Circulation: Cardiovascular Imaging 2008;1:244–56.

3. Fam NP, Verma S, Kutryk M, et al. Clinician guide to angiogenesis. Circulation 2003;108:2613–8.

4. Sasayama S, Fujita M. Recent insights into coronary collateral circulation. Circulation 1992;85:1197–204.

5. Lake Tahoe invitation meeting 2002. J Nucl Cardiol 2003;10:223–57.

6. Lee SH, Wolf PL, Escudero R, et al. Early expression of angiogenesis factors in acute myocardial ischemia and infarction. N Engl J Med 2000;342:626–33.

7. Shweiki D, Itin A, Soffer D, et al. Vascular endothelial growth factor induced by hypoxia may mediate hypoxia-initiated angiogenesis. Nature 1992;359:843–5.

8. Brogi E, Schatteman G, Wu T, et al. Hypoxia-induced paracrine regulation of vascular endothelial growth factor receptor expression. J Clin Invest 1996;97:469–76.

9. Banai S, Jaklitsch MT, Shou M, et al. Angiogenic-induced enhancement of collateral blood flow to ischemic myocardium by vascular endothelial growth factor in dogs. Circulation 1994;89:2183–9.

10. Li J, Brown LF, Hibberd MG, et al. VEGF, flk-1, and flt-1 expression in a rat myocardial infarction model of angiogenesis. Am J Physiol 1996;270:H1803–11.

11. Ferrara N, Gerber HP, LeCouter J. The biology of VEGF and its receptors. Nat Med 2003;9:669–76.

12. Xiong JP, Stehle T, Diefenbach B, et al. Crystal structure of the extracellular segment of integrin alpha Vbeta3. Science 2001;294:339–45.

13. Schwartz MA, Schaller MD, Ginsberg MH. Integrins: emerging paradigms of signal transduction. Annu Rev Cell Dev Biol 1995;11:549–99.

14. Hynes RO. Integrins: bidirectional, allosteric signaling machines. Cell 2002;110:673–87.

15. Clyman RI, Mauray F, Kramer RH. Beta 1 and beta 3 integrins have different roles in the adhesion and migration of vascular smooth muscle cells on extracellular matrix. Exp Cell Res 1992;200:272–84.

16. Brooks PC, Montgomery AM, Rosenfeld M, et al. Integrin alpha v beta 3 antagonists promote tumor regression by inducing apoptosis of angiogenic blood vessels. Cell 1994;79:1157–64.

17. Li J, Brown LF, Laham RJ, et al. Macrophage-dependent regulation of syndecan gene expression. Circ Res 1997;81:785–96.

18. Bhagwat SV, Lahdenranta J, Giordano R, et al. CD13/APN is activated by angiogenic signals and is essential for capillary tube formation. Blood 2001;97:652–9.

19. Lu E, Wagner WR, Schellenberger U, et al. Targeted in vivo labeling of receptors for vascular endothelial growth factor: approach to identification of ischemic tissue. Circulation 2003;108:97–103.

20. Rodriguez-Porcel M, Cai W, Gheysens O, et al. Imaging of VEGF receptor in a rat myocardial infarction model using PET. J Nucl Med 2008;49:667–73.

21. Wu JC, Inubushi M, Sundaresan G, et al. Positron emission tomography imaging of cardiac reporter gene expression in living rats. Circulation 2002;106:180–3.

22. Inubushi M, Wu JC, Gambhir SS, et al. Positron-emission tomography reporter gene expression imaging in rat myocardium. Circulation 2003;107:326–32.

23. Bengel FM, Anton M, Richter T, et al. Noninvasive imaging of transgene expression by use of positron emission tomography in a pig model of myocardial gene transfer. Circulation 2003;108:2127–33.

24. Wu JC, Chen IY, Wang Y, et al. Molecular imaging of the kinetics of vascular endothelial growth factor gene expression in ischemic myocardium. Circulation 2004;110:685–91.

25. Sipkins DA, Cheresh DA, Kazemi MR, et al. Detection of tumor angiogenesis in vivo by alphaVbeta3-targeted magnetic resonance imaging. Nat Med 1998;4:623–6.

26. Haubner R, Wester HJ, Weber WA, et al. Noninvasive imaging of alpha(v)beta3 integrin expression using 18F-labeled RGD-containing glycopeptide and positron emission tomography. Cancer Res 2001;61:1781–5.

27. Haubner R, Wester HJ, Burkhart F, et al. Glycosylated RGD-containing peptides: tracer for tumor targeting and angiogenesis imaging with improved biokinetics. J Nucl Med 2001;42:326–36.

28. Harris TD, Kalogeropoulos S, Nguyen T, et al. Design, synthesis, and evaluation of radiolabeled integrin alpha v beta 3 receptor antagonists for tumor imaging and radiotherapy. Cancer Biother Radiopharm 2003;18:627–41.

29. Sadeghi M, Krassilnikova S, Zhang J, et al. Imaging of avb3 integrin in vascular injury: does this reflect increased integrin expression or activation? Circulation 2008;108:404.

30. Meoli DF, Sadeghi MM, Krassilnikova S, et al. Noninvasive imaging of myocardial angiogenesis following experimental myocardial infarction. J Clin Invest 2004;113:1684–91.

31. Kalinowski L, Dobrucki LW, Meoli DF, et al. Targeted imaging of hypoxia-induced integrin activation in myocardium early after infarction. J Appl Physiol 2008;104:1504–12.

32. Su H, Hu X, Bourke B, et al. Detection of myocardial angiogenesis in chronic infarction with a novel technetium-99m labeled peptide targeted at avb3 integrin. Circulation 2003;108:278–9.

33. Makowski MR, Ebersberger U, Nekolla S, et al. In vivo molecular imaging of angiogenesis, targeting alphavbeta3 integrin expression, in a patient after acute myocardial infarction. Eur Heart J 2008;29:2201.

34. Piot C, Croisille P, Staat P, et al. Effect of cyclosporine on reperfusion injury in acute myocardial infarction. N Engl J Med 2008;359:473–81.

35. Fliss H, Gattinger D. Apoptosis in ischemic and reperfused rat myocardium. Circ Res 1996;79:949–56.

36. Yellon DM, Hausenloy DJ. Myocardial reperfusion injury. N Engl J Med 2007;357:1121–35.

37. Yaoita H, Ogawa K, Maehara K, et al. Attenuation of ischemia/reperfusion injury in rats by a caspase inhibitor. Circulation 1998;97:276–81.

38. Dumont EA, Reutelingsperger CP, Smits JF, et al. Real-time imaging of apoptotic cell-membrane changes at the single-cell level in the beating murine heart. Nat Med 2001;7:1352–5.

39. Hayakawa Y, Chandra M, Miao W, et al. Inhibition of cardiac myocyte apoptosis improves cardiac function and abolishes mortality in the peripartum cardiomyopathy of Galpha(q) transgenic mice. Circulation 2003;108:3036–41.

40. Thimister PW, Hofstra L, Liem IH, et al. In vivo detection of cell death in the area at risk in acute myocardial infarction. J Nucl Med 2003;44:391–6.

41. Wyllie AH. Glucocorticoid-induced thymocyte apoptosis is associated with endogenous endonuclease activation. Nature 1980;284:555–6.

42. Kerr JF, Wyllie AH, Currie AR. Apoptosis: a basic biological phenomenon with wide-ranging implications in tissue kinetics. Br J Cancer 1972;26:239–57.

43. Wyllie AH, Kerr JF, Currie AR. Cell death: the significance of apoptosis. Int Rev Cytol 1980;68:251–306.

44. Danial NN, Korsmeyer SJ. Cell death: critical control points. Cell 2004;116:205–19.

45. Green DR, Kroemer G. The pathophysiology of mitochondrial cell death. Science 2004;305:626–9.

46. Riedl SJ, Shi Y. Molecular mechanisms of caspase regulation during apoptosis. Nat Rev Mol Cell Biol 2004;5:897–907.

47. Tait JF. Imaging of apoptosis. J Nucl Med 2008;49:1573–6.

48. Martin SJ, Reutelingsperger CP, McGahon AJ, et al. Early redistribution of plasma membrane phosphatidylserine is a general feature of apoptosis regardless of the initiating stimulus: inhibition by overexpression of Bcl-2 and Abl. J Exp Med 1995;182:1545–56.

49. Koopman G, Reutelingsperger CP, Kuijten GA, et al. Annexin V for flow cytometric detection of phosphatidylserine expression on B cells undergoing apoptosis. Blood 1994;84:1415–20.

50. van Engeland M, Ramaekers FC, Schutte B, et al. A novel assay to measure loss of plasma membrane asymmetry during apoptosis of adherent cells in culture. Cytometry 1996;24:131–9.

51. Dumont EA, Hofstra L, van Heerde WL, et al. Cardiomyocyte death induced by myocardial ischemia and reperfusion: measurement with recombinant human annexin-V in a mouse model. Circulation 2000;102:1564–8.

52. Khaw BA. The current role of infarct avid imaging. Semin Nucl Med 1999;29:259–70.

53. Flotats A, Carrio I. Non-invasive in vivo imaging of myocardial apoptosis and necrosis. Eur J Nucl Med Mol Imaging 2003;30:615–30.

54. Blankenberg FG, Katsikis PD, Tait JF, et al. In vivo detection and imaging of phosphatidylserine expression during programmed cell death. Proc Natl Acad Sci U S A 1998;95:6349–54.

55. Ogasawara J, Watanabe-Fukunaga R, Adachi M, et al. Lethal effect of the anti-Fas antibody in mice. Nature 1993;364:806–9.

56. Hofstra L, Liem IH, Dumont EA, et al. Visualisation of cell death in vivo in patients with acute myocardial infarction. Lancet 2000;356:209–12.

57. Hofstra L, Dumont EA, Thimister PW, et al. In vivo detection of apoptosis in an intracardiac tumor. JAMA 2001;285:1841–2.

58. Laguens RP, Meckert PM, Martino JS, et al. Identification of programmed cell death (apoptosis) in situ by means of specific labeling of nuclear DNA fragments in heart biopsy samples during acute rejection episodes. J Heart Lung Transplant 1996;15: 911–8.

59. Narula J, Acio ER, Narula N, et al. Annexin-V imaging for noninvasive detection of cardiac allograft rejection. Nat Med 2001;7:1347–52.

60. Tokita N, Hasegawa S, Tsujimura E, et al. Serial changes in 14C-deoxyglucose and 201Tl uptake in autoimmune myocarditis in rats. J Nucl Med 2001; 42:285–91.

61. Faust A, Wagner S, Law MP, et al. The nonpeptidyl caspase binding radioligand (S)-1-(4-(2-[18F]Fluoroethoxy)-benzyl)-5-[1-(2-methoxymethylpyrrolidinyl)s ulfonyl]isatin ([18F]CbR) as potential positron emission tomography-compatible apoptosis imaging agent. Q J Nucl Med Mol Imaging 2007;51:67–73.

62. Zhou D, Chu W, Rothfuss J, et al. Synthesis, radiolabeling, and in vivo evaluation of an 18F-labeled isatin analog for imaging caspase-3 activation in apoptosis. Bioorg Med Chem Lett 2006;16: 5041–6.

63. Corbett JR, Lewis M, Willerson JT, et al. 99mTc-pyrophosphate imaging in patients with acute myocardial infarction: comparison of planar imaging with single-photon tomography with and without blood pool overlay. Circulation 1984;69:1120–8.

64. Orlandi C, Crane PD, Edwards DS, et al. Early scintigraphic detection of experimental myocardial infarction in dogs with technetium-99m-glucaric acid. J Nucl Med 1991;32:263–8.

65. Narula J, Petrov A, Pak KY, et al. Very early noninvasive detection of acute experimental nonreperfused myocardial infarction with 99mTc-labeled glucarate. Circulation 1997;95:1577–84.

66. Mariani G, Villa G, Rossettin PF, et al. Detection of acute myocardial infarction by 99mTc-labeled D-glucaric acid imaging in patients with acute chest pain. J Nucl Med 1999;40:1832–9.

67. Peters AM, Danpure HJ, Osman S, et al. Clinical experience with 99mTc-hexamethylpropylene-amineoxime for labelling leucocytes and imaging inflammation. Lancet 1986;2:946–9.

68. Peters AM, Saverymuttu SH. The value of indium-labelled leucocytes in clinical practice. Blood Rev 1987;1:65–76.

69. Lavender JP, Lowe J, Barker JR, et al. Gallium 67 citrate scanning in neoplastic and inflammatory lesions. Br J Radiol 1971;44:361–6.

70. Mochizuki T, Tsukamoto E, Kuge Y, et al. FDG uptake and glucose transporter subtype expressions in experimental tumor and inflammation models. J Nucl Med 2001;42:1551–5.

71. Kubota R, Yamada S, Kubota K, et al. Intratumoral distribution of fluorine-18-fluorodeoxyglucose in vivo: high accumulation in macrophages and granulation tissues studied by microautoradiography. J Nucl Med 1992;33:1972–80.

72. Johnson LL, Seldin DW, Becker LC, et al. Antimyosin imaging in acute transmural myocardial infarctions: results of a multicenter clinical trial. J Am Coll Cardiol 1989;13:27–35.

73. Khaw BA, Gold HK, Yasuda T, et al. Scintigraphic quantification of myocardial necrosis in patients after intravenous injection of myosin-specific antibody. Circulation 1986;74:501–8.

74. Yasuda T, Palacios IF, Dec GW, et al. Indium 111-monoclonal antimyosin antibody imaging in the diagnosis of acute myocarditis. Circulation 1987;76:306–11.

75. Dec GW, Palacios I, Yasuda T, et al. Antimyosin antibody cardiac imaging: its role in the diagnosis of myocarditis. J Am Coll Cardiol 1990;16:97–104.

76. Narula J, Khaw BA, Dec GW, et al. Diagnostic accuracy of antimyosin scintigraphy in suspected myocarditis. J Nucl Cardiol 1996;3:371–81.

77. Sato M, Toyozaki T, Odaka K, et al. Detection of experimental autoimmune myocarditis in rats by 111In monoclonal antibody specific for tenascin-C. Circulation 2002;106:1397–402.

78. Ford-Hutchinson AW. Regulation of leukotriene biosynthesis. Cancer Metastasis Rev 1994;13:257–67.

79. Yokomizo T, Izumi T, Shimizu T. Leukotriene B4: metabolism and signal transduction. Arch Biochem Biophys 2001;385:231–41.

80. Serhan CN, Prescott SM. The scent of a phagocyte: advances on leukotriene b(4) receptors. J Exp Med 2000;192:F5–8.

81. Brouwers AH, Laverman P, Boerman OC, et al. A 99Tcm-labelled leukotriene B4 receptor antagonist for scintigraphic detection of infection in rabbits. Nucl Med Commun 2000;21:1043–50.

82. Riou LM, Ruiz M, Sullivan GW, et al. Assessment of myocardial inflammation produced by experimental coronary occlusion and reperfusion with 99mTc-RP517, a new leukotriene B4 receptor antagonist that preferentially labels neutrophils in vivo. Circulation 2002;106:592–8.

83. van Eerd JE, Oyen WJ, Harris TD, et al. A bivalent leukotriene B(4) antagonist for scintigraphic imaging of infectious foci. J Nucl Med 2003;44:1087–91.

84. Weber KT. Extracellular matrix remodeling in heart failure: a role for de novo angiotensin II generation. Circulation 1997;96:4065–82.

85. Sutton MG, Sharpe N. Left ventricular remodeling after myocardial infarction: pathophysiology and therapy. Circulation 2000;101:2981–8.

86. Creemers EE, Cleutjens JP, Smits JF, et al. Matrix metalloproteinase inhibition after myocardial infarction: a new approach to prevent heart failure? Circ Res 2001;89:201–10.

87. Spinale FG. Matrix metalloproteinases: regulation and dysregulation in the failing heart. Circ Res 2002;90:520–30.

88. Ducharme A, Frantz S, Aikawa M, et al. Targeted deletion of matrix metalloproteinase-9 attenuates left ventricular enlargement and collagen accumulation after experimental myocardial infarction. J Clin Invest 2000;106:55–62.

89. Rohde LE, Ducharme A, Arroyo LH, et al. Matrix metalloproteinase inhibition attenuates early left ventricular enlargement after experimental myocardial infarction in mice. Circulation 1999;99: 3063–70.

90. Lindsey ML, Gannon J, Aikawa M, et al. Selective matrix metalloproteinase inhibition reduces left ventricular remodeling but does not inhibit angiogenesis after myocardial infarction. Circulation 2002;105:753–8.

91. Yarbrough WM, Mukherjee R, Escobar GP, et al. Selective targeting and timing of matrix metalloproteinase inhibition in post-myocardial infarction remodeling. Circulation 2003;108:1753–9.

92. Nahrendorf M, Hu K, Frantz S, et al. Factor XIII deficiency causes cardiac rupture, impairs wound healing, and aggravates cardiac remodeling in mice with myocardial infarction. Circulation 2006;113: 1196–202.

93. Nahrendorf M, Aikawa E, Figueiredo JL, et al. Transglutaminase activity in acute infarcts predicts healing outcome and left ventricular remodelling: implications for FXIII therapy and antithrombin use in myocardial infarction. Eur Heart J 2008;29:445–54.

94. Shirani J, Dilsizian V. Imaging left ventricular remodeling: targeting the neurohumoral axis. Nat Clin Pract Cardiovasc Med 2008;5(Suppl 2):S57–62.

95. Aras O, Messina SA, Shirani J, et al. The role and regulation of cardiac angiotensin-converting enzyme for noninvasive molecular imaging in heart failure. Curr Cardiol Rep 2007;9:150–8.

96. Su H, Spinale FG, Dobrucki LW, et al. Noninvasive targeted imaging of matrix metalloproteinase activation in a murine model of postinfarction remodeling. Circulation 2005;112:3157–67.

97. Dilsizian V, Eckelman WC, Loredo ML, et al. Evidence for tissue angiotensin-converting enzyme in explanted hearts of ischemic cardiomyopathy using targeted radiotracer technique. J Nucl Med 2007;48:182–7.

98. Shirani J, Narula J, Eckelman WC, et al. Early imaging in heart failure: exploring novel molecular targets. J Nucl Cardiol 2007;14:100–10.

Radiotracer Imaging of Atherosclerotic Plaque Biology

Maysoon Elkhawad, MA, MB, BChir, MRCS *,
James H.F. Rudd, PhD, MRCP

KEYWORDS

- Atherosclerosis • Nuclear medicine
- PET • Tracer • Imaging

It is commonly accepted that atherosclerosis is a chronic inflammatory systemic disease characterized by accumulation of lipids, inflammatory cells, and connective tissue within the arterial wall.[1] Traditional imaging modalities used in the assessment of atherosclerotic plaque have focused on anatomic characteristics of size and luminal encroachment. The ability to identify plaques at risk for rupture that may go on to cause clinical events remains limited, however. By labeling tracer compounds capable of identifying important cellular or molecular processes involved in plaque vulnerability with radioactive isotopes, there is now potential for the noninvasive identification of vulnerable plaques. This article discusses several radiotracers that can report on high-risk plaque pathophysiology.

BIOLOGY OF ATHEROSCLEROSIS

Atherosclerosis is a lifelong, systemic inflammatory condition. It has origins that can be detected within the arterial wall in childhood. The etiology of the disease is believed to be multifactorial, incorporating complex interactions between innate genetic predisposition and acquired risk factors (smoking, elevated cholesterol). The stepping-off point seems to be an increase in endothelial permeability resulting in lipids, monocytes, and inflammatory cells infiltrating the subintimal space, which results in a chronic inflammatory reaction. This chronic inflammatory response also serves to activate a cytokine cascade, resulting in the recruitment of smooth muscle cells from the media

and the formation of a necrotic lipid pool. The smooth muscle cells and their secreted proteoglycans establish a protective smooth muscle fibrous cap over the lipid core. The cap protects the artery from thrombus that would likely result from contact between the thrombogenic, tissue factor–rich lipid core and the circulating luminal blood. A balance is achieved between the reparative smooth muscle cells and the destructive inflammatory cycle perpetuated by macrophages within the plaque. It is this balance that determines plaque vulnerability and consequent rupture and clinical events.[2] The ability to quantify and identify inflammation within plaque should allow better patient risk stratification, treatment monitoring, and novel drug development.

THE PRINCIPLES OF NUCLEAR IMAGING IN RELATION TO IMAGING ATHEROSCLEROSIS

The expectation for nuclear imaging in relation to atherosclerosis follows the rationale that a radiolabeled molecule, known as a radiotracer, will colocalize with a cell or receptor of interest in the plaque. In nuclear imaging, radiotracers emit γ rays, which can be detected by imaging with either single photon emission computed tomography (SPECT) or positron emission tomography (PET). Compared with nuclear imaging of the heart or lungs, however, the imaging of atherosclerotic plaque presents several challenges. First, most plaques are very small (less than 5 mm) and close to the limit of resolution of either SPECT or PET scanners. Additionally, plaques often lie close to

Work in this paper was partly funded by the NIHR Comprehensive Cambridge Biomedical Research Centre.
Division of Cardiovascular Medicine, Addenbrooke's Hospital, Box 110, Hills Road, Cambridge CB2 0QQ, UK
* Corresponding author.
E-mail address: me204@cam.ac.uk (M. Elkhawad).

Cardiol Clin 27 (2009) 345–354
doi:10.1016/j.ccl.2008.12.006

other structures that also accumulate the radiotracer, consequently reducing the signal-to-noise ratio of the resulting image. Some arteries of interest, such as the aorta and coronaries, are deep within the body cavity, which may result in radiation scatter and resultant image degradation. Finally, in the case of coronary artery imaging, there is cardiac and respiratory movement to overcome. A tracer/target combination that can overcome these hurdles has not yet been developed, but great progress has been made in addressing at least some of these fundamental requirements.

RADIOTRACERS FOR IMAGING LIPOPROTEINS

Over recent years there has been a paradigm shift in the concept of atherogenesis, from the accumulation of lipid in the artery wall to a systemic chronic disease driven by inflammation.[3–6] Low-density lipoprotein (LDL), particularly when oxidized, does still play a key pathogenic role in the formation, progression, and destabilization of plaque. Attempts to label and detect LDL in plaque have had limited success, however.[7–12] Early studies showed that radiolabeled LDL could be taken up in experimental atherosclerosis in rabbits. Subsequent clinical studies showed that ^{99}Tc-LDL could be imaged in coronary, carotid, iliac, or femoral arteries in 7 of 17 patients who had documented atherosclerosis. Analysis of carotid endarterectomy specimens 1 day after imaging revealed fourfold greater uptake into macrophage-rich lesions than into more fibrous plaque.[10,11] Because of slow radiotracer clearance from the blood, however, the authors concluded that radiolabels with improved kinetics were needed to provide useful clinical information.

Macrophages play a key role in atherogenesis and take up oxidized LDL by way of surface scavenger receptors more readily than LDL. It is logical to attempt to label this as a marker of plaque macrophage activity.[13–15] In a study of seven patients who had symptomatic carotid artery disease, the uptake of labeled oxidized LDL was detected at 150% higher level in 10 of 11 plaques, compared with normal arterial segments.[16] Oxidized LDL also has a more rapid blood clearance that native LDL.

Radiolabeled antibodies raised against epitopes on the LDL particle itself, such as antibody MDA2, have also been studied. MDA2 recognizes malondialdehyde lysine epitopes on oxidized LDL particles and has been studied in LDL receptor–deficient Watanabe heritable hyperlipidemic (WHHL) rabbits.[17] Seven WHHL and two normal New Zealand rabbits were injected intravenously with ^{125}I-MDA2, and aortic plaque uptake was found to be 17 times higher in the WHHL rabbits.

There was preferential radiotracer uptake within the diseased segments of the artery. Imaging was then performed using ^{99}Tc-MDA2 in a similar group of rabbits but this revealed visible signal in only 50% of hyperlipidemic rabbits. This finding was probably due to suboptimal imaging technique, but no other studies have been done and because of the mutagenic possibility of metabolites human studies have not been performed.

Lectin-like LDL receptor 1 (LOX-1), a cell surface receptor for oxidized LDL, has been implicated in vascular cell dysfunction related to plaque instability. A recent study was undertaken using ^{99}Tc-labeled anti-LOX1 monoclonal IgG in WHHL myocardial infarction–prone and control rabbits. There was a 10-fold greater accumulation of ^{99}Tc-anti-LOX-1 mIgG in the aorta of WHHL rabbit than in the control. Autoradiographic and histologic examination revealed a significant correlation between ^{99}Tc-anti-LOX-1 mIgG accumulation and LOX-1 receptor density and plaque vulnerability index. Vulnerability index is an index of morphologic destabilization characteristics and was calculated for each lesion in the WHHLMI rabbits by the method of Shiomi and colleagues.[18] The vulnerability index was defined as the ratio of the lipid component area (macrophages and extracellular lipid deposits) to the fibromuscular component area (smooth muscle cells and collagen fibers).

Peptides are cleared rapidly from the circulation theoretically, improving the target (atherosclerotic plaque) to background (blood pool) ratio in imaging studies. Radiotracers based on the apo-B portion of LDL were the first peptides to be evaluated. Using WWHL rabbits, Hardoff and colleagues[19] found significant uptake of the radioiodinated synthetic apo-B analog SP-4 into experimental atherosclerotic lesions. A human pilot study[10] showed uptake in carotid lesions; however, there are no large studies published. Radiolabeled endothelin peptides have also been investigated. Endothelin production in the endothelium and smooth muscle cells is up-regulated in the presence of endothelial dysfunction, a key mechanism in atherogenesis.[20] Both iodinated and radiolabeled endothelin accumulate in experimental atheromatous lesions; human studies are awaited.[21,22]

RADIOTRACERS FOR IMAGING MONOCYTES

Macrophages are central to atherogenesis and drive inflammation within the plaque. Resident macrophages express cell surface Fc receptors. Indium 111 (^{111}In)–labeled polyclonal human IgG contains an Fc subunit capable of binding to these macrophage receptors. Studies in WHHL rabbits were limited because of adverse target-to-background ratio. There was also no detectable change in uptake after lipid-lowering therapy.[23] This tracer has also been studied in patients who have carotid disease and detected in 86% of lesions subsequently identified using ultrasound. Uptake did not correlate well with morphology that suggested a large lipid core on ultrasound. Ultrasound is not a well-validated method of delineating plaque composition, however, and the lack of correlation is as likely to represent the shortcomings of ultrasound as it is the failings of the immunoglobulin binding.[24] Taken together, these two studies suggest that ^{111}In-labeled polyclonal human IgG is not appropriate as a tracer to identify unstable atherosclerotic lesions.

Radiolabels have been produced with the potential to provide an indirect measure of macrophage content. An example is a radioiodinated monoclonal antibody against amino malonic acid, a molecule vital for monocyte recruitment and foam cell production.[25] Although studies in rabbits showed significant uptake, slow tracer clearance from the circulation meant that in vivo imaging was not as successful. Other antibodies directed at cells and antigens have been studied but with limited success.[26,27]

Chemotactic peptides, such as monocyte chemotactic protein-1 (MCP-1), play a key role in the development and progression of the inflammatory process in atherosclerotic disease.[28] MCP-1 is overexpressed at the site of inflammation and mediates the transendothelial migration of mononuclear cells by way of chemokine receptor 2 (CCR-2) receptors expressed at their cell surface.[29–31] MCP-1 labeled with iodine-125 (^{125}I) has been shown to accumulate selectively in lipid-rich, macrophage-dense regions of experimental atherosclerosis in rabbits. The uptake correlated closely with lesion severity.[32] Furthermore, there was a strong correlation between the injected dose per gram accumulation of ^{125}I-MCP-1 in the atherosclerotic lesions and quantitative estimates of the number of macrophages per unit area.

A recent study examined dynamic monocyte trafficking in live animals using ^{111}In-oxyquinoline, (^{111}In-oxine) labeling with noninvasive micro SPECT. The authors showed substantial reduction in monocyte recruitment to existing atherosclerotic plaque in response to statin drug administration.[33]

POSITRON-EMITTING RADIOTRACERS

Imaging macrophage activity using fluorine-18-fluorodeoxyglucose (^{18}F-FDG) with PET has also been studied. ^{18}F-FDG is an analog of glucose and is considered the gold standard in tumor staging and for monitoring the response of tumors to therapy.[34] PET, in which paired 511 keV gamma rays are detected by a ring of specialized scintillation detectors, offers several advantages over SPECT, including superior 4- to 5-mm spatial resolution compared with 1 to 1.5 cm. PET is now usually combined in a single scanner with an anatomic imaging modality, such as CT. This method allows coregistration of images and accurate anatomic localization of activity. The first human study to use FDG imaged eight patients shortly after transient ischemic attack. Significantly more ^{18}F-FDG accumulated within the clinically symptomatic carotid plaques than in the contralateral asymptomatic arteries (P<.01). Subsequent autoradiography revealed most of the FDG had accumulated within plaque macrophages. Subsequent studies have also found correlation between ^{18}F-FDG uptake and macrophage activity.[35–37] The aorta, iliac, vertebral, and femoropopliteal arteries have also been imaged successfully,[38] and recently the technique has been shown to be reproducible, with little change in arterial FDG signal over a 2-week period.[39] The technique has demonstrated its use as a novel way of assessing drug therapy. Tahara and colleagues[39,40] showed an approximate 10% reduction in plaque inflammation in response to low-dose statin therapy (simvastatin 20 mg daily) over a 3-month period, compared with placebo (Fig. 1). Currently, FDG PET arterial imaging is being used in several trials of novel anti-atherosclerosis therapies as a surrogate marker of efficacy. There are no studies that have correlated ^{18}F-FDG PET/CT findings with clinical events in a prospective manner, however. This deficit will be addressed by the publication of the BioImage study in 2011 (http://www.bg-medicine.com/content/initiatives/hrp). This collaborative trial will track a group of 7300 asymptomatic but high-risk patients for 3 years after baseline imaging tests, including arterial FDG PET imaging. Imaging findings will be correlated with both clinical events and the results of other arterial imaging modalities.

RADIOTRACERS FOR IMAGING APOPTOSIS

Overt apoptosis is a common feature seen in resident macrophages and smooth muscle cells within the atherosclerotic plaque and is commonly observed in fibrous caps of ruptured plaque.[41] The process seems to be a surrogate for plaque vulnerability and rupture.[42] Annexin A5 is a molecule that recognizes apoptotic cells by their surface expression of phosphatidylserine. ^{99}Tc-labeled annexin A5 has shown uptake in the atherosclerotic lesions in rabbit,[43] porcine

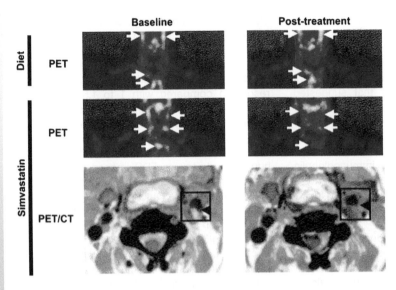

Fig. 1. Effects of simvastatin on [18]FDG uptake in atherosclerotic plaque inflammation. Representative [18]FDG-PET images at baseline and after 3 months of treatment (post-treatment) with dietary management alone (diet) or simvastatin. (*Top*) Dietary management alone had no effect on [18]FDG uptakes (*arrows*) in the aortic arch and the carotid arteries. (*Middle*) ^{18}F-FDG uptakes were attenuated by simvastatin treatment. (*Bottom*) The co-registered images of [18]FDG-PET and CT clearly show that the plaque [18]FDG uptake (*arrowheads*) was lowered after treatment with simvastatin. (*From* Tahara N, Kai H, Ishibashi M, et al. Simvastatin attenuates plaque inflammation: evaluation by fluorodeoxyglucose positron emission tomography. J Am Coll Cardiol 2006;48:1828; with permission.)

coronary arteries,[44] and apolipoprotein E-deficient mice,[45] and in patients who have carotid artery disease with SPECT imaging (**Fig. 2**).[46] There was a directly observable correlation between signal intensity and plaque macrophage content but not smooth muscle cell number, indicating a degree of cell specificity. A study has been performed using ^{99}Tc-labeled annexin A5 to asses effects of intervention, such as combination of withdrawal from high-fat diet and treatment with statin. There was clear reduction in ^{99m}Tc-labeled annexin A5 uptake that paralleled histologic regression.[47] Despite these encouraging results the use of ^{99}Tc-labeled annexin A5 to assess apoptosis is limited, due to some lack of specificity and a predilection to bind to phosphatidylserine expressed by platelets within thrombus. This limitation may not be an important failing, however, because plaque thrombosis is one of the cardinal features of vulnerability.

RADIOTRACERS FOR INTRA-ARTERIAL THROMBOSIS

The clinical consequences of atheromatous plaques are due to plaque disruption (fibrous cap rupture or erosion), subsequent adherence of platelets, and the activation of the clotting cascade. When this is not fatal, thrombus can become incorporated into the plaque and it may provide a target for imaging. Imaging studies reported have targeted three components of thrombosis: platelets, fibrinogen, and fibrinolytic molecules. Results from studies using radiolabeled autologous platelets in patients who have carotid, femoral, and aortic atherosclerosis have been conflicting.[48–50] These studies had important design differences, which could account for the different outcomes. One imaged 60 patients of whom 38 had cerebrovascular events referable to carotid disease. It could be demonstrated that ^{111}In-labeled platelets accumulated to a degree that reflected the total plaque burden and degree of carotid plaque ulceration as detected by B-mode ultrasound. In contrast, Minar and colleagues[50] found no correlation between radiotracer uptake and ultrasound findings. The crucial difference between these studies is that in the former antiplatelet medications were stopped 3 weeks before imaging, which was performed 48 hours after injection of the radiotracer, whereas antiplatelet medication continued throughout and images were obtained 24 to 26 hours after radiotracer injection in the latter.

Although this would provide explanation for the contradictory findings, the first study would have little application to patients presenting with suspected vascular events whose mainstay of treatment is antiplatelet therapy.

Radiolabeled fibrinogen has been used to detect thrombus in patients who have proven carotid disease and in patients who have venous thrombus.[51] Because of the slower accumulation of fibrinogen into arterial thrombus and its lower fibrin content compared with venous thrombus, this seriously limits its usefulness as a candidate radiotracer for rapidly imaging atheroma because of the potential poor target-to- background ratio

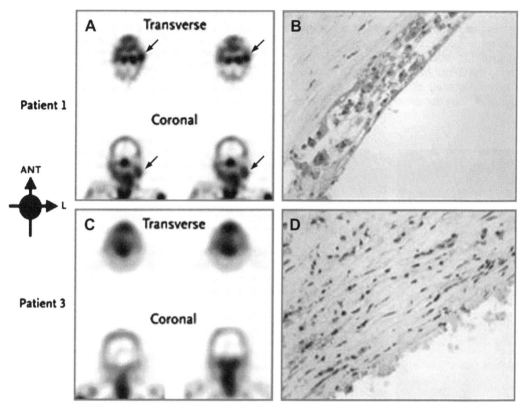

Fig. 2. Images of unstable atherosclerotic carotid artery lesions obtained with radiolabeled annexin A5. (*A*) Transverse and coronal views obtained by SPECT in Patient 1, who had a left-sided transient ischemic attack (TIA) 3 days before imaging. Although this patient had clinically significant stenosis of both carotid arteries, uptake of radiolabeled annexin A5 is evident only in the culprit lesion (*arrows*). Histopathologic analysis of an endarterectomy specimen from Patient 1 (*B*; polyclonal rabbit anti-annexin A5 antibody, ×400) shows substantial infiltration of macrophages into the neointima, with extensive binding of annexin A5 (*brown*). In contrast, SPECT images of Patient 3 (*C*), who had a right-sided TIA 3 months before imaging, do not show evidence of annexin A5 uptake in the carotid artery region on either side. Doppler ultrasonography revealed a clinically significant obstructive lesion on the affected side. Histopathologic analysis of an endarterectomy specimen from Patient 3 (*D*; polyclonal rabbit anti-annexin A5 antibody, ×400) shows a lesion rich in smooth muscle cells, with negligible binding of annexin A5. ANT, anterior; L, left. (*From* Kietselaer BL, Reutelingsperger CP, Heidendal GA, et al. Noninvasive detection of plaque instability with use of radiolabeled annexin A5 in patients with carotid-artery atherosclerosis. N Engl J Med 2004;350:1472; with permission.)

and long acquisition time. Fibrin degradation products, however, can be detected within hours of thrombus formation, offering a more promising target for thrombus detection. Fibrin fragment E1 has been labeled with both ^{123}I and ^{99}Tc and its ability to detect thrombus has been demonstrated in animals with deep vein thrombosis.[52,53] There have not been further published human or animal studies to date that have evaluated the detection of arterial thrombus associated with atheroma using labeled fibrin fragment E1.

Annexin V is a small protein that binds avidly to a phosphatidylserine moiety on the surface of activated platelets and apoptotic vascular smooth muscle cells (VSMCs) in the fibrous cap.[54,55] In a porcine model, ^{99}Tc-labeled annexin V localized

to thrombus generated in the left atrium and because of rapid blood clearance yielded high target-to-background ratios.[56] In a study using a porcine model of coronary artery disease, ^{99}Tc-annexin V uptake was greater in injured vessels with focal apoptosis in smooth muscle cells.[44] No animal or human studies have confirmed uptake by intra-arterial thrombus.

Several antibodies to platelet and fibrin have been identified with the potential to image thrombus on atherosclerotic plaques. Monoclonal antibodies against the glycoprotein IIb/IIIa receptor and the membrane glycoprotein GMP-140 on activated platelets have been developed. Using an animal model, s-12, an antibody against GMP140 has localized to acute thrombus within atherosclerotic plaque.[57] Several synthetic peptides that mostly target the GPIIb/IIIa receptor on activate platelets have been radiolabeled. Binding of ^{99}Tc-labeled −P748, a synthetic peptide ligand to the GPIIb/IIIa receptor within thrombus in the carotid arteries of dogs (induced by crush injury), has been demonstrated. It is less likely to raise an immune reaction than the immunoglobulin labels and because of its rapid uptake and clearance, it demonstrates a very favorable thrombus-to-blood ratio.[58] ^{99}Tc-labeled −P280 was the first GPIIb/IIIa-binding peptide to be studied in humans. A pilot study of nine patients who had carotid plaque demonstrated uptake in 11 of the 18 arteries.

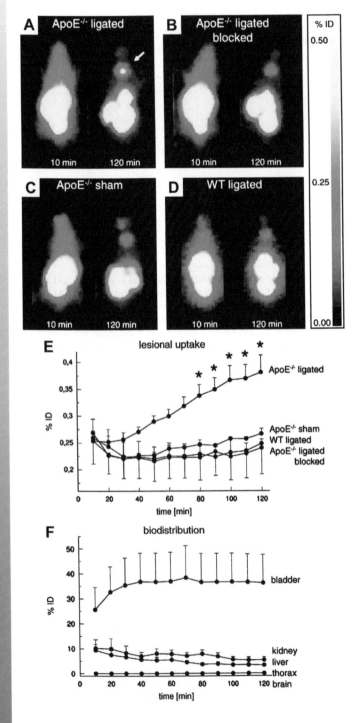

Fig. 3. In vivo scintigraphic uptake of [^{123}I]HO-CGS 27023A. Representative planar images taken 10 minutes (*left*) and 120 minutes (*right*) after injection in apolipoprotein E−deficient mice (A–C) and wild-type mice (D) 4 weeks after carotid ligation. (A) Unblocked, (B) after predosing with 6 mmol/L CGS 27023A, (C) sham-operated, and (D) wild type. (E, F) Quantitative uptake of the radioligand in the carotid lesion and tissues over time is expressed as % ID. *P<.05 between unblocked and predosed lesional uptake. The signal in the abdominal cavity is unspecific and probably reflects metabolism of the original compound, because there is no inhibition after predosing in all experiments. (*From* Schafers M, Riemann B, Kopka K, et al. Scintigraphic imaging of matrix metalloproteinase activity in the arterial wall in vivo. Circulation 2004;109:2556; with permission.)

Patients underwent injection with ^{99}Tc-labeled −P280 with SPECT imaging of the neck.[59] A GPIIb/IIIa inhibitor, DMP-444, has also been labeled with ^{99}Tc in a study of canine model coronary arteries. There were positive nuclear images and postmortem confirmation of radioactive platelet-rich thrombus.[60] There was a significantly lower postmortem nuclear count and thrombus weight in dogs that had little DMP-444 uptake. To our knowledge, there has only been one study in humans that used [99]mTc-labeled DMP-444 in patients who had infective endocarditis, and none with ^{99}Tc-labeled DMP-444 in atheroma. ^{99}Tc-labeled apcitide has been shown to have sensitivity and specificity to differentiate between acute and chronic thrombus of 92% and 86%, respectively, albeit in venous thrombus.[61]

RADIOTRACERS FOR MATRIX METALLOPROTEINASES

Matrix metalloproteinases (MMP) enzymes are responsible for the breakdown of the connective tissue matrix of the plaque leading to instability. Macrophages activated in response to oxLDL and proinflammatory cytokines secrete inactive MMP, including interstitial collagenases (MMP-1) and gelatinase B (MMP-9), which are in turn activated by plasmin.[62,63] Immunohistochemistry shows that MMP production within the atheromatous plaque is predominantly in the vicinity of macrophages.[64] Kopka and colleagues[65] have successfully synthesized several synthetic radiolabeled MMP inhibitors that bind to the active zinc(II) ion on a broad spectrum of MMPs. Schafers and colleagues[66] studied a ^{123}I-labeled molecule (HO-CGS 27023A) in apolipoprotein E null mice that had undergone carotid artery ligation followed by high-cholesterol diet to induce rapid development of atherosclerosis. They showed that after injection with ^{123}I-labeled HO-CGS 27023A, uptake into carotid lesions was significantly higher than in normal arterial tissue from the contralateral carotid artery and in carotid arteries from the sham and control mice (**Fig. 3**). Clearance of the tracer was rapid and allowed clear plaque imaging. Ex vivo imaging confirmed the findings and colocalization with MMP-9 was proved with immunostaining. A similar ^{111}In-labeled MMP inhibitor has been used to image atherosclerotic lesions in New Zealand white rabbits. After injection of the tracer, γ-camera imaging revealed greater uptake in those rabbits that had a higher-cholesterol diet compared with a normal chow diet.[67]

These preliminary studies show promise for MMP as a tracer target in the imaging of plaque instability using PET scanning, which offers greater special resolution and tracer detection.

SUMMARY

The focus in vascular imaging until relatively recently has been to define anatomic obstructions to blood flow. This definition is robustly achieved with several techniques, such as ultrasound, x-ray angiography, and CT. More recently, there has been a shift toward imaging the wall of the artery where the disease process is concentrated. Here, radionuclide imaging is already beginning to provide useful insights into the biology of the disease. Additionally, readily available techniques, such as FDG PET/CT, are now providing early, noninvasive surrogate imaging markers of drug efficacy, potentially shortening the pharmaceutical development pipeline. None of the techniques highlighted here have been shown to reliably predict plaque rupture or clinical events, however. These questions and others, including target specificity and radiation exposure, will likely be addressed over the next 5 years. Today, however, several of these imaging approaches have already yielded exciting insights into plaque structure, function, and pathogenesis.

REFERENCES

1. Naghavi M, Libby P, Falk E, et al. From vulnerable plaque to vulnerable patient: a call for new definitions and risk assessment strategies: part II. Circulation 2003;108:1772–8.

2. Davies MJ. Stability and instability: two faces of coronary atherosclerosis. The Paul Dudley White Lecture 1995. Circulation 1996;94:2013–20.

3. Binder CJ, Chang MK, Shaw PX, et al. Innate and acquired immunity in atherogenesis. Nat Med 2002;8:1218–26.

4. Li AC, Glass CK. The macrophage foam cell as a target for therapeutic intervention. Nat Med 2002; 8:1235–42.

5. Libby P. Inflammation in atherosclerosis. Nature 2002;420:868–74.

6. Libby P, Ridker PM. Inflammation and atherosclerosis: role of C-reactive protein in risk assessment. Am J Med 2004;116(Suppl 6A):9S–16S.

7. Rosen JM, Butler SP, Meinken GE, et al. Indium-111-labeled LDL: a potential agent for imaging atherosclerotic disease and lipoprotein biodistribution. J Nucl Med 1990;31:343–50.

8. Vallabhajosula S, Paidi M, Badimon JJ, et al. Radiotracers for low density lipoprotein biodistribution studies in vivo: technetium-99m low density lipoprotein versus radioiodinated low density

lipoprotein preparations. J Nucl Med 1988;29: 1237–45.

9. Pirich C, Sinzinger H. Evidence for lipid regression in humans in vivo performed by 123iodine-low-density lipoprotein scintiscanning. Ann N Y Acad Sci 1995; 748:613–21.

10. Lees AM, Lees RS, Schoen FJ, et al. Imaging human atherosclerosis with 99mTc-labeled low density lipoproteins. Arteriosclerosis 1988;8:461–70.

11. Virgolini I, Rauscha F, Lupattelli G, et al. Autologous low-density lipoprotein labelling allows characterization of human atherosclerotic lesions in vivo as to presence of foam cells and endothelial coverage. Eur J Nucl Med 1991;18:948–51.

12. Chang MY, Lees AM, Lees RS. Time course of 125I-labeled LDL accumulation in the healing, balloon-deendothelialized rabbit aorta. Arterioscler Thromb 1992;12:1088–98.

13. Steinberg D, Parthasarathy S, Carew TE, et al. Beyond cholesterol. Modifications of low-density lipoprotein that increase its atherogenicity. N Engl J Med 1989;320:915–24.

14. Steinbrecher UP, Lougheed M, Kwan WC, et al. Recognition of oxidized low density lipoprotein by the scavenger receptor of macrophages results from derivatization of apolipoprotein B by products of fatty acid peroxidation. J Biol Chem 1989;264: 15216–23.

15. Goldstein JL, Ho YK, Basu SK, et al. Binding site on macrophages that mediates uptake and degradation of acetylated low density lipoprotein, producing massive cholesterol deposition. Proc Natl Acad Sci U S A 1979;76:333–7.

16. Iuliano L, Signore A, Vallabajosula S, et al. Preparation and biodistribution of 99m technetium labelled oxidized LDL in man. Atherosclerosis 1996;126: 131–41.

17. Tsimikas S, Palinski W, Halpern SE, et al. Radiolabeled MDA2, an oxidation-specific, monoclonal antibody, identifies native atherosclerotic lesions in vivo. J Nucl Cardiol 1999;6:41–53.

18. Shiomi M, Ito T, Hirouchi Y, et al. Fibromuscular cap composition is important for the stability of established atherosclerotic plaques in mature WHHL rabbits treated with statins. Atherosclerosis 2001; 157:75–84.

19. Hardoff R, Braegelmann F, Zanzonico P, et al. External imaging of atherosclerosis in rabbits using an 123I-labeled synthetic peptide fragment. J Clin Pharmacol 1993;33:1039–47.

20. Perticone F, Ceravolo R, Pujia A, et al. Prognostic significance of endothelial dysfunction in hypertensive patients. Circulation 2001;104:191–6.

21. Dinkelborg LM, Duda SH, Hanke H, et al. Molecular imaging of atherosclerosis using a technetium-99m-labeled endothelin derivative. J Nucl Med 1998;39: 1819–22.

22. Prat L, Torres G, Carrio I, et al. Polyclonal 111In-IgG, 125I-LDL and 125I-endothelin-1 accumulation in experimental arterial wall injury. Eur J Nucl Med 1993;20:1141–5.

23. Demacker PN, Dormans TP, Koenders EB, et al. Evaluation of indium-111-polyclonal immunoglobulin G to quantitate atherosclerosis in Watanabe heritable hyperlipidemic rabbits with scintigraphy: effect of age and treatment with antioxidants or ethinylestradiol. J Nucl Med 1993;34:1316–21.

24. Sinzinger H, Rodrigues M, Kritz H. Radioisotopic imaging of atheroma. In: Fuster V, editor. Syndromes of atherosclerosis: Correlations of clinical imaging and pathology. Armonk, NY: Futura Publishing Co. Inc.; 1996. p. 369–83.

25. Chakrabarti M, Cheng KT, Spicer KM, et al. Biodistribution and radioimmunopharmacokinetics of 131I-Ama monoclonal antibody in atherosclerotic rabbits. Nucl Med Biol 1995;22:693–7.

26. Narula J, Petrov A, Bianchi C, et al. Noninvasive localization of experimental atherosclerotic lesions with mouse/human chimeric Z2D3 F(ab')2 specific for the proliferating smooth muscle cells of human atheroma. Imaging with conventional and negative charge-modified antibody fragments. Circulation 1995;92:474–84.

27. Carrio I, Pieri PL, Narula J, et al. Noninvasive localization of human atherosclerotic lesions with indium 111-labeled monoclonal Z2D3 antibody specific for proliferating smooth muscle cells. J Nucl Cardiol 1998;5:551–7.

28. Ross R. Atherosclerosis—an inflammatory disease. N Engl J Med 1999;340:115–26.

29. Yoshimura T, Leonard EJ. Identification of high affinity receptors for human monocyte chemoattractant protein-1 on human monocytes. J Immunol 1990;145:292–7.

30. Namiki M, Kawashima S, Yamashita T, et al. Local overexpression of monocyte chemoattractant protein-1 at vessel wall induces infiltration of macrophages and formation of atherosclerotic lesion: synergism with hypercholesterolemia. Arterioscler Thromb Vasc Biol 2002;22:115–20.

31. Butcher EC. Leukocyte-endothelial cell recognition: three (or more) steps to specificity and diversity. Cell 1991;67:1033–6.

32. Ohtsuki K, Hayase M, Akashi K, et al. Detection of monocyte chemoattractant protein-1 receptor expression in experimental atherosclerotic lesions: an autoradiographic study. Circulation 2001;104:203–8.

33. Kircher MF, Grimm J, Swirski FK, et al. Noninvasive in vivo imaging of monocyte trafficking to atherosclerotic lesions. Circulation 2008;117:388–95.

34. Shankar LK, Hoffman JM, Bacharach S, et al. Consensus recommendations for the use of 18F-FDG PET as an indicator of therapeutic response in patients in National Cancer Institute Trials. J Nucl Med 2006;47:1059–66.

35. Tawakol A, Migrino RQ, Bashian GG, et al. In vivo 18F-fluorodeoxyglucose positron emission tomography imaging provides a noninvasive measure of carotid plaque inflammation in patients. J Am Coll Cardiol 2006;48:1818–24.

36. Tawakol A, Migrino RQ, Hoffmann U, et al. Noninvasive in vivo measurement of vascular inflammation with F-18 fluorodeoxyglucose positron emission tomography. J Nucl Cardiol 2005;12:294–301.

37. Ogawa M, Ishino S, Mukai T, et al. (18)F-FDG accumulation in atherosclerotic plaques: immunohistochemical and PET imaging study. J Nucl Med 2004;45:1245–50.

38. Rudd JH, Fayad ZA. Imaging atherosclerotic plaque inflammation. Nat Clin Pract Cardiovasc Med 2008; 5(Suppl 2):S11–7.

39. Rudd JH, Myers KS, Bansilal S, et al. Atherosclerosis inflammation imaging with 18F-FDG PET: carotid, iliac, and femoral uptake reproducibility, quantification methods, and recommendations. J Nucl Med 2008;49:871–8.

40. Tahara N, Kai H, Ishibashi M, et al. Simvastatin attenuates plaque inflammation: evaluation by fluorodeoxyglucose positron emission tomography. J Am Coll Cardiol 2006;48:1825–31.

41. Kolodgie FD, Narula J, Burke AP, et al. Localization of apoptotic macrophages at the site of plaque rupture in sudden coronary death. Am J Pathol 2000;157:1259–68.

42. Virmani R, Ladich ER, Burke AP, et al. Histopathology of carotid atherosclerotic disease. Neurosurgery 2006;59:S219–27.

43. Ishino S, Kuge Y, Takai N, et al. 99mTc-Annexin A5 for noninvasive characterization of atherosclerotic lesions: imaging and histological studies in myocardial infarction-prone Watanabe heritable hyperlipidemic rabbits. Eur J Nucl Med Mol Imaging 2007; 34:889–99.

44. Johnson LL, Schofield L, Donahay T, et al. 99mTc-annexin V imaging for in vivo detection of atherosclerotic lesions in porcine coronary arteries. J Nucl Med 2005;46:1186–93.

45. Isobe S, Tsimikas S, Zhou J, et al. Noninvasive imaging of atherosclerotic lesions in apolipoprotein E-deficient and low-density-lipoprotein receptor-deficient mice with annexin A5. J Nucl Med 2006; 47:1497–505.

46. Kietselaer BL, Reutelingsperger CP, Heidendal GA, et al. Noninvasive detection of plaque instability with use of radiolabeled annexin A5 in patients with carotid-artery atherosclerosis. N Engl J Med 2004;350:1472–3.

47. Hartung D, Sarai M, Petrov A, et al. Resolution of apoptosis in atherosclerotic plaque by dietary modification and statin therapy. J Nucl Med 2005;46: 2051–6.

48. Smyth JV, Dodd PD, Walker MG. Indium-111 platelet scintigraphy in vascular disease. Br J Surg 1995;82: 588–95.

49. Moriwaki H, Matsumoto M, Handa N, et al. Functional and anatomic evaluation of carotid atherothrombosis. A combined study of indium 111 platelet scintigraphy and B-mode ultrasonography. Arterioscler Thromb Vasc Biol 1995;15:2234–40.

50. Minar E, Ehringer H, Dudczak R, et al. Indium-111-labeled platelet scintigraphy in carotid atherosclerosis. Stroke 1989;20:27–33.

51. Knight LC. Scintigraphic methods for detecting vascular thrombus. J Nucl Med 1993;34:554–61.

52. Knight LC, Maurer AH, Robbins PS, et al. Fragment E1 labeled with I-123 in the detection of venous thrombosis. Radiology 1985;156:509–14.

53. Knight LC, Abrams MJ, Schwartz DA, et al. Preparation and preliminary evaluation of technetium-99m-labeled fragment E1 for thrombus imaging. J Nucl Med 1992;33:710–5.

54. Flynn PD, Byrne CD, Baglin TP, et al. Thrombin generation by apoptotic vascular smooth muscle cells. Blood 1997;89:4378–84.

55. Thiagarajan P, Tait JF. Binding of annexin V/placental anticoagulant protein I to platelets. Evidence for phosphatidylserine exposure in the procoagulant response of activated platelets. J Biol Chem 1990; 265:17420–3.

56. Stratton JR, Dewhurst TA, Kasina S, et al. Selective uptake of radiolabeled annexin V on acute porcine left atrial thrombi. Circulation 1995;92:3113–21.

57. Miller D. Radionuclide labeled monoclonal antibody imaging of atherosclerosis and vascular injury. In: Fuster V, editor. Syndromes of atherosclerosis: correlations of clinical imaging and pathology. Futura Publishing Co., Inc; 1996. p. 403–16.

58. Vallabhajosula S, Moyer BR, Lister-James J, et al. Preclinical evaluation of technetium-99m-labeled somatostatin receptor-binding peptides. J Nucl Med 1996;37:1016–22.

59. Lister-James J, Knight LC, Maurer AH, et al. Thrombus imaging with a technetium-99m-labeled activated platelet receptor-binding peptide. J Nucl Med 1996;37:775–81.

60. Mitchel J, Waters D, Lai T, et al. Identification of coronary thrombus with a IIb/IIIa platelet inhibitor radiopharmaceutical, technetium-99m DMP-444: a canine model. Circulation 2000;101:1643–6.

61. Bates SM, Lister-James J, Julian JA, et al. Imaging characteristics of a novel technetium Tc 99m-labeled platelet glycoprotein IIb/IIIa receptor antagonist in patients with acute deep vein thrombosis or a history of deep vein thrombosis. Arch Intern Med 2003;163:452–6.

62. Lendon CL, Davies MJ, Born GV, et al. Atherosclerotic plaque caps are locally weakened when macrophages density is increased. Atherosclerosis 1991;87:87–90.

63. Galis ZS, Sukhova GK, Lark MW, et al. Increased expression of matrix metalloproteinases and matrix degrading activity in vulnerable regions of human atherosclerotic plaques. J Clin Invest 1994;94: 2493–503.

64. Narula J, Virmani R, Zaret B. Radionuclide imaging of atherosclerotic lesions. In: Braunwald E, Dilsizian V, Narula J, editors. Atlas of nuclear cardiology. Philadelphia, PA; 2003. p. 217–35.

65. Kopka K, Breyholz HJ, Wagner S, et al. Synthesis and preliminary biological evaluation of new radioiodinated MMP inhibitors for imaging MMP activity in vivo. Nucl Med Biol 2004;31:257–67.

66. Schafers M, Riemann B, Kopka K, et al. Scintigraphic imaging of matrix metalloproteinase activity in the arterial wall in vivo. Circulation 2004;109: 2554–9.

67. Kolodgie FD, Edwards S, Petrov A, et al. Noninvasive detection of matrix metalloproteinase upregulation in experimental atherosclerotic lesions and its abrogation by dietary modification. Circulation 2004;104:694 [Ref type: abstract].

Role of Nuclear Imaging in Regenerative Cardiology

Riikka Lautamäki, MD, PhD[a,b], Frank M. Bengel, MD[b,*]

KEYWORDS

- PET • SPECT • Stem cells • Cell labeling
- Nuclear cardiology

BACKGROUND OF STEM CELL THERAPY FOR MYOCARDIAL REGENERATION AND OPEN ISSUES

Preliminary animal studies of cardiac stem cell therapy suggested significant improvements in left ventricular (LV) function and a decrease in infarct size. These positive observations resulted in a series of clinical trials (**Tables 1** and **2**), from which the results have been often contradictory and somewhat inconclusive. It is still unclear how the cells operate, what the actual mechanism of action is, and whether modifications can be made to enhance therapeutic effects.

Various different cell types of autologous or nonautologous origin have been studied, but no consensus on the optimal type has been achieved. The major advantage of autologous cells is that they do not trigger immune responses because of self-recognition; thus, there is no rejection against them. Cell types, such as bone marrow–derived stem cells,[1] embryonic stem cells,[2,3] skeletal myoblasts,[4,5] and adipose tissue stem cells,[6] have been tested as potential candidates for regeneration. One of the key concerns regarding such nonresiding cells is whether they are able to transdifferentiate into functional cardiac cells. There are some positive reports,[1] but other study results have not been in line with those.[7,8] In addition to this process of cell plasticity, fusion of stem cells with resident cardiomyocytes[7] and neovascularization[9] have been offered as alternative explanations. Also, paracrine effects have been suggested to be a major mechanistic factor.[10] Recently cardiac-derived stem cells were introduced as an attractive option because of their early commitment to the cardiac lineage,[11] but experience is still limited.

In addition to the cell type, there are additional open issues that need to be addressed. The method of delivery should be optimized to be minimally invasive but still efficient. Systemic delivery would be preferable with regard to its convenience; however, no significant cell homing has been observed after intravenous injection,[12–17] and localized intracoronary[16–19] or intramyocardial[20–22] injections have yielded significantly better cell retention. Also, it is probable that the number of cells and especially the time point of delivery play a crucial role.

Noninvasive imaging modalities may provide answers to these fundamental questions of stem cell therapy. Using nuclear imaging, in vivo cell tracking may be combined with a functional and physiologic analysis of the myocardial environment. This article summarizes the current status of nuclear imaging in cardiac stem cell therapy. Basic molecular imaging techniques and clinical trials are reviewed.

Dr. Lautamäki is supported by grants from The Finnish Cardiac Research Foundation, The Finnish Medical Foundation, The Instrumentarium Foundation for Science, Paavo Nurmi Foundation, and by the Bracco/SNM Research Fellowship in Cardiovascular Molecular Imaging kindly provided by the Cardiovascular and Radiopharmaceutical Sciences Councils, the Society of Nuclear Medicine, and Bracco.

a Turku PET Centre, Turku University Hospital, P.O. Box 52, FIN-20521 Turku, Finland
b Division of Nuclear Medicine, Department of Radiology, Johns Hopkins Medical Institutions, 601 North Caroline Street, JHOC 3225, Baltimore, MD 21210, USA
* Corresponding author.
E-mail address: fbengel1@jhmi.edu (F.M. Bengel).

Table 1
Imaging in clinical trials in acute myocardial infarction

Study	Patient Group	Patient Group	Cell Type	Randomization	Route of Delivery	Time of Follow-up	Efficacy	Technique
Assmus et al[40] Britten et al[59] Schächinger et al[41] (TOPCARE-AMI)	29 (BMC) versus 30 (CPC) versus 11 control	Acute MI	BMC CPC	Yes	Intracoronary	4–12 mo	↑ ejection fraction[a,b] ↑ wall motion[b] ↑ end-systolic volume[a,b] ↑ flow reserve[b] ↑ viability[b] ↓ infarct size[b]	LV angiography, intracoronary Doppler, dobutamine echocardiography, [18F]FDG-PET, MRI
Bartunek et al[43]	19 versus 15 control	Acute MI	BMC	No	Intracoronary	4 mo	↑ ejection fraction[b] ↓ infarct size[b] ↑ viability[b]	LV angiography 99mTc-MIBI SPECT, [18F]FDG-PET
Chen et al[44]	34 versus 35 control	Acute MI	BMC	Yes	Intracoronary	6 mo	↑ wall motion[b] ↓ infarct size[b]	[18F]FDG-PET Echocardiography
Döbert et al[42] (TOPCARE-AMI substudy)	15 (BMC) versus 11 (EPC)	Acute MI	BMC CPC	Yes	Intracoronary	4 mo	↑ viability[b] ↑ ejection fraction[b]	201Tl-SPECT [18F]FDG-PET
Fernández-Avilés et al[60]	20 versus 13 control	Acute MI	BMC	No	Intracoronary	6 mo	↓ end-systolic volume[b] ↑ ejection fraction[b] ↑ wall motion[b]	Stress echocardiography MRI LV angiography
Ge et al[61] (TCT-STAMI)	10 versus 10 control	Acute MI	BMC	Yes	Intracoronary	6 mo	↑ ejection fraction[b] ↑ perfusion[b]	201Tl-SPECT Echocardiography
Janssens et al[45]	33 versus 34 control	Acute MI	BMC	Yes	Intracoronary	4 mo	↔ LV function[a] ↔ perfusion[a] ↔ metabolism[a] ↓ infarct size[a]	MRI Echocardiography 11C-acetate PET
Kang et al[62] (MAGIC)	7 cells versus 3 growth factor versus 1 control	Acute and chronic MI	CPC	Yes	Intracoronary	6 mo	↑ restenosis[b] ↑ ejection fraction[b] ↓ end-systolic volume[b] ↑ coronary flow reserve[b] ↓ infarct size[b]	201Tl-99mTc-MIBI dual SPECT LV angiography Intracoronary Doppler Stress echocardiography

Study	N	Condition	Cell type	Randomized	Delivery	Follow-up	Outcomes	Imaging modality
Kaminek et al[47]	31 versus 31 control	Acute MI	BMC	Yes	Intracoronary	3 mo	↑ ejection fraction[a,b] ↓ end-systolic volume[a,b] ↔ infarct size	Echocardiography Stress echocardiography 99mTc-MIBI-SPECT [18F]FDG-PET
Lunde et al[46] (ASTAMI)	50 versus 50 control	Acute MI	BMC	Yes	Intracoronary	6 mo	↑ (↔a) LV function[b] ↓ (↔a) infarct size[b]	Gated SPECT, echocardiography, MRI
Meluzin et al[39]	20 high dose versus 20 low dose versus 20 control	Acute MI	BMC	Yes	Intracoronary	12 mo	↑ LV function[a] ↔ infarct size	99mTc-MIBI Echocardiography Stress echocardiography [18F]FDG-PET
Schächinger et al[63]	101 versus 103 control	Acute MI	BMC	Yes	Intracoronary	4 mo	↑ ejection fraction[a,b] ↓ end-systolic volume[a,b] ↑ wall motion	LV angiography
Strauer et al[64]	10 versus 10 control	Acute MI	BMC	No	Intracoronary	3 mo	↓ infarct size[a] ↔ ejection fraction[a] ↑ perfusion[b] ↓ end-systolic volume[b]	LV angiography, 201Tl-SPECT
Wollert et al[38] Meyer et al[65] (BOOST)	30 versus 30 control	Acute MI	BMC	Yes	Intracoronary	6–18 mo	↑ ejection fraction[a,b] (↔ at 18 months[a]) ↑ wall motion (border zone)[a,b]	MRI

Abbreviations: BMC, Bone marrow–derived cells; CPC, Circulating progenitor cells; EPC, Endothelial progenitor cells; MI, Myocardial infarction.
↔ indicates no change.
[a] versus control group.
[b] versus baseline.

Table 2
Imaging in clinical trials in chronic coronary artery disease

Study	Patient Group	Patient Group	Cell Type	Randomization	Route of Delivery	Time of Follow-up	Efficacy	Technique
Assmus et al[66] (TOPCARE-CHD)	28 (BMC) versus 24 (CPC) versus 23 control	Chronic CAD with previous MI	BMC CPC	Yes	Intracoronary	3 mo	↑ ejection fraction[a] ↑ wall motion (BMC group) ↔ infract size	LV angiography MRI
Beeres et al[48,49,67]	25	Chronic CAD/AP	BMC	—	Intramyocardial	3–12 mo	↑ ejection fraction[b] ↓ end-systolic volume[b] ↑ wall motion[b] ↑ perfusion[b] ↔ viability	99mTc-tetrofosmin SPECT [18F]FDG-SPECT MRI
Erbs et al[51]	13 versus 13 control	Chronic CAD/coronary occlusion	CPC	Yes	Intracoronary	3 mo	↑ coronary flow reserve[a] ↑ viability[a] ↑ ejection fraction[b] ↓ end-systolic volume[b]	Intracoronary Doppler MRI [18F]FDG-PET 99mTc-tetrofosmin SPECT
Fuchs et al[56,68]	27	Chronic CAD/AP	BMC	—	Intramyocardial	3 mo	↓ inducible ischemia[b] ↔ ejection fraction ↔ wall motion	201Tl-99mTc-MIBI dual SPECT Echocardiography
Herreros et al[52] Gavira et al[53]	12 versus 14 controls	Chronic CAD/CABG	MYO	No	Intramyocardial	3–12 mo	↑ ejection fraction[b] ↑ viability[b] ↑ perfusion[b]	Echocardiography [18F]FDG-PET 13N-ammonia-PET
Ince et al[69]	6 versus 6 control	Chronic CAD/HF	MYO	No	Intramyocardial	6 mo	↑ ejection fraction[a] ↑ wall motion[a]	Stress echocardiography

Study	Patients	Patient type	Cell type	Previous MI	Delivery	Follow-up	Results	Imaging
Katritsis et al[70]	11 versus 11 control	Chronic CAD with previous MI	BMC	No	Intracoronary	4 mo	↔ LV function[a] ↑ wall motion[a] ↑ viability[b]	Rest and stress echocardiography 99mTc-MIBI
Menasche et al[71] (MAGIC)	33 versus 30 cell groups with different doses; versus 34 control	Chronic CAD/HF	MYO	Yes	Intramyocardial	6 mo	↔ ejection fraction[a] ↓ end-diastolic volume[a] ↓ end-systolic volume[a]	Echocardiography
Mocini et al[55]	18 versus 18 control	Chronic CAD/CABG	BMC	Yes	Intramyocardial	12 mo	↔ ejection fraction[a]	Echocardiography
Perin et al[57,58]	14 versus 7 control	Chronic CAD/HF	BMC	No	Intramyocardial	2–12 mo	↔ ejection fraction[a] ↓ end-systolic volume[a] ↓ inducible ischemia[a]	LV angiography Echocardiography 99mTc-MIBI-SPECT
Stamm et al[54]	22 versus 21 control	Chronic CAD/CABG	BMC (CD133+)	Yes	Intramyocardial	6 mo	↑ ejection fraction[a] ↑ perfusion[a]	Echocardiography 201Tl-SPECT
Strauer et al[50] (IACT)	18 versus 18 control	Chronic CAD with previous MI	BMC	Yes	Intracoronary	3 mo	↓ infarct size[b] ↑ ejection fraction[b] ↑ wall motion[b] ↑ 99mTc-tetrofosmin uptake[b] ↑ [18F]FDG uptake[b]	LV angiography, 99mTc-tetrofosmin SPECT, [18F]FDG-PET

Abbreviations: AP, angina pectoris; BMC, bone marrow–derived cells; CABG, coronary artery bypass grafting; CAD, coronary artery disease; CPC, circulating progenitor cells; HF, heart failure; MYO, skeletal myoblasts.
↔ indicates no change.
[a] versus control group.
[b] versus baseline.

IN VIVO TRACKING OF STEM CELLS

Currently, it is not clear how the benefits of stem cell therapy are achieved. Use of techniques to follow stem cell fate early and late after injection may help to improve understanding of therapeutic mechanisms. An ideal technique should be highly sensitive and specific for the labeled cells and should allow for long-term follow-up, but should not be toxic or have any significant effects on the cellular environment.[23] MRI and iron-based contrast material have been successfully applied for cell detection.[24–27] Ferrous particles may be introduced into cells and do not have any known side effects on cell viability.[24] MRI provides morphologic information with excellent spatial resolution and thus iron labeling and MRI have been considered attractive for cell tracking. But a significant drawback of this technique was shown in a recently published study, which suggested that the iron-dependent cell signal may still be seen after cell death.[27] Alternative methods that allow for more specific cell tracking with a signal linked to cell viability are therefore sought.

Nuclear imaging provides alternative options. Although it has lower spatial resolution compared with MRI, its sensitivity is excellent and many tracers are already approved for use in clinical practice to label other target structures.[28]

Direct Labeling Techniques

The most straightforward method for stem cell imaging is direct labeling with an agent that is detectable by an imaging system (**Fig. 1**). Iron-oxide particles for MRI and several radionuclides for SPECT and PET have been used in the experimental setting. MRI has high spatial resolution, but the sensitivity is low. In contrast, direct labeling with a radionuclide is highly sensitive with lower

background signal, but it provides inferior spatial resolution. Another disadvantage of this technique is that cells may only be visualized as long as the radiolabel has not decayed. Potential adverse effects of any labeling technique on cell integrity need to be carefully assessed in vitro before any in vivo deliveries.

One of the first tracers used for direct cell labeling is [111]indium-oxine. In clinical practice, it is commonly used for leukocyte labeling and detection of inflammation. It is an attractive option for cell labeling because it has a relatively long half-life (67.3 hours); thus, serial imaging may be performed over a longer period of time. For the purpose of stem cell detection, it was first used to label endothelial progenitor cells for subsequent injection either into the tail vein or directly into the left ventricular cavity in a rat model of myocardial infarction.[14] Cells were scintigraphically detected at various time points. Intracavital injection resulted in a significantly higher number of cells homing to the infarct site. The total amount of radioactivity was only 4.7% of the injected dose, however,[29] confirming high sensitivity of the technique but poor homing of the cells after systemic delivery. Similar findings were reported in another study in which intravenous injection of ^{99m}Tc exametazime (HMPAO)–labeled cells did not result in a significant signal from the heart.[12] A study in a porcine model of myocardial infarction showed no significant myocardial retention of mesenchymal stem cells after intravenous injection.[13] It was concluded that intravenous injection might have caused an entrapment of the cells in the lungs and intracavital injection might improve the delivery to the myocardium. Another SPECT-CT study with ^{111}In oxine–labeled mesenchymal stem cells in a dog model confirmed a high amount of intravenously injected cells in the lungs.[15] In a human study, bone marrow cells were labeled with ^{99m}Tc-HMPAO and intracoronarily injected after acute and chronic infarction.[18] Significant homing of the cells to the area of acute infarction was shown, but not to chronic infarction. Moreover, only three patients out of five who had acute infarction had a cell signal persisting 20 hours after injection. This finding suggests that inflammation may partly work as a chemoattractant for stem cells in some cases, and cells home to the site of inflammation, but a stimulus for longer-term engraftment may be missing. It is still unknown whether this is important with regard to functional benefits (ie, whether stem cell integration is an essential process for restoration of contractile function or whether potential paracrine effects and recruitment of residing cardiac stem cells are sufficient).

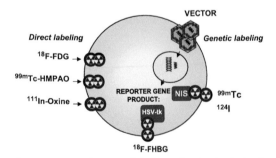

Fig. 1. Direct and genetic labeling of transplanted cells for nuclear imaging. FDG, fluorodeoxyglucose; FHBG, fluoro-hydroxymethylbutylguanine; HMPAO, exametazime; HSV-tk, herpes simplex virus thymidine kinase; I, iodine; In, indium; NIS, sodium-iodide symporter; Tc, technetium.

A most attractive option for direct cell labeling is PET. Using state-of-the-art hybrid PET-CT systems, cell tracking may be combined with quantitative assessment of myocardial perfusion and metabolism and with noninvasive coronary angiography. A limitation, however, is that currently only [18F]-fluorodeoxyglucose ([18F]FDG) has been successfully applied for direct labeling of cells for cardiac regeneration. Despite the high sensitivity, the half-life of [18F]-fluoride is 110 minutes; thus, only the immediate fate of the stem cells can be interrogated.

Several studies have used [18F]FDG-PET for cell detection (**Fig. 2**). Autologous bone marrow cells were labeled with [18F]FDG and injected either by peripheral vein or by coronary artery in patients who had myocardial infarction.[16] Again, intravenously injected cells did not home to the myocardium and better myocardial signal was obtained with an intracoronary injection. Moreover, a combination of preselection of CD34 positive cells (hematopoietic stem cells) and intracoronary injection yielded the highest signal, which was specifically localized in the infarct border zone.[16] Another study also investigated different types of intracoronary delivery with PET-CT.[19] [18F]FDG-labeled circulating progenitor cells were injected into a coronary artery in a porcine model of myocardial infarction with or without the help of balloon occlusion at the injection site. Balloon occlusion turned out to be less effective and most cells were trapped in lungs. In a human study, peripheral stem cells (CD34-positive) were labeled with [18F]FDG and injected by coronary artery or peripheral vein in patients who had acute or chronic infarction.[17] There was no significant effect of the age of infarction on early stem cell retention in this study, and no myocardial activity was observed after intravenous injection.

In summary, direct labeling provides a good option for immediate cell tracking. Catheter-based, targeted delivery may be crucial for cell therapy because no cell signal was found in the target area after systemic delivery in several cell tracking studies.

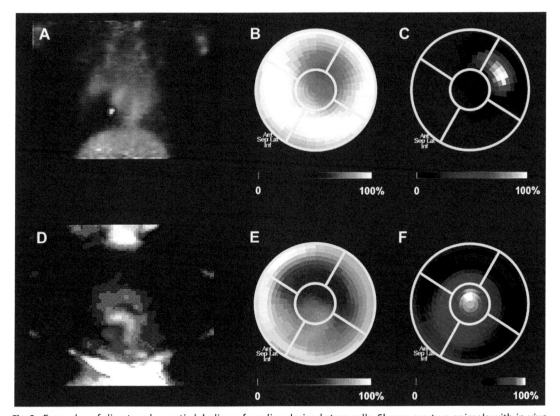

Fig. 2. Examples of direct and genetic labeling of cardiac-derived stem cells. Shown are two animals with in vivo PET scan at day 1 (*A–C*) and SPECT scan at day 3 (*D–F*). A total of 3×10^6 cardiac-derived stem cells (*bright yellow*) were injected intramyocardially in a rat model of experimental myocardial infarction (permanent ligation of the left coronary artery). Gray color represents myocardial perfusion scan with [13N]-ammonia for PET (*B*) and with [201]thallium for SPECT (*E*). Polarmap images for the left ventricle show that with both animals the stem cells are located within the infarct border zone.

Indirect (Genetic) Labeling Techniques

Reporter genes and labeled reporter probes have been successfully applied for monitoring cardiac cell therapy in experimental models.[30,31] The technique is based on a vector-mediated transfection of the cells with a reporter gene of choice, which produces a protein that may be targeted by a radiotracer (see **Fig. 1**). Expression of these proteins may be successfully detected in a living animal.[32,33] The most significant benefit of this technique is the potential for serial imaging at various time points, although there are reports that without any intervention reporter gene silencing may cause problems in the long run.[34] For imaging, the radiolabeled probe, which is specific for the reporter gene, is administered intravenously and only viable cells are detected because expression of the gene product is needed for the imaging signal; this is a significant benefit compared with direct labeling.[27]

Proof of principle studies showed successful detection of in vitro transfected stem cells in living animals.[20] Cardiomyoblasts were transfected with herpes simplex virus type 1 thymidine kinase (HSV1-sr39tk) reporter gene and 9-(4-[18F]-fluoro-3hydroxymethylbutyl)guanine ([18F]-FHBG) was used as a probe to detect cells. The study used perfusion images to delineate the myocardium and thus to localize cells in the heart. Cells were visible up to 2 weeks and results were confirmed with optical imaging and with ex vivo histology. In another study, embryonic stem cells were transfected, and the cells were injected into intact rat myocardium.[21] Because HSV-thymidine kinase is not present in host tissue, its expression in transplanted cells was readily detected, with an increasing signal over weeks after transplantation. This finding shows that the gene was successfully transferred to daughter cells; however, it also confirms a problem with embryonic stem cells (ie, the uncontrolled growth of these cells).

A recent study used the human sodium-iodide symporter gene (NIS) as a reporter gene for stem cell tracking.[22] Cardiac-derived stem cells were transfected with NIS and injected in a rat model of myocardial infarction (see **Fig. 2**). [99m]Tc (pertechnetate) or [124]I were injected intravenously and cells were successfully detected by SPECT and PET, respectively. This approach might be more easily transformed into clinical practice because first, NIS is normally expressed in some of the tissues (thyroid, stomach, choroid plexus, and salivary gland)[35] making it nonimmunogenic, and because there is no NIS expression in the myocardium the signal is highly specific for cells in the heart. Second, [99m]Tc (pertechnetate) is in routine clinical use for SPECT and readily and broadly available.

Taken together, genetic labeling holds promise for future clinical studies, because if proven safe and efficient it may be used for longer-term cell tracking and the cell signal may be correlated with functional therapeutic effects. There are still essential issues that need to be resolved, however. Genetic labeling uses highly manipulated cells; thus, transfection techniques must be optimized to be safe but efficient enough for high protein expression. At the same time, the protein itself should not negatively affect the tissue environment. Also, the systemically administered tracer for protein detection needs to be safe and provide low nonspecific binding for good cell detection sensitivity. Currently, genetic cell labeling is still limited to small animal models, and further studies are essential to show its applicability in large animals and then in humans.

INTEGRATION OF CELL TRACKING AND LEFT VENTRICULAR FUNCTION

The ultimate goal for any study investigating the effects of cardiac cell therapy is to combine the cell fate with therapeutic effects on LV function and physiology. This goal has been challenging because an optimal labeling technique for follow-up studies has been difficult to find. In an experimental study, the fate of the different stem cell types was investigated with optical imaging and several ex vivo techniques and then combined with functional data obtained with echocardiography and invasive hemodynamic measurements.[36] It was found that after 3 to 6 weeks from cell transplantation, mononuclear bone marrow cells were more favorable than mesenchymal stem cells, skeletal myoblasts, and fibroblasts with regard to cell engraftment and cardiac function. In human trials, a long-term evaluation of cell fate has not been possible because of a lack of long-term labeling techniques. But a recent study in patients who have acute and chronic myocardial infarction evaluated ^{111}In-Oxine–labeled preselected circulating progenitor cell homing within the limitation of tracer decay.[37] Serial scintigraphic imaging of ^{111}In activity was performed at 1 hour, 24 hours, and 3 to 4 days after intracoronary injection. The authors found a substantial amount of cell signal even after 4 days and the signal was higher in patients who had acute myocardial infarction. These results are not conclusive with regard to the long-term effects but emphasize the potential of cell tracking to improve understanding of clinical myocardial regenerative therapy.

NUCLEAR IMAGING IN CLINICAL TRIALS OF STEM CELL THERAPY

Although the human application of direct labeling techniques is still limited, functional imaging with established techniques, such as perfusion scintigraphy or MRI of LV function, is a key factor in evaluating stem cell therapy clinically. Optimal methods in the follow-up of any therapy should be noninvasive, fast, and reliable, and allow for high patient throughput. Currently, clinical trials of stem cell therapy have included several invasive and noninvasive imaging modalities, which are summarized in **Tables 1** and **2**.

Nuclear Imaging in Studies After Acute Myocardial Infarction

Clinical studies in the acute infarct setting are summarized in **Table 1**. All studies used intracoronary injections and follow-up time varied between 3 and 18 months. Most studies used bone marrow–derived mononuclear cells, but the effects of circulating progenitor cells have also been investigated.

Improvements in LV function have been reported in many studies. Out of 14 studies, 11 studies reported beneficial effects of cell therapy on LV function. In 5 studies, LV function improved significantly compared with controls, but 3 studies could not find any change in cell-treated patients. What causes the difference between the findings is unknown. One of the reasons may be different times for follow-up. In the BOOST trial, the first results reported improvement in LV function at 3 months, but the change was not significant any more at 18 months.[38] Another study showed that the amount of injected cells is critical for functional benefits.[39] Also, the effect of different cell types may be important, because both TOPCARE-AMI and MAGIC trials reported positive effects of circulating progenitor cells. No definite conclusions may be drawn at the moment, however, because only 2 studies reported the use of circulating progenitor cells, and when those cells were directly compared with bone marrow–derived cells, no significant difference was observed.[40–42]

[18F]FDG-PET is a gold standard for myocardial viability studies and it has been used in several stem cell studies to investigate metabolism in the infarct region. TOPCARE-AMI reported increased [18F]FDG uptake in the infarct region suggesting improved viability after treatment with bone marrow cells or circulating progenitor cells at 4 months.[40,42] Bartunek and coworkers[43] evaluated the effect of preselected CD133-positive bone marrow cells on viability by FDG-PET. They also observed increased viability in the infarct region,

which was in agreement with a study by Chen and colleagues.[44] In contrast, Janssens and coworkers[45] reported that the increase in perfusion and metabolism in the infarct area as measured with ^{11}C-acetate PET in patients who were treated with autologous bone marrow–derived stem cells was similar compared with that of a conventionally treated patient group. Similar findings were reported in ASTAMI, in which 50 patients who had acute myocardial infarction were treated with intracoronary injection of autologous bone marrow–derived cells.[46] LV function and infarct size were evaluated with gated SPECT, echocardiography, and MRI. LV function improved and infarct size decreased during follow-up, but the change was not different compared with controls. Kaminek and coworkers[47] found that only 39% of patients responded positively to therapy and found that an increased baseline ^{99m}Tc-MIBI uptake was a significant predictor for responsiveness to therapy.

Nuclear Imaging in Studies in Chronic Coronary Artery Disease or Heart Failure

Table 2 summarizes results of clinical trials in patients who have chronic CAD or heart failure. Intracoronary and intramyocardial injections were used and follow-up time varied from 2 months to 1 year. Most of the studies used bone marrow–derived stem cells, but the effects of circulating progenitor cells and skeletal myoblasts were investigated in some studies.

Beeres and coworkers[48,49] evaluated the effect of autologous bone marrow–derived cells on LV function, infarct size, and the amount of stress-induced ischemia in patients who had ischemic coronary disease with ^{99m}Tc-tetrofosmin SPECT and [18F]-FDG SPECT. Gated ^{99m}Tc-tetrofosmin SPECT showed a significant increase in ejection fraction and decrease in end-systolic volume after 3 and 12 months from therapy. There was also a decrease in the amount of ischemic segments, which was found both in injected and in noninjected segments; however, they did not find any significant change in the [18F]FDG uptake by SPECT in the infarct region. On the other hand, the IACT study investigators reported a 5% to 15% increased tetrofosmin and [18F]FDG uptake in the infarct region compared with baseline in the cell therapy group.[50]

Stem cell therapy has been combined with other interventions in some studies with chronic coronary disease. The effect of circulating progenitor cell therapy was evaluated after recanalization of chronic coronary occlusion.[51] Myocardial perfusion and metabolism were studied with

^{99m}Tc-tetrofosmin SPECT and by [^{18}F]FDG-PET and the results were compared with a control group. At 3 months, coronary flow reserve was improved and the amount of perfusion-metabolism mismatch was decreased. Stem cells have also been applied during coronary bypass grafting by intramyocardial injections. LV function and myocardial viability were increased in most of the studies,[52–54] but controversial results were obtained in one study, in which there was no effect of therapy on LV function.[55]

Intramyocardial cell injections have also been used without other concomitant interventions. Bone marrow cells were intramyocardially injected, and myocardial perfusion with dual isotope SPECT imaging and LV function with conventional echocardiography were studied.[56] The study results showed a significant decrease in reversible ischemia in the injected areas. A similar study was performed by Perin and coworkers,[57,58] who evaluated the effect of an intramyocardial injection of bone marrow cells on rest-dipyridamole stress ^{99m}Tc-MIBI and on LV function at 2 months. They found that there was a significant decrease in reversible ischemia in the cell treatment group compared with the control group,[57] and the changes persisted at 12 months' follow-up.[58]

FUTURE ASPECTS FOR NUCLEAR IMAGING IN REGENERATIVE THERAPY

Cardiac stem cell therapy has significantly affected cardiology. The first enthusiastic reports of functional benefits created a set of clinical trials at a relatively fast pace, some showing positive effects and some no significant effect. Existing clinical nuclear imaging modalities, which have been used in clinical trials, provide surrogate markers of success and may be used to evaluate myocardial perfusion and metabolism in addition to LV function. In the future, this may be done at even higher accuracy using novel hybrid PET-CT scanners, whereby noninvasive coronary angiography can be combined with quantitative PET imaging.

A significant limitation in currently available clinical studies is the limited information on the longitudinal fate of transplanted cells. Cell tracking is currently performed with direct labeling in selected small-scale clinical studies enabling the monitoring of cell homing and retention, and short-term follow-up within the limits of radiolabel decay. Experimental studies have proved the feasibility of genetic labeling, which may allow for monitoring over a longer period; however, more efforts are needed to confirm safety before pursuing human trials with this technique. A broader clinical application of cell tracking techniques, and combination with measures of functional outcome of therapy, are expected to refine the understanding of therapeutic mechanisms of cell delivery.

In conclusion, although there are several ongoing clinical trials in the stem cell area, there are still fundamental questions to be answered: What is the best clinical situation for therapy? What is the best method for cell delivery? And what is the best time for delivery? Currently, it is difficult to predict who will truly benefit from cell therapy. It is most probable that these answers may be found using the help of several molecular imaging techniques, some already existing, but some yet to be discovered.

REFERENCES

1. Orlic D, Kajstura J, Chimenti S, et al. Bone marrow cells regenerate infarcted myocardium. Nature 2001;410:701–5.
2. Xu C, Police S, Rao N, et al. Characterization and enrichment of cardiomyocytes derived from human embryonic stem cells. Circ Res 2002;91:501–8.
3. Kehat I, Kenyagin-Karsenti D, Snir M, et al. Human embryonic stem cells can differentiate into myocytes with structural and functional properties of cardiomyocytes. J Clin Invest 2001;108:407–14.
4. Winitsky SO, Gopal TV, Hassanzadeh S, et al. Adult murine skeletal muscle contains cells that can differentiate into beating cardiomyocytes in vitro. PLoS Biol 2005;e87:662–71.
5. Oshima H, Payne TR, Urish KL, et al. Differential myocardial infarct repair with muscle stem cells compared to myoblasts. Mol Ther 2005;12:1130–41.
6. Planat-Benard V, Menard C, Andre M, et al. Spontaneous cardiomyocyte differentiation from adipose tissue stroma cells. Circ Res 2004;94:223–9.
7. Nygren JM, Jovinge S, Breitbach M, et al. Bone marrow-derived hematopoietic cells generate cardiomyocytes at a low frequency through cell fusion, but not transdifferentiation. Nat Med 2004;10:494–501.
8. Murry CE, Soonpaa MH, Reinecke H, et al. Haematopoietic stem cells do not transdifferentiate into cardiac myocytes in myocardial infarcts. Nature 2004;428:664–8.
9. Rota M, Kajstura J, Hosoda T, et al. Bone marrow cells adopt the cardiomyogenic fate in vivo. Proc Natl Acad Sci U S A 2007;104:17783–8.
10. Fazel S, Cimini M, Chen L, et al. Cardioprotective c-kit+ cells are from the bone marrow and regulate the myocardial balance of angiogenic cytokines. J Clin Invest 2006;116:1865–77.
11. Smith RR, Barile L, Cho HC, et al. Regenerative potential of cardiosphere-derived cells expanded

from percutaneous endomyocardial biopsy specimens. Circulation 2007;115:896–908.

12. Barbash IM, Chouraqui P, Baron J, et al. Systemic delivery of bone marrow-derived mesenchymal stem cells to the infarcted myocardium: feasibility, cell migration, and body distribution. Circulation 2003;108:863–8.

13. Chin BB, Nakamoto Y, Bulte JW, et al. 111In oxine labelled mesenchymal stem cell SPECT after intravenous administration in myocardial infarction. Nucl Med Commun 2003;24:1149–54.

14. Aicher A, Brenner W, Zuhayra M, et al. Assessment of the tissue distribution of transplanted human endothelial progenitor cells by radioactive labeling. Circulation 2003;107:2134–9.

15. Kraitchman DL, Tatsumi M, Gilson WD, et al. Dynamic imaging of allogeneic mesenchymal stem cells trafficking to myocardial infarction. Circulation 2005;112:1451–61.

16. Hofmann M, Wollert KC, Meyer GP, et al. Monitoring of bone marrow cell homing into the infarcted human myocardium. Circulation 2005;111:2198–202.

17. Kang WJ, Kang HJ, Kim HS, et al. Tissue distribution of 18F-FDG-labeled peripheral hematopoietic stem cells after intracoronary administration in patients with myocardial infarction. J Nucl Med 2006;47:1295–301.

18. Penicka M, Lang O, Widimsky P, et al. One-day kinetics of myocardial engraftment after intracoronary injection of bone marrow mononuclear cells in patients with acute and chronic myocardial infarction. Heart 2007;93:837–41.

19. Doyle B, Kemp BJ, Chareonthaitawee P, et al. Dynamic tracking during intracoronary injection of 18F-FDG-labeled progenitor cell therapy for acute myocardial infarction. J Nucl Med 2007;48:1708–14.

20. Wu JC, Chen IY, Sundaresan G, et al. Molecular imaging of cardiac cell transplantation in living animals using optical bioluminescence and positron emission tomography. Circulation 2003;108:1302–5.

21. Cao F, Lin S, Xie X, et al. In vivo visualization of embryonic stem cell survival, proliferation, and migration after cardiac delivery. Circulation 2006; 113:1005–14.

22. Terrovitis J, Kwok KF, Lautamaki R, et al. Ectopic expression of the sodium-iodide symporter enables imaging of transplanted cardiac stem cells in vivo by SPECT or PET. J Am Coll Cardiol 2008;52(20): 1652–60.

23. Bengel FM, Schachinger V, Dimmeler S. Cell-based therapies and imaging in cardiology. Eur J Nucl Med Mol Imaging 2005;32(Suppl 2):S404–16.

24. Frank JA, Miller BR, Arbab AS, et al. Clinically applicable labeling of mammalian and stem cells by combining superparamagnetic iron oxides and transfection agents. Radiology 2003;228:480–7.

25. Wunderbaldinger P, Josephson L, Weissleder R. Crosslinked iron oxides (CLIO): a new platform for the development of targeted MR contrast agents. Acad Radiol 2002;9(Suppl 2):S304–6.

26. Hinds KA, Hill JM, Shapiro EM, et al. Highly efficient endosomal labeling of progenitor and stem cells with large magnetic particles allows magnetic resonance imaging of single cells. Blood 2003;102: 867–72.

27. Terrovitis J, Stuber M, Youssef A, et al. Magnetic resonance imaging overestimates ferumoxide-labeled stem cell survival after transplantation in the heart. Circulation 2008;117:1555–62.

28. Beeres SL, Bengel FM, Bartunek J, et al. Role of imaging in cardiac stem cell therapy. J Am Coll Cardiol 2007;49:1137–48.

29. Brenner W, Aicher A, Eckey T, et al. 111In-labeled CD34+ hematopoietic progenitor cells in a rat myocardial infarction model. J Nucl Med 2004;45: 512–8.

30. Bengel FM, Anton M, Avril N, et al. Uptake of radio-labeled 2′-fluoro-2′-deoxy-5-iodo-1-beta-D-arabino-furanosyluracil in cardiac cells after adenoviral transfer of the herpesvirus thymidine kinase gene: the cellular basis for cardiac gene imaging. Circulation 2000;102:948–50.

31. Miyagawa M, Beyer M, Wagner B, et al. Cardiac reporter gene imaging using the human sodium/iodide symporter gene. Cardiovasc Res 2005;65: 195–202.

32. Wu JC, Inubushi M, Sundaresan G, et al. Positron emission tomography imaging of cardiac reporter gene expression in living rats. Circulation 2002; 106:180–3.

33. Inubushi M, Wu JC, Gambhir SS, et al. Positron-emission tomography reporter gene expression imaging in rat myocardium. Circulation 2003;107: 326–32.

34. Krishnan M, Park JM, Cao F, et al. Effects of epigenetic modulation on reporter gene expression: implications for stem cell imaging. FASEB J 2006;20: 106–8.

35. Dohan O, De I V, Paroder V, et al. The sodium/iodide symporter (NIS): characterization, regulation, and medical significance. Endocr Rev 2003;24:48–77.

36. van der Bogt KE, Sheikh AY, Schrepfer S, et al. Comparison of different adult stem cell types for treatment of myocardial ischemia. Circulation 2008; 118:S121–9.

37. Schachinger V, Aicher A, Dobert N, et al. Pilot trial on determinants of progenitor cell recruitment to the infarcted human myocardium. Circulation 2008; 118:1425–32.

38. Wollert KC, Meyer GP, Lotz J, et al. Intracoronary autologous bone-marrow cell transfer after myocardial infarction: the BOOST randomised controlled clinical trial. Lancet 2004;364:141–8.

39. Meluzin J, Janousek S, Mayer J, et al. Three-, 6-, and 12-month results of autologous transplantation of

mononuclear bone marrow cells in patients with acute myocardial infarction. Int J Cardiol 2008;128: 185–92.

40. Assmus B, Schachinger V, Teupe C, et al. Transplantation of Progenitor Cells and Regeneration Enhancement in Acute Myocardial Infarction (TOPCARE-AMI). Circulation 2002;106:3009–17.

41. Schachinger V, Assmus B, Britten MB, et al. Transplantation of progenitor cells and regeneration enhancement in acute myocardial infarction: final one-year results of the TOPCARE-AMI Trial. J Am Coll Cardiol 2004;44:1690–9.

42. Dobert N, Britten M, Assmus B, et al. Transplantation of progenitor cells after reperfused acute myocardial infarction: evaluation of perfusion and myocardial viability with FDG-PET and thallium SPECT. Eur J Nucl Med Mol Imaging 2004;31:1146–51.

43. Bartunek J, Vanderheyden M, Vandekerckhove B, et al. Intracoronary injection of CD133-positive enriched bone marrow progenitor cells promotes cardiac recovery after recent myocardial infarction: feasibility and safety. Circulation 2005;112:I178–83.

44. Chen SL, Fang WW, Ye F, et al. Effect on left ventricular function of intracoronary transplantation of autologous bone marrow mesenchymal stem cell in patients with acute myocardial infarction. Am J Cardiol 2004;94:92–5.

45. Janssens S, Dubois C, Bogaert J, et al. Autologous bone marrow-derived stem-cell transfer in patients with ST-segment elevation myocardial infarction: double-blind, randomised controlled trial. Lancet 2006;367:113–21.

46. Lunde K, Solheim S, Aakhus S, et al. Intracoronary injection of mononuclear bone marrow cells in acute myocardial infarction. N Engl J Med 2006;355: 1199–209.

47. Kaminek M, Meluzin J, Panovsky R, et al. Individual differences in the effectiveness of intracoronary bone marrow cell transplantation assessed by gated sestamibi SPECT/FDG PET imaging. J Nucl Cardiol 2008;15:392–9.

48. Beeres SL, Bax JJ, bbets-Schneider P, et al. Sustained effect of autologous bone marrow mononuclear cell injection in patients with refractory angina pectoris and chronic myocardial ischemia: twelve-month follow-up results. Am Heart J 2006;152: 684–6.

49. Beeres SL, Bax JJ, Dibbets P, et al. Effect of intramyocardial injection of autologous bone marrow-derived mononuclear cells on perfusion, function, and viability in patients with drug-refractory chronic ischemia. J Nucl Med 2006;47:574–80.

50. Strauer BE, Brehm M, Zeus T, et al. Regeneration of human infarcted heart muscle by intracoronary autologous bone marrow cell transplantation in chronic coronary artery disease: the IACT Study. J Am Coll Cardiol 2005;46:1651–8.

51. Erbs S, Linke A, Adams V, et al. Transplantation of blood-derived progenitor cells after recanalization of chronic coronary artery occlusion: first randomized and placebo-controlled study. Circ Res 2005; 97:756–62.

52. Herreros J, Prosper F, Perez A, et al. Autologous intramyocardial injection of cultured skeletal muscle-derived stem cells in patients with non-acute myocardial infarction. Eur Heart J 2003;24:2012–20.

53. Gavira JJ, Herreros J, Perez A, et al. Autologous skeletal myoblast transplantation in patients with nonacute myocardial infarction: 1-year follow-up. J Thorac Cardiovasc Surg 2006;131:799–804.

54. Stamm C, Kleine HD, Choi YH, et al. Intramyocardial delivery of CD133+ bone marrow cells and coronary artery bypass grafting for chronic ischemic heart disease: safety and efficacy studies. J Thorac Cardiovasc Surg 2007;133:717–25.

55. Mocini D, Staibano M, Mele L, et al. Autologous bone marrow mononuclear cell transplantation in patients undergoing coronary artery bypass grafting. Am Heart J 2006;151:192–7.

56. Fuchs S, Satler LF, Kornowski R, et al. Catheter-based autologous bone marrow myocardial injection in no-option patients with advanced coronary artery disease: a feasibility study. J Am Coll Cardiol 2003; 41:1721–4.

57. Perin EC, Dohmann HF, Borojevic R, et al. Transendocardial, autologous bone marrow cell transplantation for severe, chronic ischemic heart failure. Circulation 2003;107:2294–302.

58. Perin EC, Dohmann HF, Borojevic R, et al. Improved exercise capacity and ischemia 6 and 12 months after transendocardial injection of autologous bone marrow mononuclear cells for ischemic cardiomyopathy. Circulation 2004;110:II213–8.

59. Britten MB, Abolmaali ND, Assmus B, et al. Infarct remodeling after intracoronary progenitor cell treatment in patients with acute myocardial infarction (TOPCARE-AMI): mechanistic insights from serial contrast-enhanced magnetic resonance imaging. Circulation 2003;108:2212–8.

60. Fernandez-Aviles F, San Roman JA, Garcia-Frade J, et al. Experimental and clinical regenerative capability of human bone marrow cells after myocardial infarction. Circ Res 2004;95:742–8.

61. Ge J, Li Y, Qian J, et al. Efficacy of emergent transcatheter transplantation of stem cells for treatment of acute myocardial infarction (TCT-STAMI). Heart 2006;92:1764–7.

62. Kang HJ, Kim HS, Zhang SY, et al. Effects of intracoronary infusion of peripheral blood stem-cells mobilised with granulocyte-colony stimulating factor on left ventricular systolic function and restenosis after coronary stenting in myocardial infarction: the MAGIC cell randomised clinical trial. Lancet 2004; 363:751–6.

63. Schachinger V, Erbs S, Elsasser A, et al. Intracoronary bone marrow-derived progenitor cells in acute myocardial infarction. N Engl J Med 2006;355:1210–21.

64. Strauer BE, Brehm M, Zeus T, et al. Repair of infarcted myocardium by autologous intracoronary mononuclear bone marrow cell transplantation in humans. Circulation 2002;106:1913–8.

65. Meyer GP, Wollert KC, Lotz J, et al. Intracoronary bone marrow cell transfer after myocardial infarction: eighteen months' follow-up data from the randomized, controlled BOOST (BOne marrOw transfer to enhance ST-elevation infarct regeneration) trial. Circulation 2006;113:1287–94.

66. Assmus B, Honold J, Schachinger V, et al. Transcoronary transplantation of progenitor cells after myocardial infarction. N Engl J Med 2006;355:1222–32.

67. Beeres SL, Bax JJ, Kaandorp TA, et al. Usefulness of intramyocardial injection of autologous bone marrow-derived mononuclear cells in patients with severe angina pectoris and stress-induced myocardial ischemia. Am J Cardiol 2006;97:1326–31.

68. Fuchs S, Kornowski R, Weisz G, et al. Safety and feasibility of transendocardial autologous bone marrow cell transplantation in patients with advanced heart disease. Am J Cardiol 2006;97:823–9.

69. Ince H, Petzsch M, Rehders TC, et al. Transcatheter transplantation of autologous skeletal myoblasts in postinfarction patients with severe left ventricular dysfunction. J Endovasc Ther 2004;11:695–704.

70. Katritsis DG, Sotiropoulou PA, Karvouni E, et al. Transcoronary transplantation of autologous mesenchymal stem cells and endothelial progenitors into infarcted human myocardium. Catheter Cardiovasc Interv 2005;65:321–9.

71. Menasche P, Alfieri O, Janssens S, et al. The Myoblast Autologous Grafting in Ischemic Cardiomyopathy (MAGIC) trial: first randomized placebo-controlled study of myoblast transplantation. Circulation 2008;117:1189–200.

Index

Note: Page numbers of article titles are in **boldface** type.

A

Absolute blood flow quantification, PET
  in clinical setting, 243–245
  in coronary artery disease
    advanced, 243–245
    preclinical, 245
  in nonischemic heart diseases, 245
Acute myocardial infarction, stem cell therapy for,
  clinical trials of, imaging in, 355–357, 363
Aging, as factor in myocardial metabolism, 296–298
Angiogenesis, 330–332
  biology of, 330
  radiotracer-based imaging of, molecular targets
    used for, 330–332
Angiotensin II type I antagonists, 338–340
Angiotensin-converting enzyme (ACE) inhibitors,
  338–340
Apoptosis
  imaging of, radiotracers for, 347–348
  necrosis vs., 332–335
Arrhythmic diseases, primary, cardiac neuronal
  imaging in, 321–322
Atherosclerosis
  biology of, 345
  imaging of, 306
    nuclear imaging, 345–346
  radiotracer imaging of, **345–354**

B

Blood flow, myocardial. See *Myocardial blood flow.*

C

Camera technology, in nuclear cardiology, **227–236**
  new trends in
    CardiArc system, 228–229
    Cardius 3 XPO system, 231
    D-SPECT system, 227–228
    IQ SPECT collimation, 231
    multi-pinhole SPECT system, 231–232
    rotating camera developments, 229–232
    ultrafast AT cardiac system, 229
    ultrafast cameras, 227–229
Carbohydrate(s), metabolism of, imaging of, 294–295
Cardiac CT. See *Computed tomography (CT),
  cardiac; Nuclear imaging, cardiac CT.*
Cardiac dyssynchrony, implications in cardiac
  resynchronization therapy, 273–275
Cardiac neuronal anatomy, 311

Cardiac neuronal imaging. See also ^{123}I-*m*IMB.
  with ^{123}I-*m*IMB, 313
    image interpretation, 313–315
  in congestive heart failure assessment, 315–316
  in diabetes mellitus, 321
  at edge of clinical application, **311–327**
  following heart transplantation, 319–320
  of parasympathetic function, 322
  post-chemotherapy, 322
  of postsynaptic receptors, 322
  in primary arrhythmic diseases, 321–322
Cardiac PET, current clinical practice, **237–255**. See
  also *Positron emission tomography (PET), cardiac.*
Cardiac resynchronization therapy, assessment of
  cardiac dyssynchrony implications in, 273–275
Cardiac sympathetic innervation, imaging of,
  radiotracers for, 311–313
CardiArc system, in nuclear cardiology, 228–229
Cardiomyopathy
  ischemic vs. nonischemic, 266–267
  nonischemic-dilated, imaging of, 301–302
Cardiovascular disorders, inflammatory, ^{18}F-FDG
  PET in, 250–251
Cardius 3 XPO system, in nuclear cardiology, 231
Chemotherapy, cardiac neuronal imaging after, 322
Commercial implementations, in nuclear cardiology,
  234–235
Computed tomography (CT), cardiac, 259
  nuclear imaging and, integration of, **257–273**. See
    also *Nuclear imaging, cardiac CT and,
    integration of.*
Congestive heart failure, assessment of, cardiac
  neuronal imaging in, 315–316
Coronary artery disease
  advanced, PET absolute blood flow quantification
    in, 243–245
  chronic, stem cell therapy for, clinical trials of,
    imaging in, 357–359, 363–364
  diagnosis of, PET myocardial perfusion imaging in,
    242–243
  preclinical, PET absolute blood flow quantification
    in, 245
  prognosis of, PET myocardial perfusion imaging
    in, 245
Coronary blood flow, regulation of, 278–280
Coronary circulatory function, targets of, 280–282
  endothelium-related coronary vasomotion,
    281–282
  epicardial conduit vessel function, 281–282
  integrated vasodilator capacity, 281
Coronary vasomotion, endothelium-related, 281–282

D

Defibrillator(s), implantable
  in heart failure management, assessment of
    cardiac innervation implications for, 270–273
  need for, assessment of, ^{123}I-*m*IMB in, 317–319
Diabetes mellitus
  cardiac neuronal imaging in, 321
  myocardial metabolic imaging of, 302–304
D-SPECT system, in nuclear cardiology, 227–228

E

Endothelium-related coronary vasomotion, 281–282
Epicardial conduit vessel function, 281–282

F

Factor XIII, 338
Fast-speed myocardial perfusion imaging, clinical
  implications of, in nuclear cardiology, 235
Fatty acids, metabolism of, imaging of, 295–296
^{18}F-FDG. See *^{18}F-Fluorodeoxyglucose.*
^{18}F-Fluorodeoxyglucose PET, clinical applications of,
  under investigation, 251
^{18}F-Fluorodeoxyglucose PET, in inflammatory
  cardiovascular disorders, 250–251
^{18}F-Fluorodeoxyglucose PET viability imaging,
  protocol for, 240–241

G

Gender, as factor in myocardial metabolism, 296–298

H

Heart disease
  ischemic, ^{123}I-*m*IBG in, 320–321
  nonischemic, PET absolute blood flow
    quantification in, 245
Heart failure
  congestive, assessment of, cardiac neuronal
    imaging in, 315–316
  morbidity and mortality associated with, 265
  nuclear imaging in, **265–276**
  prevalence of, 265
  treatment of
    ^{123}I-*m*IMB imaging in guiding, 316–317
    implantable defibrillator in, assessment of
      cardiac innervation implications for,
      270–273
    tailoring of, 265–266
Heart transplantation, cardiac neuronal imaging after,
  319–320
Hybrid imaging, **257–273**
Hypertension/left ventricular hypertrophy, imaging of,
  299–301

I

Image reconstruction advancements, in nuclear
  cardiology, 232–235
^{123}I-*m*IBG, in ischemic heart disease, 320–321
^{123}I-*m*IMB
  in assessing need for implantable defibrillator,
    317–319
  cardiac imaging with, 313
  in guiding heart failure therapy, 316–317
  image interpretation, 313–315
Implantable defibrillators
  in heart failure management, assessment of
    cardiac innervation implications for, 270–273
  need for, assessment of, ^{123}I-*m*IMB in, 317–319
Inflammation, 335–337
  vascular, PET in, 251
Insulin resistance, myocardial metabolic imaging of,
  304–306
Integrin $\alpha_v\beta_3$, 332
Intra-arterial thrombosis, radiotracers for, 348–351
IQ SPECT collimation, in nuclear cardiology, 231
Ischemia
  assessment of, 267
  imaging of, 298–299
Ischemic heart disease, ^{123}I-*m*IBG in, 320–321
Iterative techniques, in nuclear cardiology, 233–234

L

Left ventricular dysfunction, severe, viability imaging
  in, prospective outcome data on, 249
Left ventricular ejection fraction, measurement of,
  assessment of function by, cardiac PET in, 245
Left ventricular function, stem cell tracking and,
  integration of, 362
Left ventricular hypertrophy, imaging of, 299–301
Lipoprotein(s), imaging of, radiotracers for, 346
LTB$_4$ receptor, 337

M

Macrovascular disease, myocardial blood flow
  measurements in, 283
Magnetic resonance spectroscopy (MRS), of
  myocardial metabolism, 292–293
Matrix metalloproteinases, radiotracers for, 351
Metabolism, myocardial, imaging of, translation into
  clinics, **291–310.** See also *Myocardial metabolism,
  imaging of.*
Metalloproteinases, matrix, radiotracers for, 351
Microvascular disease, myocardial blood flow
  measurements in, 283–285
Molecular imaging
  approaches to, 329
  nuclear imaging, described, 329–330
  role of, 329

targets in myocardial biology characterization, **329–344**
  angiogenesis, 330–332
  apoptosis vs. necrosis, 332–335
  inflammation, 335–337
  ventricular remodeling, 337–340
Monocyte(s), imaging of, radiotracers for, 346–347
MRS. See *Magnetic resonance spectroscopy (MRS)*.
Multi-pinhole SPECT system, in nuclear cardiology, 231–232
MVO$_2$. See *Myocardial oxygen consumption (MVO$_2$)*.
Myocardial biology, characterization of, molecular imaging targets in, **329–344**. See also *Molecular imaging, targets in myocardial biology characterization*.
Myocardial blood flow
  measurements of, **277–289**
    clinical applications of, 282–285
    in coronary risk assessment, 285–286
    future developments in, 286
    in macrovascular disease, 283
    in microvascular disease, 283–285
    technical considerations of, 277–278
    in "total ischemic burden" assessment, 283
  quantification of, **277–289**
  regulation of, 278–280
Myocardial infarction, acute, stem cell therapy for, clinical trials of, imaging in, 355–357, 363
Myocardial metabolism
  imaging of
    aging as factor in, 296–298
    carbohydrate metabolism, 294–295
    diabetes mellitus, 302–304
    fatty acid metabolism, 295–296
    future needs related to, 306
    gender as factor in, 296–298
    hypertension/left ventricular hypertrophy, 299–301
    insulin resistance, 304–306
    ischemia, 298–299
    methods in, 292–296
    MRS, 292–293
    MVO$_2$, 294
    nonischemic-dilated cardiomyopathy, 301–302
    obesity, 304–306
    PET, 293–294
    SPECT, 293
    translation into clinics, **291–310**
    vascular, 306
  overview of, 291–292
Myocardial metabolism tracers, for PET, 239–240
Myocardial oxygen consumption (MVO$_2$), in myocardial metabolism, 294
Myocardial perfusion imaging, 257–259
  PET
    advantages of, 241–242

    in coronary artery disease diagnosis, 242–243
    in coronary artery disease prognosis, 245
    cost effects of, 245–248
    disadvantages of, 242
    protocols for, 240
Myocardial perfusion tracers, for PET, 237–239
Myocardial viability, assessment of, 267–270
Myocardium, processes within, 330–340
  angiogenesis, 330–332
  apoptosis vs. necrosis, 332–335
  inflammation, 335–337
  ventricular remodeling, 337–340

N

Necrosis, apoptosis vs., 332–335
Nonischemic heart diseases, PET absolute blood flow quantification in, 243–245
Nonischemic-dilated cardiomyopathy, imaging of, 301–302
Nuclear cardiology, camera and software technology in, new trends in, **227–236**. See also *Camera technology, in nuclear cardiology; Software technology, in nuclear cardiology*.
  fast-speed myocardial perfusion imaging, clinical implications of, 235
Nuclear imaging
  cardiac CT and, integration of, **257–273**
    for diagnosis and management, 259–262
    in obstructive coronary artery disease diagnosis, 259–260
    in prognosis assessment, 260
    rationale for, 257–259
  described, 329–330
  in heart disease, **265–276**
  in regenerative cardiology, **355–367**. See also *Regenerative cardiology, nuclear imaging in*.

O

Obesity, myocardial metabolic imaging of, 304–306
Obstructive coronary artery disease, diagnosis of, nuclear imaging and cardiac CT in, 259–260

P

Parasympathetic function, cardiac, cardiac neuronal imaging of, 322
PET. See *Positron emission tomography (PET)*.
Position emission tomography (PET), of myocardial metabolism, 293–294
Positron emission tomography (PET)
  cardiac. See also *Myocardial perfusion imaging, PET*.
    absolute blood flow quantification in clinical setting, 243–245

Positron (*continued*)

    in assessment of function, measurement of left ventricular ejection fraction, 245

    current clinical practice, **237–255**

    ^{18}F-FDG viability imaging, protocol for, 240–241

    myocardial metabolism tracers for, 239–240

    myocardial perfusion tracers for, 237–239

    in vascular inflammation, 251

    ^{18}F-FDG

        clinical applications of, under investigation, 251

        in inflammatory cardiovascular disorders, 250–251

    myocardial viability with

        assessment of, 248–249

        outcome-related, 248

        in severe left ventricular dysfunction, prospective outcome data on, 249

        stunning and hibernation, 248

        wall motion recovery and, 248

Positron-emitting radiotracers, 347

Postsynaptic receptors, cardiac neuronal imaging of, 322

R

Radiotracer(s)

    in apoptosis imaging, 347–348

    for cardiac sympathetic innervation imaging, 311–313

    for intra-arterial thrombosis, 348–351

    in lipoprotein imaging, 346

    for matrix metalloproteinases, 351

    in monocyte imaging, 346–347

    position-emitting, 347

Radiotracer imaging, of atherosclerotic plaque biology, **345–354**. See also *Atherosclerosis.*

Regenerative cardiology

    myocardial, stem cell therapy for

        background of, 355–357

        in vivo tracking of stem cells, 360–362

            left ventricular function and, 362

    nuclear imaging in, **355–367**

        future aspects for, 364

        stem cell therapy–related, clinical trials of, 355–357, 363–364

Resolution recovery, in nuclear cardiology, 232–233

S

Sarcoidosis, cardiac, detection of, PET in, 250–251

Single photon emission computed tomography (SPECT), of myocardial metabolism, 293

Software technology, in nuclear cardiology, **227–236**

    image reconstruction advancements, 232–235

        clinical trials of, 235

        commercial implementations, 234–235

        iterative techniques, 233–234

        resolution recovery, 232–233

SPECT. See *Single photon emission computed tomography (SPECT).*

Stem cell(s), in vivo tracking of, 360–362

    direct labeling techniques, 360–361

    indirect labeling techniques, 362

Stem cell therapy

    for acute myocardial infarction, imaging in, clinical trials of, 355–357, 363

    for chronic coronary artery disease, clinical trials of, imaging in, 357–359, 363–364

    clinical trials of, nuclear imaging in, 355–357, 363–364

T

Thrombosis(es), intra-arterial, radiotracers for, 348–351

"Total ischemic burden," assessment of, myocardial blood flow measurements in, 283

Transplantation, heart, cardiac neuronal imaging after, 319–320

U

Ultrafast AT cardiac system, in nuclear cardiology, 229

V

Vascular imaging, of atherosclerosis, 306

Vascular inflammation, PET in, 251

Vasodilator capacity, integrated, 281

Ventricular remodeling, 337–340

Vsomotion, coronary, endothelium-related, 281–282

Moving?

Make sure your subscription moves with you!

To notify us of your new address, find your **Clinics Account Number** (located on your mailing label above your name), and contact customer service at:

E-mail: elspcs@elsevier.com

800-654-2452 (subscribers in the U.S. & Canada)
314-453-7041 (subscribers outside of the U.S. & Canada)

Fax number: 314-523-5170

Elsevier Periodicals Customer Service
11830 Westline Industrial Drive
St. Louis, MO 63146

*To ensure uninterrupted delivery of your subscription, please notify us at least 4 weeks in advance of move.

Printed and bound by CPI Group (UK) Ltd, Croydon, CR0 4YY

03/10/2024

01040362-0012